ADENOSINE, CARDIOPROTECTION AND ITS CLINICAL APPLICATION

Developments in Cardiovascular Medicine

M.LeWinter. H. Suga and M.W. Watkins (eds.): *Cardiac Energetics: From Emax to Pressure-volume Area.* 1995 ISBN 0-7923-3721-2

R.J. Siegel (ed.): *Ultrasound Angioplasty.* 1995 ISBN 0-7923-3722-0

D.M. Yellon and G.J. Gross (eds.): *Myocardial Protection and the Katp Channel.* 1995 ISBN 0-7923-3791-3

A.V.G. Bruschke. J.H.C. Reiber. K.I. Lie and H.J.J. Wellens (eds.): *Lipid Lowering Therapy and Progression of Coronary Atherosclerosis.* 1996 ISBN 0-7923-3807-3

A.S.A. Abd-Elfattah and A.S. Wechsler (eds.): *Purines and Myocardial Protection.* 1995 ISBN 0-7923-3831-6

M. Morad, S. Ebashi, W. Trautwein and Y. Kurachi (eds.): *Molecular Physiology and Pharmacology of Cardiac Ion Channels and Transporters.* 1996 ISBN 0-7923-3913-4

A.M. Oto (ed.): *Practice and Progress in Cardiac Pacing and Electrophysiology.* 1996 ISBN 0-7923-3950-9

W.H. Birkenhager (ed.): *Practical Management of Hypertension. Second Edition.* 1996 ISBN 0-7923-3952-5

J.C. Chatham, J.R. Forder and J.H. McNeill(eds.):*The Heart In Diabetes.* 1996 ISBN 0-7923-4052-3

M. Kroll, M. Lehmann (eds.): *Implantable Cardioverter Defibrillator Therapy: The Engineering-Clinical Interface.* 1996 ISBN 0-7923-4300-X

Lloyd Klein (ed.): *Coronary Stenosis Morphology: Analysis and Implication.* 1996 ISBN 0-7923-9867-X

Johan H.C. Reiber, Ernst E. Van der Wall (eds.): *Cardiovascular Imaging.* 1996 ISBN 0-7923-4109-0

A.-M. Salmasi, A. Strano (eds.): *Angiology in Practice.* ISBN 0-7923-4143-0

Julio E. Perez, Roberto M. Lang, (eds.): *Echocardiography and Cardiovascular Function: Tools for the Next Decade.* 1996 ISBN 0-7923-9884-X

Keith L. March (ed.): *Gene Transfer in the Cardiovascular System: Experimental Approaches and Therapeutic Implications.* 1997 ISBN 0-7923-9859-9

Anne A. Knowlton (ed.): *Heat Shock Proteins and the Cardiovascular System.* 1997 ISBN 0-7923-9910-2

Richard C. Becker (ed.): *The Textbook of Coronary Thrombosis and Thrombolysis.* 1997 ISBN 0-7923-9923-4

Robert M. Mentzer, Jr., Masafumi Kitakaze, James M. Downey, Masatsugu Hori, (eds): *Adenosine, Cardioprotection and its Clinical Application* ISBN 0-7923-9954-4

ADENOSINE, CARDIOPROTECTION AND ITS CLINICAL APPLICATION

Edited by

Robert M. Mentzer, Jr.
University of Kentucky

Masafumi Kitakaze
Osaka University School of Medicine

James M. Downey
University of South Alabama

Masatsugu Hori
Osaka University School of Medicine

Springer Science+Business Media, LLC

Library of Congress Cataloging-in-Publication Data

A C.I.P. Catalogue record for this book is available
from the Library of Congress.

ISBN 978-1-4613-4676-0 ISBN 978-1-4419-8736-5 (eBook)
DOI 10.1007/978-1-4419-8736-5

Printed on acid-free paper.

CONTENTS

CONTRIBUTING AUTHORS

ARAKAWA, Naoshi, Second Department of Internal Medicine, Iwate Medical University, 19-1 Uchimaru, Morioka, Iwate 020, Japan

BIRNBAUM, Yochai, The Heart Institute, Good Samaritan Hospital, 1225 Wilshire Blvd., Los Angeles, CA 90017, U.S.A.

BOLLI, Roberto, University of Louisville School of Medicine, ACB Third Floor, 550 South Jackson Street, Louisville, KY 40292, U.S.A.

CARR, Cornelia, The Hatter Institute, University College London, Grafton Way, London, WC1E 6DB, United Kingdom

DOWNEY, James, Department of Physiology, MSB 3024, University of South Alabama, College of Medicine, Mobile, AL 36688, U.S.A.

FUKAMI, Ken-ichi, Second Department of Internal Medicine, Iwate Medical University, 19-1 Uchimaru, Morioka, Iwate/020, Japan

FUNAYA, Hiroharu, The First Department of Medicine, Osaka University School of Medicine, 2-2 Yamadaoka, Suita 565, Japan

GAO, Wei Dong, Department of Medicine, Johns Hopkins University, 720 Rutland Ave., Ross 844, Baltimore, MD 21205, U.S.A.

GROSS, Garrett, Department of Pharmacology and Toxicology, Medical College of Wisconsin, P.O. Box 26509, Milwaukee, WI 53226-0509, U.S.A.

HIRAMORI, Katsuhiko, Second Department of Internal Medicine, Iwate Medical University, 19-1 Uchimaru, Morioka, Iwate 020, Japan

HONYE, Junko, The 2nd Department of Medicine, Nihon University School of Medicine, Oyaguchi-Kami 30-1, Itabashi-ku, Tokyo 173, Japan

HORI, Masatsugu, The First Department of Medicine, Osaka University School of Medicine, 2-2 Yamadaoka, Suita 565, Japan

HOSHIDA, Shiro, Department of Medicine and Pathophysiology, Osaka University School of Medicine, 2-2 Yamadaoka, Suita, Osaka 565, Japan

KANMATSUSE, Katsuo, The 2nd Department of Medicine, Nihon University School of Medicine, Oyaguchi-Kami 30-1, Itabashi-ku, Tokyo 173, Japan

KITAKAZE, Masafumi, The First Department of Medicine, Osaka University School of Medicine, 2-2 Yamadaoka, Suita 565, Japan

KLONER, Robert A., The Heart Institute, Good Samaritan Hospital, 1225 Wilshire Blvd., Los Angeles, CA 90017, U.S.A.

KODAMA, Kazuhisa, Division of Cardiology, National Cardiovascular Center, 5-7-1 Fujishirodai, Suita, Osaka 565, Japan

KOMAMURA, Kazuo, Division of Cardiology, National Cardiovascular Center, 5-7-1 Fujishirodai, Suita, Osaka 565, Japan

KUZUYA, Tsunehiko, Department of Medicine and Pathophysiology, Osaka University School of Medicine, 2-2 Yamadaoka, Suita, Osaka 565, Japan

LASLEY, Robert D., University of Kentucky Medical Center, 800 Rose Street, Room MN-260, Lexington, KY 40536-0084, U.S.A.

LIU, Yongge, Department of Medicine, Johns Hopkins University, 720 Rutland Ave., Ross 844, Baltimore, MD 21205, U.S.A.

MARBAN, Eduardo, Department of Medicine, Johns Hopkins University, 720 Rutland Ave., Ross 844, Baltimore, MD 21205, U.S.A.

MENASCHÈ, Philippe, Department of Cardiovascular Surgery, Hôpital Lariboisière, 2 rue Ambroise Paré, 75010, Paris, France

MENTZER, Jr., Robert M., University of Kentucky Medical Center, 800 Rose Street, Room MN-264, Lexington, KY 40536-0084, U.S.A.

MIKI, Takayuki, Second Department of Internal Medicine, Sapporo Medical University School of Medicine, South-1 West-16, Chuo-ku, Sapporo 060, Japan

MINAMINO, Tetsuo, The First Department of Medicine, Osaka University School of Medicine, 2-2 Yamadaoka, Suita 565, Japan

MIURA, Tetsuji, Second Department of Internal Medicine, Sapporo Medical University School of Medicine, South-1 West-16, Chuo-ku, Sapporo 060, Japan

MIZUMURA, Tsuneo, The 2nd Department of Medicine, Nihon University School of Medicine, Oyaguchi-Kami 30-1, Itabashi-ku, Tokyo 173, Japan

MORIUCHI, Masahito, The 2nd Department of Medicine, Nihon University School of Medicine, Oyaguchi-Kami 30-1, Itabashi-ku, Tokyo 173, Japan

NAKAMURA, Motoyuki, Second Department of Internal Medicine, Iwate Medical University, 19-1 Uchimaru, Morioka, Iwate 020, Japan

NISHIDA, Masashi, Department of Medicine and Pathophysiology, Osaka University School of Medicine, 2-2 Yamadaoka, Suita, Osaka 565, Japan

NODE, Koichi, The First Department of Medicine, Osaka University School of Medicine, 2-2 Yamadaoka, Suita 565, Japan

O'ROURKE, Brian, Department of Medicine, Johns Hopkins University, 720 Rutland Ave., Ross 844, Baltimore, MD 21205, U.S.A.

OZAWA, Yukio, The 2nd Department of Medicine, Nihon University School of Medicine, Oyaguchi-Kami 30-1, Itabashi-ku, Tokyo 173, Japan

PARK, Seong-Wook, University of Louisville School of Medicine, ACB Third Floor, 550 South Jackson Street, Louisville, KY 40292, U.S.A.

PERRAULT, Louis P., Department of Cardiovascular Surgery, Hôpital Lariboisière, 2 rue Ambroise Paré, 75010, Paris, France

QIU, Yumin, University of Louisville School of Medicine, ACB Third Floor, 550 South Jackson Street, Louisville, KY 40292, U.S.A.

SAITO, Satoshi, The 2nd Department of Medicine, Nihon University School of Medicine, Oyaguchi-Kami 30-1, Itabashi-ku, Tokyo 173, Japan

SAKAMOTA, Jun, Second Department of Internal Medicine, Sapporo Medical University School of Medicine, South-1 West-16, Chuo-ku, Sapporo 060, Japan

SCHULTZ, Jo El, Department of Pharmacology and Toxicology, Medical College of Wisconsin, P.O. Box 26509, Milwaukee, WI 53226-0509, U.S.A.

TADA, Michihiko, Department of Medicine and Pathophysiology, Osaka University School of Medicine, 2-2 Yamadaoka, Suita, Osaka 565, Japan

TAKAYAMA, Tadateru, The 2nd Department of Medicine, Nihon University School of Medicine, Oyaguchi-Kami 30-1, Itabashi-ku, Tokyo 173, Japan

TANG, Xian-Liang, University of Louisville School of Medicine, ACB Third Floor, 550 South Jackson Street, Louisville, KY 40292, U.S.A.

VAN BELLE, Herman, Janssen Research Foundation, Turnhoutseweg 30, B-2340, Beerse, Belgium

VINTEN-JOHANSEN, Jakob, Section of Cardiothoracic Surgery, Carlyle Fraser Heart Center of Emory University, Cardiothoracic Research Laboratory, Atlanta, GA 30365-2225, U.S.A.

WEINBRENNER, Christof, Department of Physiology, MSB 3024, University of South Alabama, College of Medicine, Mobile, AL 36688, U.S.A.

YAMASHITA, Nobushige, Department of Medicine and Pathophysiology, Osaka University School of Medicine, 2-2 Yamadaoka, Suita, Osaka 565, Japan

YELLON, Derek,The Hatter Institute, University College London, Grafton Way, London, WC1E 6DB, United Kingdom

ZHAO, Zhi-Qing, Section of Cardiothoracic Surgery, Carlyle Fraser Heart Center of Emory University, Cardiothoracic Research Laboratory, Atlanta, GA 30365-2225, U.S.A.

PREFACE

It has been almost 15 years since the first reports appeared indicating that adenosine exerted a protective effect in ischemic and reperfused myocardium. Numerous experimental studies have shown that adenosine (both exogenous and endogenous adenosine) delays the onset of ischemic contracture, modulates myocardial metabolism during ischemia, attenuates reversible postischemic ventricular dysfunction (myocardial stunning), and reduces myocardial infarct size. Initial studies on adenosine's cardioprotective effect were based on its ability to stimulate postischemic ATP resynthesis, increase coronary blood flow, and reduce heart rate. Although these actions of adenosine are undoubtedly beneficial to the ischemic/reperfused heart, it now appears that adenosine's cardioprotective effect may be exclusive of these properties.

The immense growth in the number of articles on adenosine cardioprotection in the last several years has been related in large part to the hypothesis that adenosine plays a role in ischemic preconditioning. Ischemic preconditioning is the phenomenon in which a brief period of ischemia (and reperfusion) prior to a more prolonged occlusion reduces myocardial infarct size. This form of myocardial protection has received much interest because ischemic preconditioning has been shown to be the most potent means of reducing infarct size in all animal models thus far tested. In fact prior to studies implicating adenosine's role in ischemic preconditioning, adenosine's infarct reducing effect was not well recognized.

Since 1990, the principal focus of adenosine cardioprotection research has centered on the role of adenosine receptors. It is currently thought that adenosine protects the ischemic heart primarily via the activation of adenosine A_1 receptors located on the cardiac myocytes. There are some reports however that adenosine A_2 receptor activation during reperfusion may reduce the extent of myocardial infarction. Still other reports suggest that adenosine may exert its protective effects via stimulation of an adenosine A_3 receptor subtype. Although the majority of evidence suggests involvement of the A_1 receptor, the intracellular signal transduction pathway(s) responsible for adenosine's beneficial effect in ischemic/reperfused myocardium remains unknown. There is evidence for the involvement of ATP-sensitive potassium (K_{ATP}) channels, however there appear to be species differences. There is also evidence for the modulation of calcium dependent protein kinase (PKC), however there are also controversies regarding this potential mechanism. There are also some differences between ischemic preconditioning, and treatments with K_{ATP} channel openers and adenosine.

Adenosine is used clinically for terminating supraventricular tachycardia, as a diagnostic tool in coronary imaging, and has been used postoperatively for blood pressure control after heart surgery. There are also recent reports that adenosine may be safely tolerated and a potentially beneficial additive to cardioplegic solutions during open heart surgery in humans. There is even evidence that ischemic preconditioning may occur in humans under various clinical situations.

This book contains chapters from contributors to the first three symposia on "Adenosine, Cardioprotection, and its Clinical Application". All aspects of adenosine cardioprotection and ischemic preconditioning, including potential mechanisms and clinical applications, are discussed by experts in these areas. The reader will find this book to be both an excellent source of information on these topics, as well a guide to future experiments.

The editors would like to thank the contributors for their chapters and the symposia attendees for their interest in these topics. We would also like to thank the sponsors and supporters who made these symposia possible. The editors would also like to express their gratitude to Steve Thomas for his assistance in preparing this book.

Robert M. Mentzer, Jr.
Masafumi Kitakaze
James M. Downey
Masatsugu Hori

ACKNOWLEDGEMENTS

The editors of this book would like to thank Chugai Pharmaceuticals for their generous underwriting support for this book. Without their assistance, this book and the Symposia would not have been possible.

The First, Second, and Third International Symposia on Adenosine, Cardioprotection and Its Clinical Application were supported by the following:

Chugai Pharmaceuticals

KOWA Company

Medco Research, Inc.

Fujisawa USA, Inc.

Bayer Corporation

Sanofi Pharmaceuticals

Cardiothoracic and Vascular Surgery Coucil and the Circulation Council of the American Heart Association

---

The editors gratefully acknowledge the assistance of Stephen K. Thomas in editing, formatting, and assembling the finished book.

Special thanks also to Mr. Thomas, Penelope Cook, and Joann Slack for their tireless efforts in coordinating the Symposia.

I. ADENOSINE AND CARDIOPROTECTION

1. Adenosine and Cardioprotection

Robert M. Mentzer, Jr.
Robert D. Lasley

Myocardial Ischemia

Myocardial ischemia is characterized by reduced ventricular function and altered myocardial metabolism. Metabolic consequences of ischemia include a net breakdown of the high energy phosphates creatine phosphate (CrP), and adenosine triphosphate (ATP), and the accumulation of metabolites such as inorganic phosphate (P_i), fatty acids, lactate, H^+, and NADH. As the ischemic period progresses leak of calcium from intracellular stores and/or reduced reuptake of calcium by the sarcolemmal and sarcoplasmic reticulum (SR) Ca^{2+}-ATPases results in increased free intracellular calcium concentration ($[Ca^{2+}]_I$.[1-3] If coronary blood flow is restored within 15-20 minutes ischemia-induced injury is reversible, but myocardial contractility may remain depressed for hours to days. This prolonged ventricular contractile dysfunction has been termed myocardial stunning.[4] Longer periods of myocardial ischemia (> 20 minutes) are associated with the activation of phospholipases and proteases resulting in irreversible myocyte injury or myocardial infarction.[5]

Myocardial protection during heart surgery and reperfusion are thus designed to prevent irreversible injury and minimize postischemic ventricular dysfunction. Clinically, myocardial stunning is seen in patients who have undergone revascularization by coronary artery bypass surgery, coronary thrombolytic therapy or angioplasty, and heart transplantation.[6,7] This may delay the benefits of myocardial reperfusion, and consequently has stimulated considerable research aimed at elucidating the mechanisms of stunning and developing therapeutic interventions to minimize cardiac ischemic injury. Myocardial protection during heart surgery is typically achieved with hypothermic, hyperkalemic cardioplegic arrest. However, the realization that current cardioplegic solutions may not provide optimal myocardial protection has led to the search for new therapeutic agents and modalities to limit myocardial ischemia reperfusion injury.

Cardioprotective Properties of Adenosine

One agent which has received much therapeutic interest is the endogenous purine adenosine. When administered prior to or during ischemia, we and others have shown that adenosine retards the rate of ATP depletion and prolongs the time to onset of ischemic contracture,[8,9] enhances postischemic ventricular function,[8,10] and reduces infarct size.[11,12] Treatment of the ischemic myocardium with agents that inhibit transport and/or metabolism of endogenously produced adenosine is associated with increased myocardial adenosine levels, improved postischemic ventricular function, and decreased infarct size.[13-15]

Adenosine possesses several properties which could be considered cardioprotective. It has negative chronotropic, negative dromotropic, and anti-adrenergic effects, increases coronary blood flow, and is a precursor for adenine nucleotide resynthesis. This latter property in fact provided the basis for the initial interest in adenosine as a cardioprotective agent. Postischemic myocardium is characterized by high levels of adenosine in the coronary venous outflow, reduced ATP levels, and prolonged ventricular dysfunction.[16] Since exogenous adenosine is rapidly incorporated into the myocardial adenine nucleotide pool,[17,18] it was proposed that treatment of the ischemic myocardium with exogenous adenosine alleviated postischemic dysfunction by stimulating ATP resynthesis.

Although adenosine treatment may enhance the resynthesis of postischemic adenine nucleotides, it is unlikely that this is a mechanism for adenosine attenuation of myocardial stunning. When adenosine is administered after global myocardial ischemia in isolated perfused hearts, ATP repletion is facilitated, but there is little, if any, effect on postischemic function.[19,20] In addition it is now well recognized that postischemic recovery of function is not determined by total tissue ATP content.[21,22]

Endogenous adenosine has been shown to mediate, in part, ischemia- and hypoxia-induced decreases in atrio-ventricular conduction and heart rate.[23,24] Exogenous adenosine produces rapid reductions in heart rate,[24] and there is a report that adenosine even accelerates the time to cardiac arrest induced with hyperkalemic cardioplegia.[25] Reductions in heart rate during ischemia could contribute to adenosine's cardioprotective effect, however adenosine mediated reductions in myocardial stunning and infarct size have been achieved under conditions in which adenosine did not decrease heart rate or hearts were paced to exclude this effect.

Adenosine-induced increases in coronary blood flow (CBF) are beneficial to the ischemic and reperfused heart by supplying additional substrates and enhancing washout of deleterious metabolites. However, the majority of adenosine cardioprotection studies have been conducted under conditions of complete occlusions, excluding adenosine's effects on blood flow during ischemia as a protective mechanism. Although adenosine-induced increases in CBF do not appear to play a direct role in adenosine cardioprotection, adenosine-induced hyperemia does produce transient changes in ventricular function in stunned myocardium. Figure 1.1 illustrates the different effects of adenosine on regional ventricular function in normal and stunned myocardium in an in situ pig preparation. Regional myocardial contractility was determined by the slope of the end systolic pressure-thickness relationship (ESPTR) generated during brief caval occlusions The slope (defined as E_{es}) of the ESPTR provides a load-insensitive index of cardiac contractility, analogous to E_{max} derived from pressure-volume loops. As shown in Figure 1.1A, the ESPTR loops prior to and during an intracoronary adenosine (50 µg/kg/min) in normal myocardium completely overlap. However, after 10 minutes coronary artery occlusion and 30 minutes reperfusion, adenosine infusion was associated with a significant change in the ESPTR. Once the adenosine infusion was terminated and the hyperemia subsided, contractile function returned to pre-adenosine levels. It is not known why

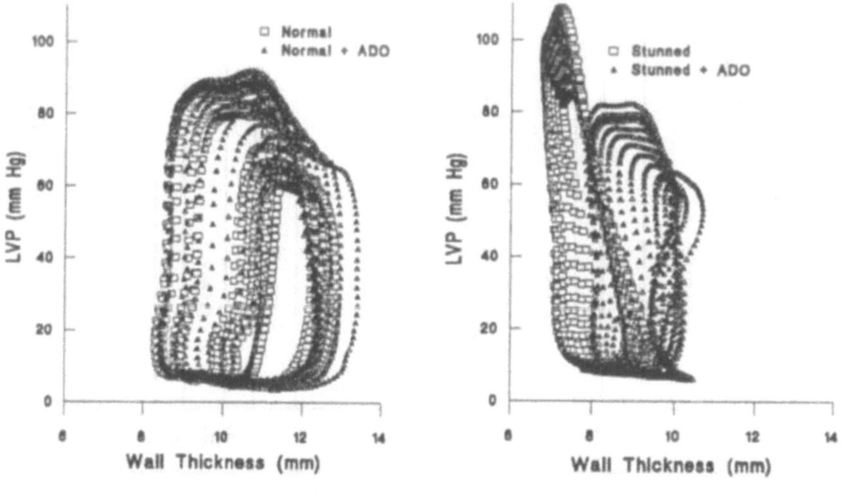

FIGURE 1-1. Effects of intracoronary adenosine infusion (50 µg/kg/min) on regional myocardial contractility in normal (1A) and stunned (1B) in vivo porcine myocardium. Contractility was determined by the slope (E_{es}) of the end systolic pressure-thickness relationship (ESPTR) generated during brief caval occlusions. Stunning was induced by 10 minutes coronary artery occlusion and 30 minutes reperfusion.

adenosine exerts this effect in the stunned heart but not the normal heart. This could be related to the Gregg phenomenon or garden-hose effect but the adenosine infusion in the normal heart produced a similar increase in CBF.

Adenosine Receptor Actions in Ischemic Myocardium

The recognition that adenosine exerts various effects in the normal heart via activation of specific receptors has facilitated efforts to determine adenosine's beneficial effects in ischemic myocardium. Adenosine increases coronary blood flow by activating vascular smooth muscle and endothelial A_2 receptors, whereas its negative chronotropic and anti-adrenergic effects are mediated by stimulation of A_1 receptors located on cardiac myocytes.[26] The results of isolated heart and in situ ischemia-reperfusion studies suggest that adenosine enhances postischemic function via the activation of myocyte adenosine A_1 receptors.[27,28] The results of isolated heart studies performed in our laboratory[27] are summarized in Figure 1.2. In isolated rat hearts treatment with adenosine (100 μM) and the adenosine A_1 receptor agonist cyclohexyladenosine (CHA, 0.25μM) prior to 30 minutes global

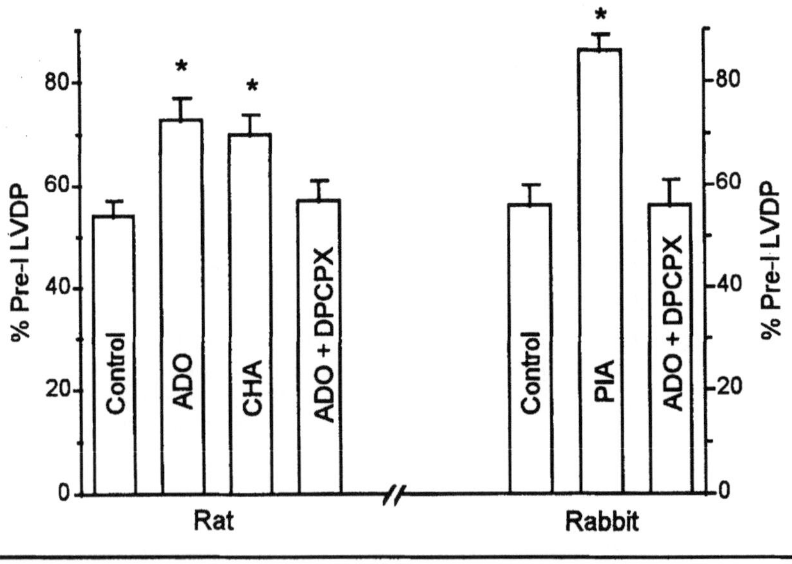

FIGURE 1-2. Summary of the effects of adenosine (ADO) and adenosine A_1 receptor agonists on postischemic function in isolated perfused rat and rabbit hearts. Postischemic left ventricular developed pressure (LVDP) is expressed as percent of preischemic values. Values are expressed as mean ± SEM, * $p < 0.05$ vs control hearts. CHA, cyclohexyladenosine; PIA, phenylisopropyladenosine; DPCPX, 8-cyclopently-1,3-dipropylxanthine.

ischemia (37°C) significantly improved postischemic left ventricular developed pressure (LVDP), whereas treatment with the adenosine A_2 receptor agonist phenylaminoadenosine (PAA, 0.25 μM) had no protective effect. In the isolated rabbit heart preparation similar protection was observed with adenosine and the A_1 receptor agonist phenylisopropyladenosine (PIA, 1 μM) infused immediately prior to 45 minutes global normothermic ischemia. The protective effects of adenosine and PIA were blocked by the adenosine A_1 selective antagonist 8-cyclopently-1,3-dipropylxanthine (DPCPX). Additional studies from our laboratory indicate that adenosine-mediated cardioprotection in the isolated rat heart is dependent upon A_1 receptor coupling to pertussis toxin sensitive inhibitory guanine nucleotide (G_i) binding proteins.[29]

Additional indirect evidence supporting the role of the A_1 receptor in adenosine-mediated cardioprotection is provided by the results of studies with cardiac microdialysis. This technique permits the sampling of myocardial interstitial fluid (ISF) adenosine, and is the only technique currently available for estimating changes in ISF metabolites during complete coronary occlusions. Adenosine levels in the ISF determine the effective concentration of adenosine in the vicinity of the extracellular A_1 receptor. The results of studies in our laboratory and others indicate that interventions that increase ISF adenosine prior to ischemia attenuate myocardial stunning[13,14] and reduce infarct size.[12,15] These interventions typically increase ISF adenosine 3-4 fold prior to ischemia, and adenosine metabolism/transport inhibitors also increase ischemic adenosine levels 10-20 fold. Our initial hypothesis was that the increase in adenosine during ischemia was the most important factor in adenosine-induced myocardial protection. However, based on studies in models of both reversible[10] and irreversible injury,[12] it appears that the preischemic increase in ISF adenosine may be more important. In an in situ canine model,[10] in which adenosine pretreatment attenuated regional myocardial stunning, intracoronary adenosine (50 μg/kg/min) increased preischemic ISF adenosine from 0.55 ± 0.12 μM to 1.25 ± 0.30 μM. However ISF adenosine levels during ischemia were identical in control and adenosine treated hearts. Similarly, in an in situ rabbit model,[12] in which a transient intravenous adenosine infusion (140 μg/kg/min) 15 minutes prior to coronary occlusion reduced infarct size by 40%, ISF adenosine was only elevated during the 5 minute treatment period. At the onset of ischemia and for the duration of the occlusion, ISF adenosine levels were not different from control ischemic values. These results suggest that the preischemic increase in adenosine levels is more important than adenosine levels during ischemia.

Metabolic Effects of Adenosine in Ischemic Myocardium

Although it is generally accepted that adenosine does not attenuate stunning or reduce infarct size by enhancing ATP resynthesis, adenosine does exert other metabolic effects which may play a role in its cardioprotective action. In fact we observed one of these effects in our initial studies. Adenosine pretreatment reduced the rate of ATP degradation during zero flow global ischemia in ischemic rat and canine myocardium.[8,30] This effect was not due simply to elevated preischemic ATP levels, and because it occurred during ischemia, not reperfusion, it could not be ascribed to purine salvage. Additional experiments revealed that this effect of adenosine could be mimicked by adenosine A_1 receptor agonists, while an adenosine receptor antagonist accelerated ATP catabolism.[9] These latter results suggested that adenosine receptor activation exerted effects on myocardial metabolism during ischemia which may mediate, in part its cardioprotective effects.

Subsequent studies indicated that adenosine exerted other metabolic effects during ischemia.[31] We observed that during low flow ischemia (0.6 ml/min) adenosine and adenosine + erythro-9-(2-hydroxy-3-nonyl)adenine (EHNA, an adenosine deaminase inhibitor) treatments in isolated rat hearts increased myocardial lactate release from 1.67 ± 0.19 μmol/min/g in control hearts to 2.20 ± 0.09 and 2.35 ± 0.31 μmol/min/g, respectively, after 20 minutes ischemia and maintained increased lactate release throughout ischemia. Adenosine and adenosine + EHNA prolonged time to onset of ischemic contracture (TOIC) from 11.6 ± 0.5 min to 13.6 ± 0.5 and 13.5 ± 0.3 min, respectively. Treatment with the adenosine A_1 receptor antagonist BW A1433U reduced TOIC (8.7 ± 0.2 min), markedly reduced lactate release, and increased adenosine release. When glucose was omitted from the perfusate, adenosine + EHNA treatment had no effect on TOIC. Lactate release during glucose-free perfusion was similar to that in hearts treated with the adenosine receptor blocker. Since it is unlikely that adenosine stimulates glycogen mobilization during ischemia, these findings suggest that during low flow ischemia adenosine exerts its beneficial effects, at least in part, via the modulation of glucose metabolism and/or myocardial lactate elimination.

To further elucidate the glucose dependent effect of adenosine we investigated the metabolic effects of adenosine during low flow ischemia in isolated guinea-pig hearts.[32] Hearts, perfused with 5 mM glucose (-insulin) at constant pressure and constant heart rate, were subjected to 15 minutes low flow (1 ml/min/g wet wt) ischemia and 20 minutes reperfusion. Treatment with 100 μM adenosine increased fructose-6-phosphate levels and lactate release during both preischemia and reperfusion. Adenosine increased hexose monophosphates but had little effect on fructose-6-phosphate/fructose diphosphate and 3-phosphoglycerate/dihydroxyacetone phosphate ratios, suggesting that adenosine may have increased glucose transport. A subsequent series of experiments addressed this possible mechanism. Normoxic isolated guinea-pig hearts were perfused with glucose in the absence of insulin, which renders glucose uptake transport limited. Glucose uptake was calculated from coronary flow and arterio-venous glucose concentration differences. Adenosine infusion (100 μM) significantly increased glucose uptake by 256 ± 77 nmol/min/g wet wt from a control glucose uptake of 317 ± 64 nmol/min/g wet wt; insulin (5 U/l) increased glucose uptake by 119 ± 18 nmol/min/g wet wt. Since the profiles of glycolytic intermediates observed with adenosine and insulin treatment are different, it is likely that adenosine and insulin act via different mechanisms. Adenosine could be altering glucose metabolism via an adenosine A_1 receptor dependent or independent pathway to facilitate glucose transport.

Since adenosine cardioprotection during low flow ischemia appears to require active glucose metabolism, and since the agent alters glycolytic profiles in reperfused myocardium, we next investigated whether adenosine enhanced cytosolic phosphorylation potential in the stunned heart.[32] Isolated perfused guinea pig hearts were submitted to low flow ischemia and reperfusion as described above. Treatment with adenosine (100 μM) had no effect on ATP or total adenylate (ATP + ADP + AMP) content after reperfusion; however, adenosine increased ATP concentration, CrP/Cr ratio, and CrP/P_i ratio during reperfusion. Adenosine increased the phosphorylation state of CrP, by 55% during reperfusion, suggesting a possible mechanism for adenosine's cardioprotective effect. Interestingly, adenosine treatment did not increase phosphorylation state in nonischemic hearts, consistent with observations that adenosine has no effect on ventricular function in normally perfused myocardium. Adenosine attenuation of in situ porcine regional myocardial stunning is also associated with improved myocardial phosphorylation potential at the end of reperfusion.[33] As shown in Figure 1-3 adenosine increased the (CrP)/(Cr)x(P_i) ratio, but not ATP content, in stunned myocardium. The exact role of adenosine's effects on myocardial energetics in the reversibly injured heart remain unclear.

Mechanisms of Adenosine Receptor-Mediated Cardioprotection

Although activation of adenosine A_1 receptors appears to be involved in adenosine-mediated cardioprotection there is little additional definitive information known concerning the mechanism. This difficulty is due in part to the fact that adenosine exerts little, if any, direct effects in normal ventricular myocardium. In fact the only known effect of adenosine in ventricular myocardium is the attenuation of the contractile and metabolic effects of b_1 adrenergic receptor stimulation.[34,35] Similar

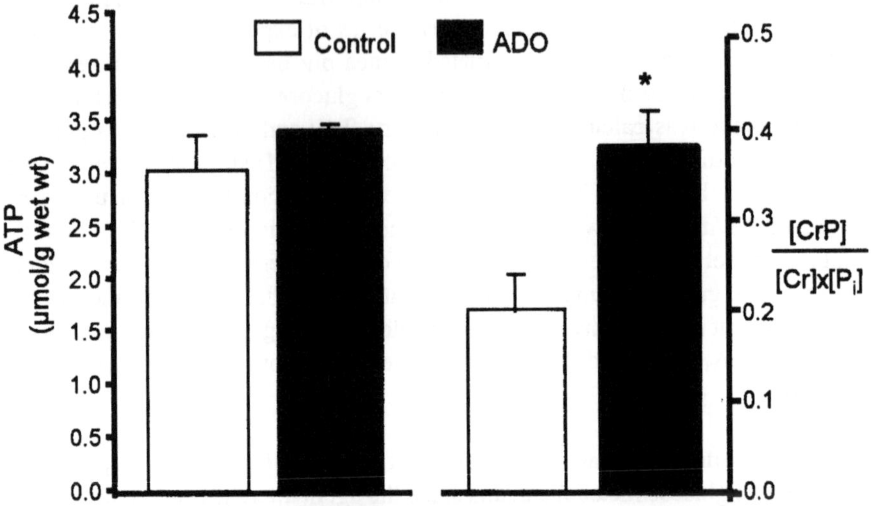

FIGURE 1-3. Adenosine (ADO) pretreatment effects on myocardial ATP contents and the CrP/CrxP$_i$ ratio in regionally stunned porcine myocardium. Tissue samples were obtained from the LAD bed after 90 minutes reperfusion following 10 minutes LAD occlusion. Adenosine treated hearts were administered intracoronary adenosine (50 µg/kg/min) for 20 minutes immediately prior to ischemia. Values are expressed as mean ± SEM, * $p < 0.05$ vs control hearts.

to the cardioprotective effect of adenosine, the anti-adrenergic effect of adenosine is mediated via activation of ventricular myocyte A_1 receptors coupled to a pertussis toxin sensitive G_i protein.[34] Since catecholamines are released during ischemia and are thought to play some role in myocardial ischemia-reperfusion injury, it is possible that the cardioprotective effect of adenosine is related to its anti-adrenergic effects. There is evidence to support this hypothesis as exogenous adenosine inhibits catecholamine release in normoxic myocardium,[36] and endogenous adenosine inhibits catecholamine release during myocardial ischemia.[37] In fact myocardial catecholamine release has been implicated in ischemia-induced increases in adenosine.[38] Two recent studies in intact[39] and isolated hearts[40] concluded that adenosine receptor activation was cardioprotective by exerting an anti-adrenergic effect during the period of ischemia.

Other mechanisms proposed for adenosine cardioprotection include attenuation of ischemia-induced intracellular Ca overload[41] and inhibition of oxygen free radical release and/or damage.[42,43] It has been shown that adenosine inhibits catecholamine-induced increases in intracellular calcium in normal ventricular myocardium,[35] so it is entirely possible that adenosine may protect the ischemic heart by reducing increases in intracellular calcium during ischemia.

However, it is not known whether this is due to a direct effect on calcium homeostasis or mediated via adenosine-enhanced preservation of myocardial energetics. Xia et al[43] recently reported that the adenosine deaminase inhibitor EHNA, which increases endogenous adenosine levels, inhibited oxygen free radical generation (assessed by electron paramagnetic resonance) and improved postischemic ventricular function in isolated perfused rat hearts. It was proposed that this effect occurred by the inhibition of adenosine metabolism to hypoxanthine and xanthine, substrates for xanthine oxidase. However it remains to be determined whether this mechanism occurs in other species, including man, which have much less myocardial xanthine oxidase activity than the rat.

In addition to reducing intracellular calcium overload during ischemia adenosine may modulate intracellular calcium homeostasis during reperfusion. There are reports that myocardial ischemia and reperfusion are associated with reductions in sarcoplasmic reticulum (SR) Ca^{2+} uptake and altered ryanodine-sensitive Ca^{2+} release channel (RyR) function.[44-46] Recent experiments in our laboratory tested whether adenosine-mediated attenuation of stunning is associated with restoration of SR function.[47] Tissue samples were obtained from the left anterior descending (LAD) coronary artery perfused bed and the nonischemic left circumflex (LC) bed of porcine myocardium after 10 minutes LAD occlusion and 2 hours reperfusion. Using heavy SR-enriched cardiac microsomes, SR Ca^{2+} uptake was estimated by measuring $^{45}Ca^{2+}$ uptake, and RyR function was assessed by the dissociation constant (K_D) and maximal binding capacity (B_{max}) of [^{3}H]-ryanodine from saturation curves. This analysis is based on the fact that ryanodine binds only to the open state of the SR Ca^{2+} release channel. $^{45}Ca^{2+}$ uptake rates in the stunned bed were decreased by 30% compared to the control nonstunned bed. Animals treated immediately prior to LAD occlusion with intracoronary adenosine (50 µg/kg/min) exhibited significantly improved regional ventricular function, however SR $^{45}Ca^{2+}$ uptake rates were depressed similarly to control stunned hearts (approx. 30%). Similar results were obtained in hearts treated with the adenosine A_1 receptor agonist CCPA, i.e., reduced stunning, but no effect on SR Ca^{2+} uptake. Myocardial stunning was associated with no change in the K_D of [^{3}H]-ryanodine binding but B_{max} was decreased 22% compared to nonstunned LC tissue from the same animal. The decreased ryanodine binding could be due to either a structural alteration of the channel or a decrease in the open state of the Ca^{2+} release channel. Pretreatments with either adenosine or the adenosine A_1 receptor agonist chlorocyclopentyladenosine (CCPA) attenuated stunning and completely prevented the decrease in [^{3}H]-ryanodine B_{max} in the stunned bed. Whether the adenosine and CCPA effects on the SR RyR in stunned myocardium are causally related to attenuation of stunning or merely a result of their beneficial effects remains to be determined.

Although the final common pathway in adenosine cardioprotection may involve maintenance of intracellular calcium homeostasis, the specific signal transduction pathway(s) responsible for this effect remain unresolved. There is some evidence that adenosine may protect the ischemic heart by modulating the activity of ATP dependent K^+ (K_{ATP}) channels,[28,48] and K_{ATP} channel openers have been shown to protect the ischemic heart.[49,50] However, there are few measurements of adenosine effects on K_{ATP} channel currents in normal or hypoxic adult ventricular myocytes. Kirsch et al[51] reported that adenosine A_1 receptors were coupled to K_{ATP} channels in 1-3 day old neonatal rat ventricular myocytes, but these results were obtained in only 7 of 16 experiments. In addition there appear to be some species and preparation differences in the ability of K_{ATP} blockers to the effects of adenosine in ischemic and hypoxic myocardium.[28,48,52,53]

Adenosine and Myocardial Infarct Size Reduction

The majority of the above described cardioprotective effects of adenosine are related to attenuation of reversible myocardial ischemic injury, since this is the injury most often occurring following cardiac surgery in humans.[6,7] However, adenosine has been shown to also reduce infarct size via an A_1 receptor mechanism similar to its anti-stunning effect,[11-13,15] and the majority of this protection, at least with exogenous adenosine, appears to be due to reduction of ischemic injury. However, there appear to be some differences between adenosine's anti-stunning and anti-infarct effects. Adenosine infusion during reperfusion does not attenuate stunning,[10,54] but there are conflicting reports on whether adenosine administered during reperfusion reduces infarct size.[15,55,56] We observed in our laboratory that elevation of endogenous adenosine levels with the nucleoside transport inhibitor draflazine increased coronary venous plasma and ISF adenosine levels during reperfusion in the intact pig, but did not reduce infarct size.[15] Draflazine administered prior to coronary occlusion was cardioprotective.

A second important difference between adenosine's protective effects in reversible and irreversible myocardial ischemic injury is related to preischemic treatment regimens. Adenosine pretreatment, in which the adenosine infusion is not terminated until the onset of ischemia reduces both myocardial stunning[8,10,13] and infarct size.[57] However, adenosine preconditioning, in which the infusion of adenosine is terminated 5-10 minutes prior to ischemia, reduces infarct size,[11,12,53,57] but does not attenuate stunning.[54,57] These differences between adenosine pretreatment and adenosine preconditioning are puzzling since the A_1 receptor appears to be involved in reduction of both types of injury.

Conclusion

In summary, significant progress has been made in the elucidation of the role of adenosine in the protection of the ischemic myocardium. Based on our work and on studies by others, we believe that there is substantial evidence to indicate that ischemic protection afforded by adenosine is via activation of myocyte adenosine A_1 receptors and possible modulation of intracellular calcium homeostasis. While we have learned the optimal timing for adenosine administration is just prior to and during the early onset of ischemia and have been successful in achieving a sustained 50% attenuation of myocardial stunning and infarct size, the ultimate objective is to provide 100% protection.

References

1. Marban E, Kitakaze M, Kusuoka H et al. Intracellular free calcium concentration measured with ^{19}F NMR spectroscopy in intact ferret hearts. Proc Natl Acad Sci USA 1987;84:6005-6009.
2. Steenbergen C, Murphy E, Levy L et al. Elevation in cytosolic free calcium concentration early in myocardial ischemia in perfused rat heart. Circ Res 1987;60:700-707.
3. Kihara Y, Grossman W, Morgan JP. Direct measurement of changes in intracellular calcium transients during hypoxia, ischemia, and reperfusion of the intact mammalian heart. Circ Res 1989;65:1029-1044.
4. Braunwald E, Kloner RB. The stunned myocardium: Prolonged postischemic ventricular dysfunction. Circulation 1982;60: 1146-1149.
5. Jennings RB, Reimer KA. The cell biology of acute myocardial ischemia. Ann Rev Med 1991;42:225-246.
6. Scott BD, Kerber RE. Clinical and experimental aspects of myocardial stunning. Prog Cardiovasc Dis 1991;35:61-76.
7. Bolli R. Myocardial stunning in man. Circulation 1992;86:1671-1691.
8. Ely SW, Mentzer RM, Lasley RD et al. Functional and metabolic evidence of enhanced myocardial tolerance to ischemia and reperfusion with adenosine. J Thorac Cardiovasc Surg 1985;90:549-556.
9. Lasley RD, Rhee JW, Van Wylen DGL et al. Adenosine A_1 receptor mediated protection of the globally ischemic isolated rat heart. J Mol Cell Cardiol 1990;22:39-47.
10. Randhawa MPS Jr, Lasley RD, Mentzer RM Jr. Salutary effects of exogenous adenosine on canine myocardial stunning in vivo. J Thorac Cardiovasc Surg 1995;110:63-74.
11. Thornton JD, Liu GS, Olsson RA et al. Intravenous pretreatment with A_1-selective adenosine analogues protects the heart against infarction. Circulation 1992;85:659-665.
12. Lasley RD, Konyn PJ, Hegge JO et al. The effects of ischemic and adenosine preconditioning on interstitial fluid adenosine and myocardial infarct size. Am J Physiol 1995;269:H1460-H1466.
13. Dorheim TA, Hoffman A, Van Wylen DGL et al. Enhanced interstitial fluid adenosine attenuates myocardial stunning. J Surg 1991;110:136-145.
14. Hudspeth DA, Williams MW, Zhao ZQ et al. Pentostatin-augmented interstitial adenosine prevents postcardioplegia injury in damaged hearts. Ann Thorac Surg 1994;58:719-727.
15. Martin BJ, Lasley RD, Mentzer RM Jr. Infarct size reduction with the nucleoside transport inhibitor R75231 in swine. Am J Physiol (In Press), 1997.

16. Benson ES, Evans GT, Hallaway BE et al. Myocardial creatine phosphate and nucleotides in anoxic cardiac arrest and recovery. Am J Physiol 1961;201:687-693.
17. Namm DH. Myocardial nucleotide synthesis from purine bases and nucleosides. Comparison of the rates of formation of purine nucleotides from various precursors and identification of the enzymatic routes for nucleotide formation in the isolated rat heart. Circ Res 1973;33:686-965.
18. Liu MS, Feinberg H. Incorporation of adenosine-8-^{14}C and inosine-8-^{14}C into rabbit heart adenine nucleotides. Am J Physiol 1971;220:1242-1284.
19. Reibel DK, Rovetto MJ. Myocardial adenosine salvage rates and restoration of ATP content following ischemia. Am J Physiol 1979;237:H247-H252.
20. Ambrosio G, Jacobus WE, Mitchell MC et al. Effects of ATP precursors on ATP and free ADP content and functional recovery of postischemic hearts. Am J Physiol 1989;256:H560-H566.
21. Neely JR, Grotyohann LW. Role of glycolytic products in damage to ischemic myocardium. Dissociation of adenosine triphosphate levels and recovery of function of reperfused ischemic hearts. Circ Res 1984;55:816-824.
22. Mallet RT, Hartman DA, Bünger R. Glucose requirement for postischemic recovery of perfused working heart. Eur J Biochem 1990;188:481-493.
23. Headrick JP, Willis RJ. Effects of adenosine antagonism and beta-blockade during low-flow ischaemia in rat heart. Clin Exper Pharmacol Physiol 1989;16:885-891.
24. Froldi G, Belardinelli L. Species-dependent effects of adenosine on heart rate and atrioventricular nodal conduction. Mechanism and physiological implications. Circ Res 1990;67:960-78.
25. Schubert T, Vetter H, Owen P et al. Adenosine cardioplegia. Adenosine versus poassium cardioplegia: effects on cardiac arrest and postischemic recovery in he isolated rat heart. J Thorac Cardiovasc Surg 1989;98:1057-1065.
26. Belardinelli L, Linden J, Berne RM. The cardiac actions of adenosine. Prog Cardiovasc Dis 1989;22:73-97.
27. Lasley RD, Mentzer RM Jr. Adenosine improves the recovery of postischemic myocardial function via an adenosine A_1 receptor mechanism. Am J Physiol 1992;263:H1460-H1465.
28. Yao Z, Gross GJ. Glibenclamide antagonizes adenosine A1 receptor-mediated cardioprotection in stunned canine myocardium. Circulation 1993;88:235-244.
29. Lasley RD, Mentzer RM Jr. Pertussis toxin blocks adenosine A_1 receptor mediated protection of the ischemic rat heart. J Mol Cell Cardiol 1993;25:815-821.
30. Wyatt DA, Ely SW, Lasley RD et al. Purine-enriched asanguineous cardioplegia retards adenosine triphosphate degradation during ischemia and improves postischemic ventricular function. J Thorac Cardiovasc Surg 1989;97:771-778.
31. Lasley RD, Mentzer RM Jr. Adenosine increases lactate release and delays onset of contracture during global low flow ischaemia. Cardiovasc Res 1993;27:96-101.
32. Mentzer RM Jr, Bünger R, Lasley RD. Adenosine enhanced preservation of myocardial function and energetics. Possible involvement of the adenosine A_1 receptor system. Cardiovasc Res 1993;27:28-35.
33. Zhou Z, Bünger R, Lasley RD et al. Adenosine pretreatment increases cytosolic phosphorylation potential and attenuates postischemic cardiac dysfunction in swine. Surg Forum 1993;44:249-252.
34. Dobson JG, Fenton RA, Romano FD. The antiadrenergic actions of adenosine in the heart. In: Gerlach, E and Becker, BF, eds. Topics and Perspectives in Adenosine Research. Berlin, Heidelberg: Springer-Verlag, 1987:356-368.
35. Fenton RA, Moore EDW, Fay FS et al. Adenosine reduces the Ca^{2+} transients of isoproterenol- stimulated rat ventricular myocytes. Am J Physiol 1991;261:C1107-C1114.

36. Wennmalm M, Fredholm BB, Hedqvist P. Adenosine as a modulator of sympathetic nerve-stimulation-induced release of noradrenaline from the isolated rabbit heart. Acta Physiol Scand 1988;132:487-494.
37. Richardt G, Waas W, Kranzhofer R et al. Adenosine inhibits exocytotic release of endogenous noradrenaline in rat heart: a protective mechanism in early myocardial ischemia. Circ Res 1987;61:117-123.
38. Richardt G, Blessing R, Schomig A. Cardiac noradrenaline release accelerates adenosine formation in the ischemic rat heart: role of neuronal noradrenaline carrier and adrenergic receptors. J Mol Cell Cardiol 1994;26:1321-1328.
39. Rynning SE, Brunvand H, Birkeland S et al. Endogenous adenosine attenuates myocardial stunning by antiadrenergic effects exerted during ischemia and not during reperfusion. J Cardiovasc Pharmacol 1995;25:432-439.
40. Fenton RA, Galeckas KJ, Dobson JG Jr. Endogenous adenosine reduces depression of cardiac function induced by beta-adrenergic stimulation during low flow perfusion. J Mol Cell Cardiol 1995;27:2373-2383.
41. Fralix, TA, Murphy E, London RE. Protective effects of adenosine in the perfused rat heart: changes in metabolism and intracellular ion homeostasis. Am J Physiol 1993;264:C986-C994.
42. Karmazyn M, Cook MA. Adenosine A_1 receptor activation attenuates cardiac injury produced by hydrogen peroxide. Circ Res 1992;71:1101-1110.
43. Xia Y, Khatchikian G, Zweier JL. Adenosine deaminase inhibition prevents free radical-mediated injury in the postischemic heart. J Biol Chem 1996;271:10096-10102.
44. Krause FM, Jacobus WE, Becker LC. Alterations in cardiac sarcoplasmic reticulum calcium transport in the postischemic "stunned" myocardium. Circ Res 1989;65:526-530.
45. Wu QY, Feher J. Effect of ischemia and ischemia-reperfusion on ryanodine binding and Ca^{2+} uptake of cardiac sarcoplasmic reticulum. J Mol Cell Cardiol 1995;27:1965-1975.
46. Zucchi R, Ronca-Testoni S, Yu G et al. Effects of ischemia and reperfusion on cardiac ryanodine receptors sarcoplasmic reticulum Ca^{2+} channels. Circ Res 1994;74:271-280.
47. Valdivia CR, Lasley RD, Hegge JO et al. Adenosine pretreatment prevents myocardial stunning-induced reduction of ryanodine receptor function. Circulation 1996;94(Suppl I):I-185.
48. Yao Z, Gross GJ. A comparison of adenosine-induced cardioprotection and ischemic preconditioning in dogs. Efficacy, time course, and role of KATP channels. Circulation 1994;89:1229-1236.
49. Grover GJ, Dzwonczyk S, Parham CS et al. The protective effects of cromakalim and pinacidil on reperfusion function and infarct size in isolated perfused hearts and anesthetized dogs. Cardiovasc Drugs Ther 1990;4:465-474.
50. Yao Z, Gross GJ. Effects of the KATP channel opener bimakalim on coronary blood flow, monophasic action potential duration, and infarct size in dogs. Circulation 1994;89:1769-1775.
51. Kirsch GE, Codina J, Birnbaumer L et al. Coupling of ATP-sensitive K^+ channels to A_1 receptors by G proteins in rat ventricular myocytes. Am J Physiol 1990;259:H820-H826.
52. Grover GJ, Baird AJ, Sleph PG. Lack of a pharmacologic interaction between ATP-sensitive potassium channels and adenosine A(1) receptors in ischemic rat hearts. Cardiovasc Res 1996;31:511-517.
53. Xu J, Wang L, Hurt CM et al. Endogenous adenosine does not activate ATP-sensitive potassium channels in the hypoxic guinea pig ventricle in vivo. Circulation 1994;89:1209-1216.
54. Sekili S, Jeroudi MO, Tang XL et al. Effect of adenosine on myocardial 'stunning' in the dog. Circ Res 1995;76:82-94.
55. Todd J, Zhao ZQ, Williams MW et al. Intravascular adenosine at reperfusion reduces infarct size and neutrophil adherence. Ann Thorac Surg 1996;62:1364-1372.

56. Vander Heide RS, Reimer KA. Effect of adenosine therapy at reperfusion on myocardial infarct size in dogs. Cardiovasc Res 1996;31:711-8.
57. Lasley RD, Noble MA, Konyn PJ et al. Different effects of an adenosine A_1 analogue and ischemic preconditioning in isolated rabbit hearts. Ann Thorac Surg 1995;60:1698-1703.

In: Mentzer, R.M., Jr., Kitakaze, M., Downey, J.M., Hori, M, eds. Adenosine, Cardioprotection and Clinical Application. Kluwer Academic Publishers, Norwell, MA, USA, 1997.

II. CARDIOPROTECTION AND MECHANISMS OF ISCHEMIC AND REPERFUSION INJURY

2. Concept of Cardioprotection Against Myocardial Ischemia

Masatsugu Hori

Introduction

When the oxygen supply to the myocardium is restricted by an occlusion or narrowing of the coronary artery, ischemic changes are induced and eventually irreversible injury occurs after some critical period of ischemia. To salvage the ischemic myocardium, early restoration of blood supply is most effective. Accumulating evidence, however, suggests that appropriate techniques of reperfusion may salvage more myocytes than the simple reperfusion since reperfusion itself may cause the additional irreversible injury.[1] Accumulation of toxic substances such as hydrogen ions, lactate, fatty acid derivatives, free radicals and intracellular calcium overload may cause the transition from reversible to irreversible injury. Microvascular injuries during ischemia and reperfusion also accelerate the ischemic damage and disturb the restoration of blood perfusion after recanalization. Preservation of microvascular integrity and acceleration of collateral development are protective against the ischemic damage. Various interventions which could scavenge free radicals and inhibit calcium overload after reperfusion have been reported. During cardiac surgery cardioplegia are commonly used to protect the myocardium from the ischemic injury. In prophylactic view, acquisition of ischemic tolerance against irreversible injury is also important. Since certain stress such as brief reversible ischemia, hypoxia, heat and oxidative stress could render the heart tolerable against myocardial infarction and functional deterioration. Ischemic preconditioning could markedly attenuate infarct size and postischemic dysfunction and arrhythmia. A delayed protective action of ischemic preconditioning is also observed. Although the precise mechanisms of this phenomenon are not clarified yet, clinical application may provide a great benefit for patients with ischemic heart disease.

In aerobic condition, myocardium depends on oxygen delivered by the arterial blood to support high-energy phosphate production. When the blood supply is insufficient to meet the requirements for mitochondrial respiration, high-energy phosphate production by anaerobic glycolysis is not enough, and accordingly, the contractile function is reduced and lactate is accumulated. In the early period of ischemia, cellular dysfunction is reversible, but eventually damage occurs to some critical subcellular organelles. When ischemia is of sufficient severity and persists long enough, myocytes become "irreversibly injured" and undergo cellular necrosis. Ischemic microvascular injury also occurs exacerbating the severity of ischemia. However, the severity of ischemia varies depending on the extent of myocardial oxygen demand and myocardial blood supply through collateral circulation. Thus, the duration to the onset of irreversible change is not uniform even with an abrupt and complete occlusion of the coronary artery. The time course of ischemic cell death during myocardial infarction cannot be easily established in humans, however, the 3- to 6-hr time limit of salvageability observed in awake dogs could be applied to patients with acute myocardial infarction.

To salvage the ischemic myocardium, early restoration of blood supply to the myocardium is critically important. Since the subendocardial myocardium is susceptible to ischemia, a transmural "wavefront" of cell death progresses from the subendocardium to the subepicardium. In canine experiments, reperfusion at 3 hrs can limit the transmural extent of the infarct by about 10%, but by 6 hrs, infarcts have reached their full size and are not influenced by reperfusion at this time. In clinical setting also, early reperfusion either by thrombolysis (PTCR) and coronary angioplasty (PTCA) of less than 6 hrs could limit the infarct size, whereas late reperfusion later than 6 hrs could not reduce the infarct size although it could attenuate ventricular remodeling.

Another important aspect of reperfusion is the microvascular damage since restoration of arterial pressure to damaged microvasculature may result in myocardial edema because of increased capillary permeability and intramyocardial hemorrhage. Intravascular obstruction by swollen endothelial cells, sticky white cells or platelet-fibrin microthrombi is also accelerated, leading to "no-reflow" phenomenon. Presence of no-reflow is demonstrated by myocardial contrast echocardiography in humans after coronary recanalization in acute myocardial infarction. Thus, prevention of no-reflow after coronary recanalization is an important target of the therapy.

Whether reperfusion injury occurs after recanalization is still debatable. Recent accumulating evidence, however, suggests that some myocytes still viable at the instant of reperfusion are killed by the added detrimental consequences of reperfusion. Since early reperfusion limits infarct size by salvaging some ischemic myocytes, it is clear that for the total population of ischemic myocytes, early reperfusion is better than no reperfusion. Possible mechanisms for reperfusion injury include: 1) a burst of free-radical production, mainly derived from activated neutrophils, 2) calcium overload due to increased calcium permeability of sarcolemma and/or enhanced Na/Ca exchange, 3) massive myocyte swelling due to impairment of volume-regulating mechanisms, and 4) apoptosis of myocardial cells characterized by disrupture of DNA and shrinkage of cells.[2,3] Reperfusion injury, however, does not only accelerate the cell death but also induce reperfusion arrhythmia and functional abnormality, termed as "myocardial stunning".

Characteristics of reperfusion injury

Reperfusion injury means that the act of reperfusion itself has some deleterious effects. There is still concern whether reperfusion injury exists in humans. If it is a case, there may be an optimal treatment or adjunctive therapies at the time of reperfusion that could prevent these deleterious effects and further improve the outcome of the patients with myocardial infarction. From the therapeutic view, the concept of reperfusion injury is attractive, because therapeutic action of clinicians usually start only after ischemic event has already begun.

The types of reperfusion injury has been documented in animal experiments and probably in humans; lethal injury, functional injury, reperfusion arrhythmia and vascular injury. Lethal reperfusion injury is described as cell death due to reperfusion itself rather than to the preceding ischemia. In this form of injury, myocardial cells become irreversibly injured by reperfusion. Demonstration of the direct evidence for the existence of lethal reperfusion injury is difficult; the only way to demonstrate the existence of reperfusion injury is to show the infarct-limiting effect of some adjunctive therapies at the time of reperfusion. A number of studies have examined the effects of oxygen radical scavengers, iron chelators, calcium channel blockers, fluosol, adenosine and angiotensin-converting enzyme inhibitors. Although not all agents reduce the infarct size, some interventions could reduce the irreversible injury in animal models with ischemia and reperfusion. We also observed that inhibition of intrinsic production of adenosine only during reperfusion by AOPCP significantly attenuates the infarct-size limiting effect of ischemic preconditioning. This indicates that intrinsic adenosine released during reperfusion could contribute to the inhibition of lethal reperfusion injury. Recent reports demonstrate that reperfusion induces apoptosis of myocardial cells in animal experiments; nucleosomal ladders of DNA fragments are observed in ischemic/reperfused animal hearts. The occurrence of apoptosis in ischemic myocytes only when they are subjected to reperfusion suggests a reperfusion-specific process that could lead to delayed cell death.

Another form of reperfusion injury is ventricular dysfunction after reperfusion, i.e., myocardial stunning which often persists for several days. It is reported that intracoronary infusion of the cell-permeable antioxidant MPG (N-[2-mercaptopropionyl]glycine) 1 min before reperfusion significantly attenuated the stunning in a canine model subjected to 15 min-ischemia and reperfusion. We also demonstrated that staged reperfusion and acidotic reperfusion which inhibit the abrupt recovery of tissue acidosis at reperfusion could attenuate myocardial stunning, indicating that Ca overload through Na/H and Na/Ca exchangers may contribute to functional abnormality of the heart after perfusion. There is substantial evidence suggesting that the stunned myocardium occurs in humans, following coronary recanalization, cardiopulmonary bypass surgery and exercise-induced ischemia.

Reperfusion arrhythmia is another type of reperfusion injury. Reperfusion arrhythmia may be defined as ventricular arrhythmias that develop within a short period after coronary reperfusion. Although ventricular arrhythmia occur in patients with acute myocardial infarction, it remains debatable whether these arrhythmias are exacerbated by reperfusion. A recent report demonstrates no difference in the incidence of ventricular fibrillation, ventricular tachycardia or premature ventricular contraction between patients who did or did not receive thrombolytic therapy. Evidence that reperfusion has no deleterious long-term consequences on arrhythmia comes from several multicenter trials. Therefore, at least from clinical view point, reperfusion arrhythmia is uncommon in patients with acute myocardial infarction. However, reperfusion arrhythmia may be more important after short episodes of myocardial ischemia, e.g., vasospastic angina, unstable angina and silent myocardial ischemia.

Microvascular reperfusion injury is present at the end of an ischemic period, however, it is suggested that further damage to the vasculature occurs with progression of reperfusion; the size of no-reflow area is increased with time after reperfusion, and coronary blood flow and flow reserve are progressively decreased for several hours. These findings indicate that some damage to the vasculature occurs during reperfusion. Contracture or swelling of neighboring myocytes, endothelial cell swelling and plugging of activated neutrophils and platelets may cause the microvascular injury. Recent clinical studies using myocardial contrast echocardiography demonstrate perfusion defects even after coronary reperfusion in one-third of the patients with acute myocardial infarction who had successful coronary recanalization. Since presence of no reflow is closely correlated with abnormal wall motion at the remote period, microvascular injury is also important among reperfusion injuries.

Protection of the ischemic myocardium against irreversible injury

It is widely accepted that larger infarcts are associated with a greater loss of contractility and greater susceptibility to life threatening arrhythmia, and hence greater risk in survival. This is attributable to absence of regeneration ability of the myocardium; irreversibly injured myocardium is replaced by scar that cannot be regenerated. The loss of myocardial cells is usually compensated by hypertrophy of the residual myocardial cells but not by hyperplasia of the myocytes. Adaptive myocardial hypertrophy could compensate the loss of contractile ability of the heart, however, excessive hypertrophy of the myocytes associated with tissue fibrosis causes various alterations in proteins, ion channels and receptors, and thus, metabolic functions of the cells are also altered probably due to increased mechanical stress, neurohumoral activation and relative myocardial ischemia. These changes result in remodeling of the heart and eventually shift to failing heart in a long period. Thus, prevention of irreversible injury or preservation of the ischemic myocardium is a primary goal of therapy for the ischemic heart. This may be possible since the ischemic myocytes do not die instantaneously or simultaneously and infarct size can be limited for a period of time after the onset of ischemia.

Early recanalization to limit the infarct size

Limitation of infarct size or prevention of infarct expansion from subendocardial to transmural infarction is entirely dependent on early restoration of adequate coronary blood flow to the ischemic region. Such restoration of blood flow can be achieved by active interventions, e.g. thrombolytic therapy (PTCR), angioplasty (PTCA) or surgical revascularization. Earlier reperfusion achieves better outcome; infarct size is limited and survival rate is improved by a timely restoration of the blood flow, mostly within 4 hrs after the onset of infarction. Limitation of infarct size is clearly dependent on the time before recanalization. Late reperfusion usually defined as a reperfusion after 6 hrs, however, also has a potential benefit to prevent the dilation of the ventricle, i.e., remodeling of the heart in a remote period although the infarct size could not be limited. Currently available thrombolytic agents are clinically very useful, but have several limitations in their efficacy. Better outcome could be obtained by direct PTCA than thrombolytic therapy alone or PTCR combined with rescue or immediate PTCA mostly due to earlier and adequate recanalization by direct PTCA. New types of thrombolytic agents that are more potent, and more specific to thrombus and less bleeding risk are developed, such as TNK-rTPA, anisoylated plasminogen streptokinase activator complex, two-chain urokinase-type plasminogen activator (UPA), recombinant single-chain UPA (prourokinase), and more recently, recombinant staphylokinase and derivatives. Accordingly, the outcome of thrombolytic therapy may be improved in next decade with these new agents. Acute reocclusion after thrombolytic therapy or angioplasty could be prevented by intracoronary stents in some cases, however, reocclusion within 24 hrs and restenosis within 6 months are current limitations of recanalization therapy. Intravenous administration of selective thrombin inhibitors (heparin and hirudin) and/or antibody against platelet glycoproteins IIb/IIIa (7E3) for several days after recanalization followed by anticoagulant or antiplatelet therapy is a promising regimen to keep the patency of the coronary flow.[4]

Collateral flow and myocardial salvage

Collateral anastomoses which supply the blood to ischemic regions largely contribute to maintain the viability and function of the ischemic myocardium. In normal human hearts, coronary collaterals are present but poorly developed. In patients with frequent ischemic episodes or previous myocardial infarction, collateral anastomoses are often developed well and visualized by coronary angiography. Although the incidence of myocardial infarction is not altered, the incidence of Q waves or pump failure has been lower in several studies of patients with myocardial infarction if the collaterals are well developed. Thus, collateral flow may be protective to prevent the transition of infarct expansion from subendocardial to subepicardial layers since collateral flow is predominantly distributed to the epicardial layers. Myocardial perfusion even via collateral vessels could wash out the accumulated metabolites in the ischemic regions and thus, slow the progression of ischemic metabolic changes. It is well known that collateral vessels are developed by repeated occlusions of the coronary artery in dogs. Although chemical mediators such as EGF and bFGF and TGF-β are known to contribute to angiogenesis, therapeutic application has not been established. Frequent episodes of myocardial ischemia and exercise training especially with administration of heparin accelerates the development of collateral vessels. Recently surgical procedures that construct multiple transmural channels across the ventricular wall by laser technique (TAR) are applied clinically to make the heart tolerable against the ischemia.

Intraoperative cardioprotection using cardioplegia

Cardiac interventions during cardiac surgery may cause the ischemic injury. Myocardial damage from inadequate protection of the heart leads to low output syndrome causing delayed myocardial fibrosis. To minimize the intraoperative ischemic injury, cardioplegia has been widely used for protection of the heart.

Initial challenge for the cardioprotection was hypothermia since it slows cardiac metabolism and preserves the high energy phosphates while limiting ischemic injury during aortic cross-clamping. Hypothermia, however, has certain adverse consequences; shifting the oxygen-hemoglobin dissociation curve leftward, promoting edema, increasing blood viscosity and activating platelets, leukocytes and complements. To avoid these disadvantages of hypothermia, warm blood cardioplegia without hypothermia was introduced; the patients and the heart are maintained at 37^0 C and the cardioplegic flow is delivered continually when feasible. The rationale of this technique is based on the hypotheses that cardiac arrest substantially decreases myocardial oxygen demand and that systemic normothermia could limit the detrimental effects of hypothermic cardiopulmonary bypass on coagulation and other organ systems. Recent experimental results, however, do not support the superiority of the warm blood cardioplegia; intermittent cold antegrade and antegrade/retrograde blood cardioplegic techniques are superior to continuous warm antegrade or retrograde cardioplegia.[5] There are also a number of issues to be answered in the technique using warm blood cardioplegia including optimal flow rate and ideal cardioplegic composition. Thus, before establishment of warm blood cardioplegia, either as a standard therapy or as an adjunctive therapy to hypothermic techniques, more comprehensive clinical testings and further experimental studies are necessary.

Inhibition of Ca overload during reperfusion

Inhibition of reperfusion injury is another important target of cardioprotection in treatment of ischemic heart disease and preservation of donor heart in cardiac transplantation. Functional reperfusion injury, i.e., myocardial stunning is frequently observed after reperfusion both in patients with acute ischemic syndrome and after cardiopulmonary bypass. Ca overload and free radical production immediately after reperfusion play an important role in pathogenesis of myocardial stunning. A volume of evidence indicate that Ca overload is induced by Na/Ca exchange. During ischemia hydrogen ions are accumulated, and consequently Na influx is augmented via Na/H exchange, whereas Na/Ca exchange is inhibited by hydrogen ions during ischemia. Upon reperfusion, however, rapid recovery of acidosis releases the inhibition of Na/Ca exchange and thus, Ca influx is augmented through this ion exchange mechanism, leading to Ca overload. Inhibitors of Na/H exchange, amiloride and its derivatives significantly attenuate the Na accumulation during ischemia and Ca overload after reperfusion. It is demonstrated that ischemic ventricular arrhythmia and myocardial stunning are markedly inhibited by Na/H exchange inhibitor in animal experiments. Since Ca influx upon reperfusion is not through voltage dependent Ca channels, calcium antagonist administered immediately before reperfusion could not attenuate myocardial stunning. Instead, reperfusion with low [Ca^{2+}] solution attenuates Ca accumulation and hence, functional recovery is improved. Gradual opening of the occluded coronary artery (staged reperfusion) also slows the recovery of acidosis and prevents Ca overload after reperfusion. Potassium channel openers, e.g., cromakalim, pinacidil and nicorandil attenuated Ca influx, preventing myocardial stunning. Administration of adenosine also attenuates Ca influx and improves the functional recovery after reperfusion. Augmentation of intrinsic adenosine production by administration of AICA-riboside or stimulation of α_1-adrenoceptors attenuates myocardial stunning.

Free radical scavengers

There is a large body of evidence that reactive oxygen species (free radicals) are generated during ischemia-reperfusion of the myocardium and may cause the cellular injury. The myocardium has endogenous antioxidant system which could metabolize free radicals generated in the normal cellular activity, however, the scavenging capacity is not sufficient during reperfusion at which excessive free radicals are generated from xanthine-xanthine oxidase reaction, mitochondrial reduction of oxygen, respiratory burst of activated neutrophils, auto-oxidation of catecholamines and metabolism of arachidonic acid. To scavenge the excessive free radicals and reduce the reperfusion injury, exogenous antioxidants have been applied to the ischemic/reperfused hearts. Many studies support the hypothesis that exogenous administration of antioxidants could reduce the infarct size after prolonged ischemia; SOD, catalase, allopurinol, perfluochemical and MPG were reported to be effective to limit the infarct size. On the other hand, there is a considerable number of reports that failed to demonstrate the positive effects. The reason why exogenous antioxidants have limited success in prevention of lethal reperfusion injury may be partly attributed to the inaccessibility of large molecules to key intracellular sites of free radical generation.[6] However, it is clear that free radicals contribute to pathogenesis of functional reperfusion injury (myocardial stunning) and reperfusion arrhythmia. In animal experiments SOD, SOD+catalase, dimethylthiourea, desferrioxamine, α-tocopherol, oxypurinol, MPG, allopurinol and spin trap agents have been reported to attenuate myocardial stunning after reperfusion. All of these antioxidants could also attenuate reperfusion arrhythmia. Intravenous administration of human-recombinant SOD before coronary thrombolysis reduced the incidence of ventricular premature contractions during first one hour of reperfusion in patients with acute myocardial infarction.

Ischemic tolerance against myocardial necrosis

Some stress such as brief ischemia, hypoxia, heat and oxidative stress may render the myocardium tolerable against irreversible injury. Ischemic preconditioning was first reported in 1986; four times of 5 min ischemia before sustained (40 min) ischemia markedly reduced the infarct size. There is increasing evidence that adenosine plays an important role in this phenomenon. After the first report that adenosine A_1-receptors are involved in ischemic preconditioning, however, a number of studies proposed other endogenous substances, e.g., acetylcholine, bradykinin, norepinephrine, angiotensin II, endothelin, Ca^{2+} and free radicals as a mediator of this cardiac protection. The current consensus is that the endogenous chemical mediators may not be a single but several mediators may contribute synergistically, however, activation of protein kinase C is important in the signal transduction. It is of note that protective effect of ischemic preconditioning against infarct persists no longer than two hrs, and there must be some "memory" mechanism in the signal transduction. More recently, a delayed protective response ("second window of protection") has been observed 24 hrs after periods of brief ischemia in dogs and rabbits. In the dog hearts this delayed response of protection is associated with an induction of an antioxidant enzyme, MnSOD, whereas in rabbit hearts it is reported that expression of HSPs may contribute to the delayed effect of protection. Accumulating evidence supports the hypothesis that some antioxidant proteins are induced by a brief ischemia imposed to the heart before sustained ischemia, and the myocardium obtains the tolerance against the ischemic injury. Protective effects of ischemic preconditioning have been also proven in humans. In patients with acute myocardial infarction who had successful coronary recanalization, infarct size assessed by serum creatine kinase levels and cardiac function was smaller if they had antecedent anginal attacks before the infarction. In TIMI-4 study also, previous angina confers a beneficial effect on in-hospital outcome after acute myocardial infarction. In open heart surgery ischemic preconditioning is applicable, and indeed, brief ischemia imposed before the open heart surgery improved the functional recovery after weaning from cardio-pulmonary bypass. A growing evidence of ischemic preconditioning in humans encourages us to investigate the precise underlying mechanisms so that considerable limiting of infarct size could be achieved by therapeutic interventions.

Conclusion

Accordingly, protection of ischemic myocardium against irreversible damage or functional impairment has a variety of aspects, i.e., 1) improvement of myocardial oxygen demand-supply relationship by attenuating oxygen demand and increasing collateral circulation to the ischemic myocardium, and applying cardioplegia and myocardial cooling during ischemia/hypoxia, 2) inhibition of accumulation of detrimental products derived from metabolic process, e.g., inhibition of intracellular Na accumulation by an inhibitor of Na/H exchanger, and inhibition of Ca accumulation by low Ca perfusion, 3) inhibition of reperfusion injury by administration of radical scavengers. Another important mean of cardioprotection is acquisition of ischemic tolerance of myocardium by preconditioning of the heart. Ischemic preconditioning could render the myocardium tolerable to ischemic damage; a marked reduction of infarct size is obtained by a precedent ischemic stress before sustained myocardial ischemia and reperfusion. This is a new area of cardioprotection to be discussed since elucidation of the underlying mechanisms may provide the therapeutic approach in the clinical settings.

References

1. Braunwald E, Kloner RA. Myocardial reperfusion: A double-edged sword? J Clin Invest 1985;80:1713-19.
2. Opie LH. The mechanism of myocyte death in ischemia. Eur Heart J 1993; 14, *Suppl* G: 31-33
3. Gottlieb RA, Burleson KO, Kloner RA et al. Reperfusion injury induces apoptosis in rabbit cardiomyocytes. J Clin Invest 1994; 94:1621-28
4. Hearse DJ, Bolli R. Reperfusion induced injury: Manifestations, mechanisms, and clinical relevance. Cardiovasc Res 1992; 26:101-8
5. Buckberg GD. Update on current techniques of myocardial protection. Ann Throrac Surg 1995; 60: 805-14
6. Kloner RA, Przyklenk K, Whittaker P. Deleterious effects of oxygen radicals in ischemia/reperfusion: Resolved and unresolved issues. Circulation 1989: 80:1115-27

In: Mentzer, R.M., Jr., Kitakaze, M., Downey, J.M., Hori, M, eds. Adenosine, Cardioprotection and Clinical Application. Kluwer Academic Publishers, Norwell, MA, USA, 1997.

3. The Late Phase of Preconditioning Against Myocardial Stunning

Roberto Bolli
Xian-Liang Tang
Yumin Qiu
Seong-Wook Park

Introduction

It has recently become apparent that there are two phases of ischemic preconditioning against myocardial stunning: an early phase, which begins within minutes, and a late phase, which begins after >6 h.[1] These two phases have different pathophysiology and probably different mechanisms. Although the early phase is somewhat controversial, most of the discrepancies can be explained by differences in the duration of the ischemic insult, as detailed in ref. 1; that is, the available evidence indicates that an episode of ischemia protects against the stunning induced by a second ischemic episode when the second episode lasts ≤5 min but not when it lasts ≥10 min. When early preconditioning does take place, the protection is limited to only a few ischemic episodes (probably less than five).[1] In addition to this early phase of protection, brief ischemia induces a late phase of preconditioning against stunning. This late phase lasts much longer and therefore is likely to be more important from a clinical standpoint.[1] The purpose of this essay is to succinctly review the existing knowledge regarding the pathophysiology and pathogenesis of late preconditioning against myocardial stunning.

The Phenomenon of Late Preconditioning Against Stunning

Although many studies have examined whether ischemic preconditioning confers immediate protection against postischemic dysfunction,[1] until recently, no information was available regarding the *late* effects of ischemic preconditioning on myocardial stunning. We hypothesized that the stress of sublethal ischemia may induce cellular adaptations that protect against the development of stunning after subsequent exposure to ischemia, but that these adaptations develop slowly and require several hours to become manifest. We initially tested this hypothesis in conscious pigs subjected to a sequence of ten 2-min coronary occlusions interspersed with 2-min reperfusion intervals.[2] We found that this sequence induced severe myocardial stunning, but when the same sequence was repeated

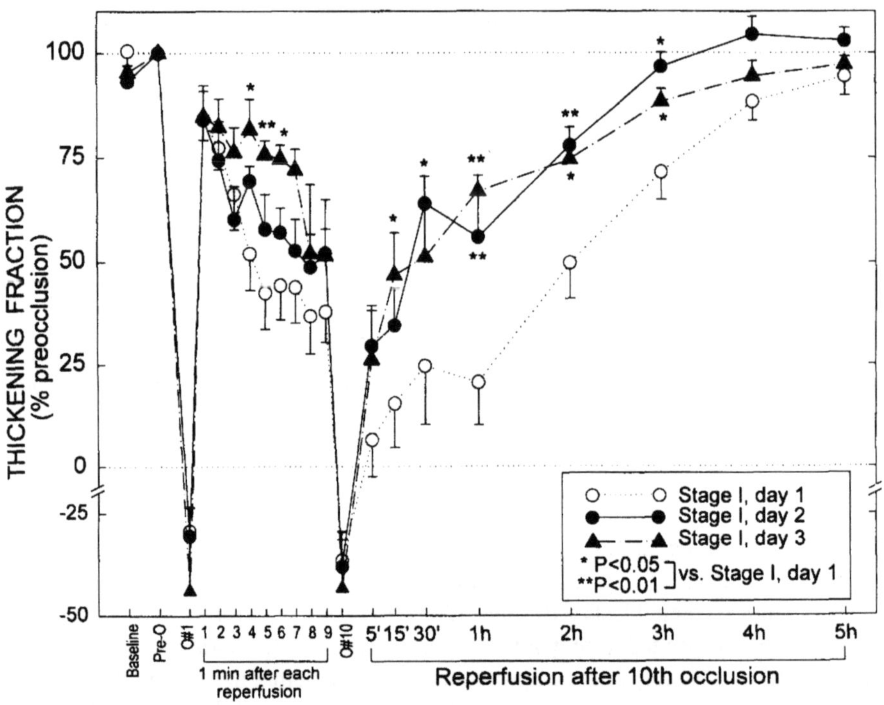

FIGURE 3-1. Systolic thickening fraction in the ischemic-reperfused region of conscious pigs subjected to a sequence of ten 2-min LAD occlusion/2-min reperfusion cycles. Shown are the measurements of thickening fraction obtained at baseline, immediately before the 1st occlusion (preocclusion, *Pre-O*), 1 min into the 1st LAD occlusion (*0#1*), 1 min into each of the first nine reperfusions, 1 min into the 10th occlusion (*0#10*), and at selected times during the 5-h reperfusion interval following the 10th coronary occlusion. (• • •O• • •) Measurements taken on day 1 (n=10); (---●---) measurements taken on day 2 (n=9); and (-• •▲• • -) measurements taken on day 3 (n=8). Thickening fraction is expressed as a percentage of preocclusion values. Data are means ±SEM.
Reprinted with permission from: Sun J-Z, Tang X-L, Knowlton AA et al.. J Clin Invest 1995; 95:388-403.

24 h later, the severity of stunning was markedly reduced (by approximately 50%) (Figs. 3-1 and 3-2). The resistance to stunning was associated with an increase in the myocardial levels of heat stress protein (HSP) 70 - a finding that is compatible with, but does not prove, a role of HSPs in the pathogenesis of the protective effect.[2] The protection dissipated within ten days after the last ischemic stress but could be reinduced by another sequence of ten 2-min occlusion/2-min reperfusion cycles (Fig. 3-2).[2]

Unlike early preconditioning against infarction, this form of protection does not appear to be mediated by activation of adenosine receptors, since it was not prevented by 8-*p*-sulfophenyl theophylline (Fig. 3-2).[2] We also assessed the time-course of this protective effect.[3] We found that preconditioning was not yet present at 6 h after the last ischemic episode, became partially manifest at 12 h, achieved full expression at 24 h, lasted for at least 3 days, and disappeared within 6 days from the preconditioning ischemia, a time-course that is consistent with the synthesis and degradation of cardioprotective proteins.[3] We have recently observed a similar preconditioning effect (with a similar time-course) in conscious rabbits

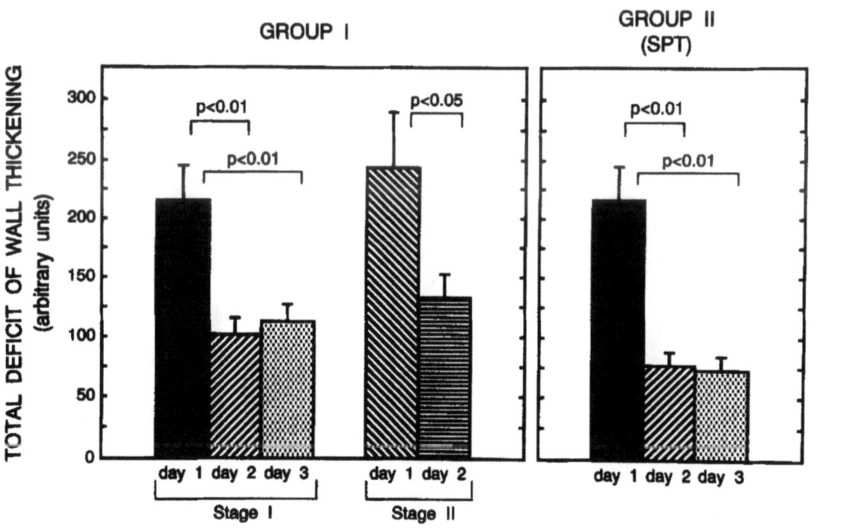

FIGURE 3-2. Total deficit of wall thickening after the 10th reperfusion in conscious pigs in group I, which did not receive SPT, and in group II, which received SPT on day 1. Conscious pigs were subjected to a sequence of ten 2-min LAD occlusion/2-min reperfusion cycles and systolic thickening fraction was measured as in Fig. 3-3. The total deficit of wall thickening was calculated in a manner similar to that shown in Fig. 3-2. SPT, 8-*p*-sulfophenyl theophylline. Data are means ±SEM.
Reprinted with permission from: Sun J-Z, Tang X-L, Knowlton AA et al. J Clin Invest 1995; 95:388-403.

subjected to a sequence of six 5-min coronary occlusion/5-min reperfusion cycles.[4] The fact that late preconditioning against stunning was observed in two different species (pigs and rabbits) suggests that this phenomenon is not peculiar to any particular animal species. It is also important to stress that late preconditioning against stunning is extremely reproducible: we have consistently observed this phenomenon in every animal studied thus far (Fig. 3-3).

In our studies in conscious rabbits, we found that when the sequence of six 5-min coronary occlusion/5-min reperfusion cycles was repeated for four consecutive days, the magnitude of the protection did not increase from the second to the fourth day, suggesting that the protection observed on the second day is maximal or near-maximal.[4] Recently, we have obtained evidence that late preconditioning against stunning is an all-or-none phenomenon. Specifically, we have found in conscious rabbits that no preconditioning effect develops on day 2

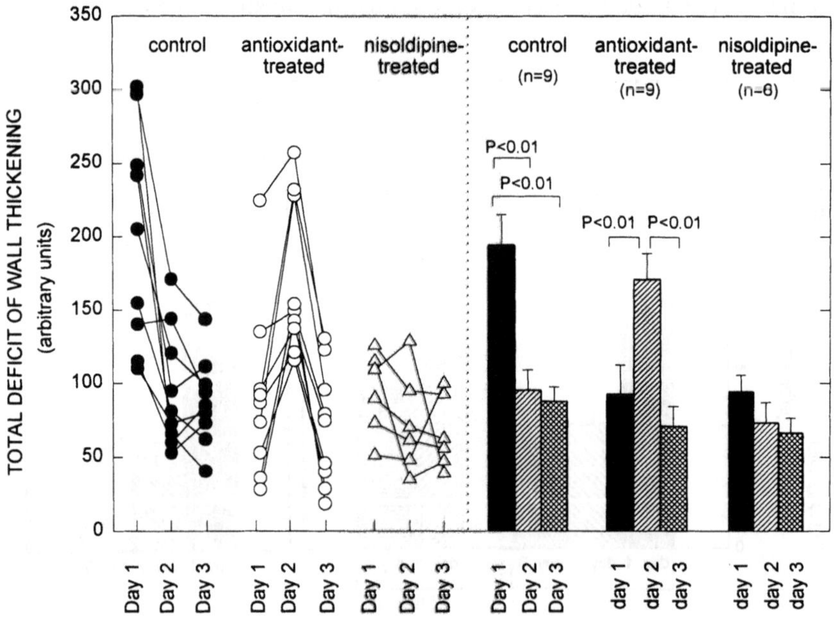

FIGURE 3-3. Total deficit of wall thickening after the 10th reperfusion in conscious pigs on days 1, 2, and 3 in the control group (n=9) and in the group treated with antioxidants (superoxide dismutase plus catalase plus mercaptopropionyl glycine) (n=9). The total deficit of wall thickening is an integrated measure of the overall severity of myocardial stunning and is expressed in arbitrary units as described in ref. 2. Note that antioxidant therapy on day 1 prevented preconditioning on day 2 in the treated group. Also note that antioxidant therapy attenuated stunning on day 1 in this group. Data are means ±SEM.
Data are from Sun J-Z, Tang X-L, Park S-W et al. J Clin Invest 1996;97:562-576.

when the animals are subjected to only one or two 4-min coronary occlusion/4-min reperfusion cycles on day 1; full protection develops when the rabbits are subjected to three 4-min coronary occlusion/4-min reperfusion cycles on day 1, and the magnitude of this protection does not increase when the rabbits are preconditioned with either six or twelve 4-min occlusion/4-min reperfusion cycles. Thus, the transition from two to three preconditioning ischemic episodes is associated with an abrupt transition from no protection to maximal protection.

In summary, studies 2-4 demonstrate, for the first time, that a brief ischemic stress induces a delayed, powerful, and long-lasting protective response that renders the myocardium relatively resistant to stunning. This protective response requires >6 h to develop, lasts for at least 60 h after its appearance, and then disappears within 6 days after the last ischemic stress but can be reinduced by another ischemic stress. When the amount of preconditioning ischemia is varied, the pattern of the protective effect is that of an all-or-none phenomenon. We have termed this response "late preconditioning against stunning." [2]

Essential Role of Reactive Oxygen Species (ROS) in Late Preconditioning Against Stunning

Recently, we have demonstrated that administration of antioxidant therapy completely prevents the development of late preconditioning against stunning, indicating that the production of ROS is the mechanism whereby ischemia induces this protective response.[5] Using the same model employed previously,[2] i.e., conscious pigs subjected to a sequence of ten 2-min occlusion/2-min reperfusion cycles for 3 consecutive days (days 1, 2, and 3), we found that administration of antioxidants (superoxide dismutase plus catalase plus mercaptopropionyl glycine) on day 1 attenuated myocardial stunning on day 1 (indicating that ROS contribute to stunning in the pig) but then resulted in complete loss of the preconditioning effect on day 2 (i.e., stunning on day 2 was much more severe than on day 1 and similar to that observed on day 1 in control pigs) (Fig. 3-3). On day 3, antioxidant-treated pigs exhibited a marked attenuation of stunning, indicating that the ischemia produced on day 2 preconditioned the heart against stunning on day 3 (Fig. 3-3).[5] Taken together, these results indicate that the oxidative stress incurred during brief ischemia and reperfusion triggers a protective response that makes the myocardium resistant to stunning 24 h later.[5] The precise mechanism whereby the exposure to oxygen radicals during the preconditioning ischemia leads to late preconditioning against stunning is unclear, but it may involve the induction of cardioprotective proteins, such as HSPs and antioxidant enzymes, possibly via activation of protein kinase C or other kinases.[5]

It could be argued that in this study antioxidants blocked late preconditioning because they attenuated myocardial stunning on day 1.[5] Perhaps it is myocardial stunning, rather than oxidative stress, that induces late preconditioning; perhaps the stimulus that triggers this protective response is the mechanical stimulation (stretch) associated with dyskinesis/hypokinesis, which is known to induce HSPs as well as early preconditioning against infarction. If this hypothesis were correct, then *any* agent that alleviates stunning should block late preconditioning. To evaluate this possibility, we studied another group of conscious pigs that underwent the same experimental protocol as the antioxidant-treated pigs except that on day 1 they received an infusion of the calcium-channel antagonist nisoldipine.[5] We found that nisoldipine was just as effective as the combination of antioxidants in alleviating stunning on day 1 but nevertheless failed to prevent preconditioning on day 2 (Fig. 3-3).[5] Thus, despite similar effects on postischemic dysfunction on day 1, antioxidant therapy and calcium antagonist therapy had divergent effects on late preconditioning, indicating that the prevention of late preconditioning by antioxidants cannot be ascribed to attenuation of myocardial stunning. We have recently obtained similar results in conscious rabbits.

This study supports a new paradigm regarding the pathophysiological role of oxygen metabolites in myocardial ischemia and reperfusion.[5] Generation of oxyradicals during reperfusion is generally viewed as a deleterious process. Our finding that oxygen radicals contribute to the genesis of myocardial stunning but, at the same time, trigger the development of late preconditioning against stunning suggests that the radical species generated after a brief ischemic episode play an injurious role in the short term (as mediators of the immediate injury) and a useful role in the long term (as triggers of a delayed, powerful, and long-lasting protective response).[5] This dual function implies that free radicals do not invariably have a detrimental effect: after a mild ischemic insult, free radical generation could serve as a "warning" signal (primordial in evolutionary terms) that activates a protective response designed to minimize further injury through the upregulation of a family of redox-sensitive genes (antioxidant enzyme genes, HSP genes, and probably other genes). In this manner, the sublethal oxidative stress associated with brief ischemic episodes could act as a transduction pathway signaling an imminent threat and the need to develop cellular defenses against it.

Conclusions

In conclusion, there are two phases of ischemic preconditioning against stunning: an early phase (which begins within minutes) and a late phase (which begins after >6 h). The duration of the early phase is unknown. The late phase of preconditioning against stunning is long-lasting (as least 72 h), is powerful (approximately 50% reduction in total dysfunction), and is mediated by the generation of reactive oxygen species during the preconditioning ischemia-reperfusion cycles. The mechanism probably involves the upregulation of cardioprotective genes. Because the late phase offers sustained protection, it is probably more important and more clinically relevant than the first phase. It is important to understand the cellular mechanisms responsible for late preconditioning against stunning, because these mechanisms could be exploited therapeutically to minimize postischemic dysfunction in patients with coronary artery disease.

Acknowledgments

Supported in part by NIH R01 Grants HL-43151 and HL-55757.

References

1. Bolli R. The early and late phases of preconditioning against myocardial stunning and the essential role of oxyradicals in the late phase: an overview. Basic Res Cardiol 1996;91:57-63.
2. Sun J-Z, Tang X-L, Knowlton AA et al. Late preconditioning against myocardial stunning: An endogenous protective mechanism that confers resistance to postischemic dysfunction 24 hours after brief ischemia in conscious pigs. J Clin Invest 1995; 95:388-403.
3. Tang X-L, Qiu Y, Park S-W, et al. Time course of late preconditioning against myocardial stunning in conscious pigs. Circ Res 1996; 79:424-434.
4. Qiu Y, Maldonado C, Tang X-L et al. Late preconditioning against myocardial stunning in conscious rabbits. Circulation 1995; (Suppl I):I-389, (Abstr.).
5. Sun J-Z, Tang X-L, Park S-W et al. Evidence for an essential role of reactive oxygen species in the genesis of late preconditioning against myocardial stunning in conscious pigs. J Clin Invest 1996;97:562-576.

In: Mentzer, R.M., Jr., Kitakaze, M., Downey, J.M., Hori, M, eds. Adenosine, Cardioprotection and Clinical Application. Kluwer Academic Publishers, Norwell, MA, USA, 1997.

4. Coronary Perfusion as the Major Determinant of Myocardial Contractility in the Heart: Implication for Myocardial Hibernation

Masafumi Kitakaze

Introduction

Coronary perfusion pressure and blood flow are closely linked to myocardial metabolic states and contractility. When coronary perfusion pressure decreases below the level of the coronary flow autoregulation, myocardial contractility is markedly decreased. Myocardial ischemia causes accumulation of H^+ and inorganic phosphates, both of which decrease the myofilament sensitivity to Ca2+ and maximal response of myofilaments to Ca^{2+}. Furthermore, adenosine and EDRF (NO), produced during ischemia, stimulate adenylate and guanulate cyclase, respectively, both of which have been reported to decrease myocardial contractility. In turn, norepinephrine is released according to the severity of myocardial ischemia, which tends to compensate the depression of myocardial contractility. On the other hand, when myocardial ischemia is not apparent due to coronary flow autoregulation during mild reduction of coronary perfusion pressure, myocardial contractility decreases, recognized as Gregg's phenomenon. There are several hypotheses to explain this phenomenon: 1) decreases in sarcomere length of the myofilaments, 2) reversal of latent myocardial ischemia, 3) release of cardiodepressive agents, and 4) decreases in either Ca^{2+} transient or Ca^{2+} sensitivity. Ca^{2+} transients were measured in the ferret Langendorff preparation at various perfusion pressure; the amplitude of Ca^{2+} transients was decreased when coronary perfusion pressure was reduced in the range of coronary flow autoregulation. Taken together, these results support the hypothesis of the tight linkage between coronary perfusion and myocardial contractility in normal and ischemic hearts. The concert interaction between myocardial perfusion and intracellular Ca^{2+}

concentration may be essential for maintaining homeostasis of myocardial cellular function.

The Mechanisms of Coronary Flow Regulation

It is critically important to prevent the myocardium from contractile dysfunction in contractility when coronary perfusion pressure is reduced. Reductions of coronary perfusion pressure may result from systemic hypotension, or narrowing of the coronary artery diameter caused by atherosclerosis, thrombus, or vasospasm in clinical settings. It is essential for the heart to regulate coronary blood flow to meet myocardial oxygen consumption because a debt of myocardial oxygen supply easily induces myocardial ischemia and cardiac pump dysfunction. Myocardial tissue is known to be less resistant to ischemia and hypoxia than the other organs except brain and kidney. Furthermore, even when myocardial ischemia is not provoked during reduction of coronary perfusion pressure, myocardial contractility is depressed, known as myocardial hibernation. In this sense, myocardial perfusion through coronary resistance vessels directly and strongly regulates myocardial contractility in the heart.

Metabolic Regulation of Coronary Blood Flow

Since myocardial oxygen demand in the heart is high relative to the other organs and tissues, the myocardium becomes easily ischemic even when coronary blood flow is only moderately decreased. When myocardial oxygen consumption is increased by exercise or sympathetic nerve stimulation, several coronary vasoactive mechanisms for the prevention of myocardial perfusion work promptly. First of all, when tissue pO_2 is decreased, coronary blood flow is increased to maintain constant tissue pO_2, suggesting that tissue pO_2 may be the sensor to regulate coronary vasomotor tones.[1-3] Increases in pCO_2 are also reported to decrease the resistance of coronary vessels. Indeed, both decreases in O_2[1] and increases in CO_2[2] may account for 23% of coronary flow autoregulation.[3] However, the mechanism how both O_2 and CO_2 regulates the tones of coronary arteries is still unknown.

On the other hand, adenosine is another vasoactive substance for mediating coronary flow autoregulation.[4] There is no doubt that adenosine is released from the heart when oxygen supply is not adequate for oxygen needs, i.e., ischemia, hypoxia and enhanced oxygen consumption.[5] Conversely, adenosine release is decreased when oxygen is excessively supplied by overperfusion.[6] These observations suggest that adenosine plays a crucial role in the local regulation of blood flow in normal and ischemic hearts. However, there are several lines of evidence against the role of adenosine in coronary flow autoregulation.[7-10] Adenosine deaminase is reported to have no effects on the coronary resistance in the unstressed heart.[7] Furthermore, adenosine deaminase does not affect coronary vascular resistance during graded reduction in perfusion pressure,[8] indicating that adenosine does not play an essential role in coronary flow autoregulation. There are other findings which suggest that the interstitial adenosine concentration might be too low for coronary vasodilation.[9] Therefore, although release of adenosine increased during reduction of coronary perfusion pressure in the range of coronary flow autoregulation,[6] adenosine does not seem to be involved in coronary flow autoregulation. Coronary flow autoregulation is re-examined to be altered by 8-phenyltheophylline, an adenosine receptor antagonist.[10] 8-Phenyltheophylline had little effect (10% attenuation of the coronary flow autoregulation) on coronary flow autoregulation, consistent with the previous results, although coronary venous adenosine concentration was increased according to the reduction of coronary perfusion pressure in the range of coronary flow autoregulation. However, regional myocardial contractility assessed by fractional shortening in the range of coronary autoregulation is markedly depressed by 8-phenyltheophylline administration. The regional flow distribution, i.e., the flow ratio between endocardial and epicardial tissue (End/Epi flow ratio), was modified by 8-phenyltheophylline in the range of coronary flow autoregulation. 8-Phenyltheophylline administration significantly decreased the End/Epi flow ratio in the range of coronary flow autoregulation. This result indicates that endogenous adenosine plays an important role in maintaining endocardial flow at the expense of epicardial flow in the range of coronary flow autoregulation.

EDRF (endothelial dependent relaxant factor) is also released due to the flow dependent mechanism and thus, adenosine may accelerate the release of EDRF due to the vasodilatory action of adenosine. Recently, Ueeda et al.[17] reported that NO synthase inhibitors potently attenuate coronary flow autoregulation, suggesting that EDRF regulates the capacity of coronary flow autoregulation. Since they employed the rat Langendorff preparation, this hypothesis needs to be tested in the experimental model of the blood-perfused hearts because the rate of the removal of EDRF in the crystalloid solution and blood may be different. There are several lines of evidence that the basal resting coronary blood flow is reduced by inhibitors of NO synthase and conflicting evidence that resting coronary flow is unaffected by inhibitors of NO synthase.[8,12] It is also noted that basal release of NO is minimal, although the release of NO is increased in the ischemic hearts.[12] Taken together, the hypothesis of EDRF for regulating the coronary autoregulation is attractive; however, further investigation is required. Recently, it has been reported that K^+ channels are involved in the regulation of coronary blood flow. Recent evidence postulates that the opening of ATP-sensitive K^+ channels plays a crucial role in coronary vasodilation during hypoxia in isolated guinea pig hearts; they observed that an ATP-sensitive K^+ channel blocker, inhibits the vasodilation during hypoxic condition.[13] Their findings suggest that the trigger of coronary vasodilation may be a decrease in intracellular ATP concentration, which augments the outward K^+ current through ATP-sensitive K^+ channels and causes hyperpolarization. Komaru et al.[14] reported that vasodilation of small coronary arteries (the diameter less than 100 mm) during reduction of coronary perfusion pressure in the range of coronary flow autoregulation is blunted by glibenclamide, suggesting that coronary flow autoregulation involves K^+ channels in the hearts. Since the stimulus to open K^+ channels during reduction of coronary perfusion pressure is not unknown, it is important to know the mechanism of opening of K^+ channels during reduction of coronary perfusion pressure in the range of coronary flow autoregulation. K^+ channels are known to open due not only to depletion of myocardial ATP content, but also acidosis and increases in intracellular Ca^{2+} concentration. However, these factors do not seem to be altered during reduction of coronary perfusion pressure in the range of coronary flow autoregulation. Interestingly, adenosine and K^+ channels are tightly linked: ATP-sensitive K^+ channels modulate adenosine-induced coronary vasodilation. Aversano et al.[15] reported that the adenosine-induced coronary vasodilation is substantially attenuated by blockade of ATP-sensitive K^+ channels. This result suggests that adenosine A_2 receptors may also be affected by ATP-sensitive K^+ channels. In the preliminary study, adenosine-induced coronary vasodilation was strongly enhanced when we additionally administered nicorandil and cromakalim, K^+ channels openers. This potentiation of adenosine-induced coronary vasodilation may be also beneficial for the ischemic myocardium, however, how this linkage is related to coronary flow autoregulation is unknown.

As the mechanical factors which may regulate autoregulation, tissue pressure and myogenic mechanism have been proposed.[16] The tissue pressure hypothesis indicates that a rise in arterial pressure transiently increases fluid exudation at the capillaries and the perivascular fluid pressure increases vascular resistance by mechanical compression. The myogenic theory postulates the intrinsic mechanism of vascular muscle tone; when vascular muscle is stretched, the muscle constricts and when intravascular pressure is lowered, the vascular muscle may relax probably due to the alteration of Ca^{2+} influx through the stretch-induced transmembrane potential changes. These two mechanisms, however, are not yet proved and additional contribution of metabolic factors may be more important.

Neural Regulation of Coronary Blood Flow

α- and β-Adrenoceptors are reported to exist in coronary arteries, and their activation mediates coronary vasoconstriction and relaxation. α-Adrenoceptor stimulation contracts the isolated coronary arteries.[17] Zuberbuhler and Bohr[17] showed that an exposure to norepinephrine under β-adrenoceptor blockade contracts isolated canine coronary artery, and exposure to norepinephrine under α-adrenoceptor blockade relaxes it. Their results suggest that α-adrenoceptor stimulation mediates coronary vasoconstriction and β-adrenoceptor stimulation mediates vasorelaxation. However, modulation of activity of β-adrenoceptor does not seem to be realistic for mediating coronary flow autoregulation, and the role of α-adrenoceptor-mediated coronary vasoconstriction is also unclear for coronary flow autoregulation. Interestingly, α-adrenoceptor-stimulation mediates redistribution of intramyocardial flow during mild reduction of coronary perfusion pressure, since it is reported that α-adrenoceptor stimulation favors an increase in endocardial flow at the expense of epicardial flow reduction during coronary hypoperfusion.[18] This effect is prominent during exercise and mild coronary hypoperfusion. Phenoxybenzamine slightly increased total coronary blood flow, but decreased endocardial flow, which may worsen overall myocardial perfusion. Recently, it was reported from our laboratory[19] that the α_1-adrenoceptor antagonist prazosin markedly attenuates the release of adenosine from the ischemic myocardium; administration of a low dose of prazosin which does not affect basal coronary blood flow reduces the coronary blood flow in response to these stimuli and further deteriorates the ischemic changes, i.e. an increase in lactate production and a decrease in regional segment shortening. Although contribution of α-adrenergic activity in release of adenine nucleotide has been reported in endothelial cells,[20] it is more likely that α_1-adrenergic activity plays a dominant role in the release of adenosine in ischemic myocardial cells via activation of protein kinase C.[21,22]

How Coronary Perfusion Regulates Myocardial Contraction

When coronary perfusion pressure is decreased, myocardial contractility is decreased due to several factors. When myocardial ischemia occurs, early contractile failure is reported to be attributable to the accumulation of P_i and H^+ in cardiomyocytes. P_i is reported to decrease both the maximal force of contraction and the Ca^{2+} sensitivity of the myofilaments, while H^+ decreases only Ca^{2+} sensitivity. During the early phase of hypoxia, contractile dysfunction correlates well with increases in P_i and H^+. However, despite no changes in P_i and H^+ in the range of coronary flow autoregulation, myocardial contraction is decreased due to decreases in coronary perfusion pressure, known as Gregg's phenomenon. In 1963,

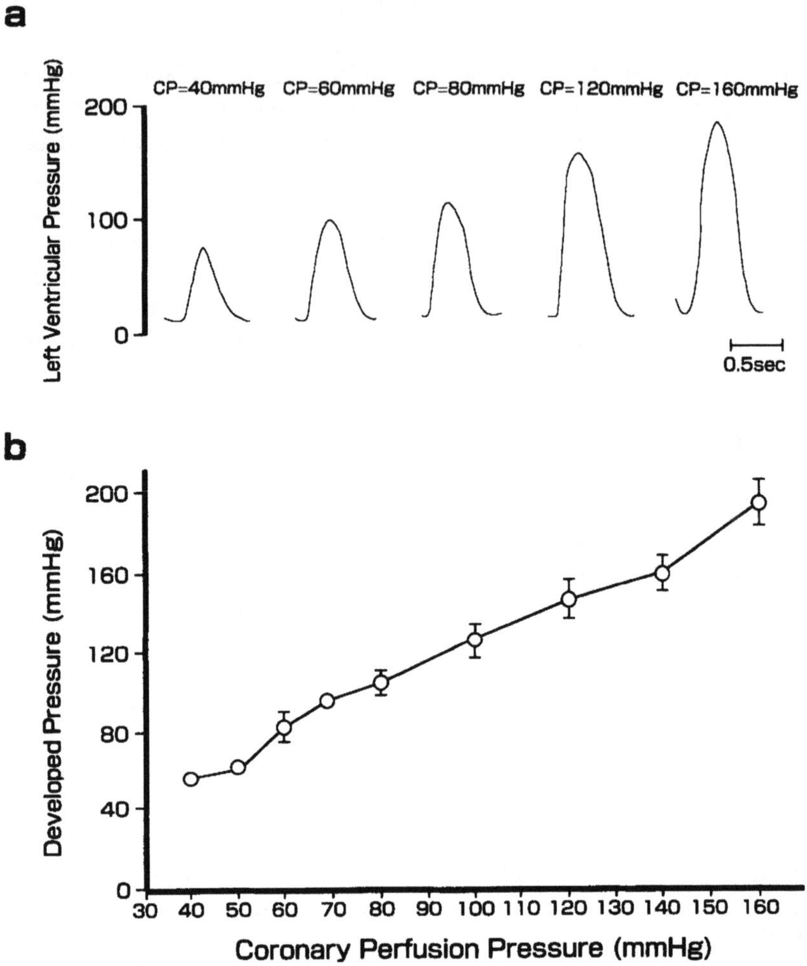

FIGURE 4-1. Dependence of contractile pressure on coronary perfusion pressure in the Langendorff perfused heart excised form the ferret. A. representative records of left ventricular pressure during twitch contractions at the value of coronary perfusion pressure indicated above each record. At each coronary perfusion pressure tested, developed pressure was allowed to reach steady state before contractile or metabolic parameters were measured. B, pooled data from eight hearts (mean ± SEM). (Ref. 24).

Gregg reported that decreases in coronary perfusion pressure decrease myocardial oxygen consumption,[23] and many researchers confirmed this observation and further observed that myocardial contraction is likewise dependent on the coronary perfusion pressure.[24,25] Figure 4-1 shows the dependence of contractile pressure on coronary arterial pressure in the ferret Langendorff preparation. This phenomenon may contribute to prevent myocardium from the occurrence of ischemia and constitute the cardioprotective mechanisms because of energy sparing effects due to decreased myocardial oxygen consumption and contractility. There are several possible mechanisms for this interesting observation[26]: 1) slight changes in P_i and H^+, 2) the presence of subtle myocardial ischemia, 3) increases in myocardial filament length (Frank- Starling mechanisms), 4) decreases in Ca^{2+} sensitivity of myofilaments due to other causes, and 5) decreases in Ca^{2+} transient. Any or all of these phenomena may well explain the decreased myocardial contractility. First of all, neither P_i nor H^+ measured by the ^{31}P NMR method changes during the mild reduction of coronary perfusion pressure in the range of coronary autoregulation. Below the range of coronary flow autoregulation, both P_i and H^+ were increased; in this range decreases in developed pressure became steeper compared with the range of coronary autoregulation. This observation suggests that although both P_i and H^+ can decrease myocardial contractility, decreases in contraction due to Gregg's phenomenon are not attributable to these metabolic changes. Decreases in coronary perfusion pressure may cause subtle subendocardial ischemia. However, when lactate release from the hearts was measured during reduction of coronary perfusion pressure in the range of coronary autoregulation, lactate release could not be detected. This observation argues against latent subendocardial ischemia during the reduction of coronary perfusion pressure when Gregg's phenomenon is clearly observed, because lactate release is a sensitive index for the detection of anaerobic glycolysis. The third possibility is the Frank-Starling mechanism - when myofilament is stretched, myocardial contractility is increased. However, this possibility is not likely. Figure 4-2 shows the results of experiments in papillary muscles by Schouten et al.[25] When perfusion pressure is altered, myocardial contractility is further increased even if the myocardium contracts and relaxes at the level of L_{max}. The fourth and fifth possibilities that modulation of Ca^{2+} sensitivity of the myofilaments and/or Ca^{2+} transients appear likely to explain Gregg's phenomenon. Figure 4-3 shows the modulation of Ca^{2+} transient during either reduction or augmentation of coronary perfusion pressure observed in the ferret heart. The heart was loaded with 5F-BAPTA and $[Ca^{2+}]o$ was increased to 8 mM prior to the gated acquisition of the ^{19}F spectra used to calculate each value of $[Ca^{2+}]i$ (A). Coronary perfusion pressure was then decreased to 60 mmHg (B) and a new set of gated spectra was obtained after contractile pressure had reached steady state. ^{31}Phosphorus spectra from the same heart revealed no significant differences at the two coronary perfusion pressures. The differences in $[Ca^{2+}]i$ were statistically significant by paired t test. When coronary perfusion pressure is decreased, the amplitude of Ca^{2+} transients is markedly decreased. This finding is consistent with the observation that ^{45}Ca uptake into perfused rat hearts is increased when coronary perfusion pressure is raised from 60 to 120 mmHg.[27] On the other hand, when coronary perfusion pressure is increased, the amplitude of Ca^{2+} transients is also increased. This observation explains the cellular mechanism for

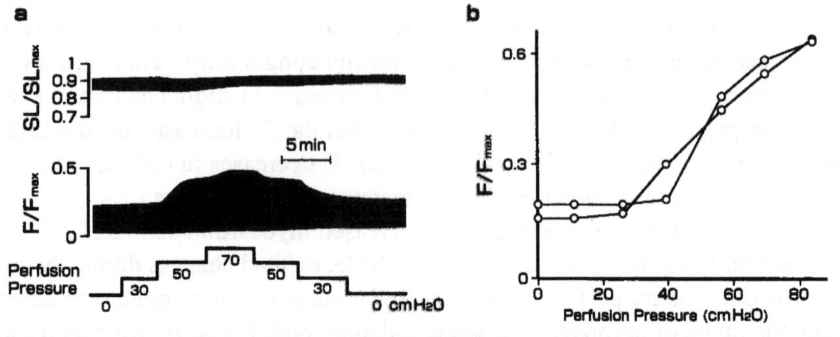

FIGURE 4-2: Influence of perfusion pressure on peak force of contraction in rat papillary muscles. A, original recording of force and segment length during stepwise changes in perfusion pressure. B, peal force-pressure relationship as obtained with a protocol comparable to that shown in A. The arrows indicate the sequence of increase in and subsequent decreasing pressure steps. When segment length was not changed as is indicated in SL/SLmax, the generated force (F/Fmax) was altered by changing perfusion pressure (Ref. 25).

Gregg's phenomenon. Furthermore, as Schouten et al.[25] suggested, we cannot negate the possibility that the myofilament sensitivity to Ca^{2+} is modulated by the changes in perfusion pressure, although maximal Ca^{2+} activated force obtained during transient myocardial tetanus is not altered by coronary perfusion pressure.[24]

The interesting issue is the subcellular mechanism for the modulation of Ca^{2+} transients at various levels of coronary perfusion pressure. Two general types of mechanism must be considered as potentially underlying the effects of an increase in perfusion pressure or flow: First, the accumulation of a positively inotropic mediator or second messenger, Second, the wash-out of negatively inotropic compounds. In the first category, a prominent candidate is cyclic AMP. Activation of adenylate cyclase occurs within 10 min of acute pressure overload in guinea pig hearts. The attendant increase in cyclic AMP concentration and cyclic AMP dependent protein kinase activity would be expected to increase Ca^{2+} transients and contractile force. If this were true, one might also expect the rate of relaxation of twitch contractions, and the spontaneous heart rate, to be accelerated. We observed neither tendency, but our experiments were not designed to detect subtle changes in either of these parameters.[24] As far as negatively inotropic compounds are concerned, adenosine may be capable of explaining at least some of the observed changes in calcium transients. Free cytosolic adenosine increases steeply when coronary perfusion pressure is decreased in the range of coronary autoregulation[24] as well as myocardial ischemia. This increase in adenosine concentration would tend to decrease Ca^{2+} current and contractile force. The negative inotropic action

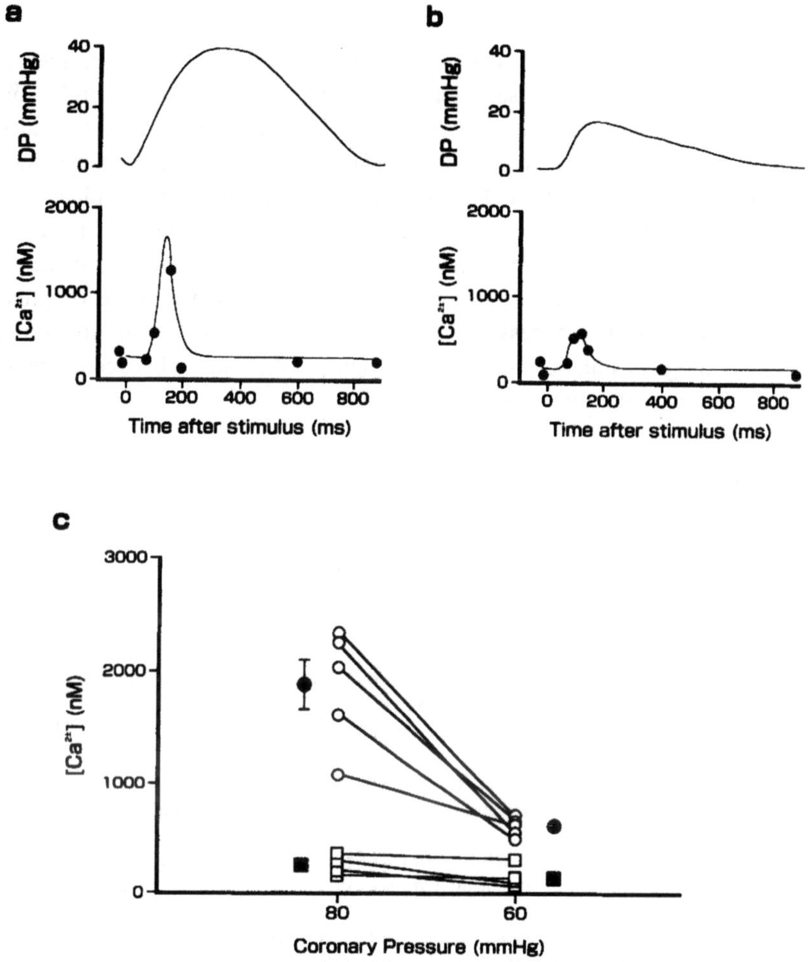

FIGURE 4-3: Changes in Ca^{2+} transients when coronary perfusion pressure is decreased. A, B: representative changes in one heart. Ventricular developed pressure (DP, upper panel) and Ca^{2+} transient (lower panel) during perfusion at 80 (A) or 60 (B) mmHg coronary perfusion pressure. Pooled data are shown in Panel C. Open circles and squares are the data during systolic and diastolic phases, respectively. Filled circles and squares represent systolic and diastolic averages, respectively. (mean ± SEM). (Ref. 24).

of adenosine is exerted only when beta adrenoceptors are stimulated; therefore, the adenosine theory cannot fully explain Gregg's phenomenon.

Clinical implication

In the clinical situation, when coronary stenosis persists for a long time, myocardial contraction remains depressed, termed as myocardial hibernation.[42] When percutaneous transluminal coronary angioplasty is performed for the fixed coronary stenosis in patients of effort angina, myocardial contraction improves markedly. This improvement may be at least partly attributable to Gregg's phenomenon. Increased coronary perfusion pressure increases myocardial contractility, although myocardial hibernation is provoked in the chronic stage with modification of myocardial properties due to sustained reduction of coronary perfusion pressure. Further investigation is necessary to learn the role of Gregg's phenomenon in the pathophysiological situation, and we need to notice the linkage between myocardial contractile force and coronary circulation.

References

1. Chang AE, Detar R. Oxygen and vascular smooth muscle contraction revisited. Am J Physiol 1980;238:H716-H718.
2. Case RB, Felix A, Wachter M et al. Relative effect of CO_2 on canine coronary vascular resistance. Circ Res 1978;42:410-418.
3. Broten TP, Feigl EO. Role of myocardial oxygen and carbon dioxide in coronary autoregulation. Am J Physiol 1992;262:H1231-H1237.
4. Hori M, Kitakaze M. Adenosine, the heart, and coronary circulation. Hypertension 1991;18:565-574.
5. Berne RM, Rubio R, Curnish RR. Release of adenosine from ischemic brain: Effect on cerebral vascular resistance and incorporation into cerebral adenine nucleotides. Circ Res 1974;35:262-271.
6. Schrader J, Haddy FJ, Gerlach E. Release of adenosine, inosine and hypoxanthine from the isolated guinea pig heart during hypoxia, flow-autoregulation and reactive hyperemia. Pflugers Arch 1977;369:1-6.
7. Kroll K, Feigl EO. Adenosine is unimportant in controlling coronary blood flow in unstressed dog hearts. Am J Physiol 1985;249:H1186-H1187.
8. Dole WP, Yamada N, Bishop VS et al. Role of adenosine in coronary blood flow regulation after reductions in perfusion pressure. Circ Res 1985;56:517-524.
9. Gidday JM, Ely SW, Esther JW et al. Progressive attenuation of coronary reactive hyperemia with increasing interstitial theophylline permeation. Fed Proc 1984;43:1084.
10. Morioka T, Kitakaze M, Minamino T et al. Role of endogenous adenosine in coronary pressure-flow relationship in dogs. J. Am. Coll. Cardiol. Special Issue 1994;262A.
11. Ueeda M, Silvia S, Olsson RA. Nitric oxide modulates coronary autoregulation in the guinea pig. Circ Res 1992;70:1296-1303.
12. Kitakaze M, Takashima S, Node K et al. Role of nitric oxide for regulation of coronary blood flow of ischemic myocardium in dogs. Am. J. Coll. Cardiol. (in press).
13. Daut J, Maier-Rudolph W, von Beckerath N et al. Hypoxic dilation of coronary arteries is mediated by ATP-sensitive potassium channels. Science 1990;247:1341-1344.
14. Komaru T, Lamping KG, Easthan CL et al. Role of ATP-sensitive potassium channels in coronary microvascular autoregulatory responses. Circ Res 1991;69:1146-1151.

15. Aversano T, Ouyang P, Silverman H. Blockade of the ATP-sensitive potassium channel modulate reactive hyperemia in the canine coronary circulation. Circ Res 1991;69:618-622.
16. Kuo L, Davis MJ, Chilian WM. Myogenic activity in isolated subepicardial and subendocardial coronary arteries. Am J Physiol 1988;255:H1558-H1562.
17. Zuberbuhler RC, Bohr DF. Responses of coronary smooth muscle to catecholamine. Circ Res 1965;16:431-440.
18. Buffington CW, Feigl EO. Effect of coronary artery pressure on transmural distribution of adrenergic coronary vasoconstriction in the dog. Circ Res 1983;53:613-621.
19. Kitakaze M, Hori M, Tamai J et al. a1-Adrenoceptor activity regulates release of adenosine from the ischemic myocardium in dogs. Circ Res 1987;60:631-639.
20. Buxton ILO, Walther J, Westfall DP. Purinergic mechanisms in cardiac blood vessels: Stimulation of endothelial cell a receptors in vitro by the neurotransmitter norepinephrine leads to the rapid release of ATP and its subsequent breakdown to adenosine (abstract). Heart and Vessel 1990;4(Suppl):27.
21. Kitakaze M, Hori M, Morioka T, et. a1-adrenoceptor activation increases ectosolic 5'-nucleotidase activity and adenosine release in rat cardiomyocytes by activing protein kinase C. Circulation 91:2226-2234, 1995
22. Kitakaze M, Hori M, Kamada T. Role of adenosine and its interaction with alpha adrenoceptor activity in ischemic and reperfusion injury of the myocardium. Cardiovasc Res 1993;27:18-27.
23. Gregg DE. Effects of coronary perfusion pressure or or coronary flow on oxygen usage of the myocardium. Circ Res 1963;13:497-500.
24. Kitakaze M, Marban E. Cellular mechanism of the modulation of contractile function by coronary perfusion pressure in ferret hearts. J Physiol 1989;414:455-472.
25. Schouten VJ, Allaart CP, Westerhof N. Effect of perfusion pressure on force contraction in thin papillary muscles and trabeculae from rat heart. J Physiol 1992;451:585-604.
26. Feigl EO. Coronary physiology. Physiol Rev 1983;63:1-205.
27. Haneda T, Morgan HE, Watson PA. Effect of calcium uptake increased by elevated aortic pressure on total and ribosomal protein synthesis in rat heart. J Mol Cell Cardiol 1988;20:Suppl(III)-S35.
28. Rahimtoola SH, Griffith GC. The hibernating myocardium. Am Heart J 1989;117:211-221.

In: Mentzer, R.M., Jr., Kitakaze, M., Downey, J.M., Hori, M, eds. Adenosine, Cardioprotection and Clinical Application. Kluwer Academic Publishers, Norwell, MA, USA, 1997.

5. Myocardial Protection From Reperfusion Injury With Adenosine

Jakob Vinten-Johansen
Zhi-Qing Zhao

Introduction

Adenosine has recently been moved into the limelight for its clinically applicable physiological effects. Certainly, its cardiovascular effects have long been recognized,[1] and its vasodilator effects have been proposed as a central mechanism of autoregulation of coronary blood flow.[2] In addition, its negative inotropic and chronotropic effects have been understood for many years.[3,4] However, it has not been until the last decade that adenosine has been appreciated for its cardioprotective potential against ischemic-reperfusion injury. Since the observations of Olafsson et al,[5] there has been a virtual explosion of research focused on unraveling the mechanisms by which this endogenous autacoid protects the heart from non-lethal as well as lethal injury after ischemia and reperfusion. As investigative efforts have progressed, the temporal dynamics and mechanisms by which adenosine exerts cardioprotection have become more intriguing, and more complex. Adenosine has potential to exert cardioprotection during all three windows of cardioprotection (pretreatment or preconditioning, ischemia and reperfusion). Therefore, adenosine has emerged as a broad-spectrum cardioprotective agent that exerts protection endogenously as well as by pharmacological application (exogenously). However, the observation of adenosine as **protagonist** of injury by its stimulation of neutrophil-mediated events, a provider of substrate for enhanced generation of superoxide anions via xanthine oxidase of its metabolites xanthine and hypoxanthine, and **antagonist** to injury via numerous mechanisms offers an intriguing challenge to investigators to elucidate its entire spectrum of physiological and molecular effects. During which of these windows adenosine exerts its effects on the participants in the injury processes will determine its optimal therapeutic use.[6] This chapter will focus on the mechanisms of myocardial protection by endogenous and exogenous adenosine, and receptor-specific analogs with specific reference to mechanisms involved in reperfusion injury; a full discussion of adenosine regulating agents is beyond its scope.

The distinction between *exogenous* adenosine and *endogenous* adenosine is an important one in several respects. 1) The physiological and therapeutic targets are confined in or constitute the various compartments (vascular, endothelial, interstitial, myocyte), and access to targets is affected by barriers between compartments. Exogenous adenosine can achieve immediate access to the intravascular compartment, with spillover into the interstitial compartment occurring when intravascular infusions exceed 5 μg/kg per minute.[7] As will be discussed in greater detail, the compartment in which adenosine is acting may be important to its overall effects in ischemic injury or reperfusion injury.[6] 2) Timing of administration: exogenous adenosine can be administered during any of the windows of protection (pretreatment, ischemia, early or late reperfusion), while endogenous adenosine is dependent largely on *release during ischemia*. 3) Therapeutic concentrations achieved: lower concentrations in both intravascular and interstitial compartments are achieved with endogenous adenosine than exogenous adenosine. However, high concentrations of parenterally administered adenosine (intravenous, intracoronary) do not ensure high interstitial concentrations because of the metabolic barrier imposed by the endothelium. 4) The vascular route allows administration of various analogs and regulating agents which may exert receptor-specific effects or increase adenosine concentrations in one compartment or the other.

Inhibition of Neutrophils And Neutrophil-endothelial Cell Interactions

Adenosine has been shown to inhibit the actions of a number of cell types activated during ischemia-reperfusion and inflammation, including neutrophils (PMNs),[8] platelets[9] and mononuclear leukocytes.[10] As reviewed in detail elsewhere, neutrophils PMNs) play an important role in ischemic-reperfusion injury.[11-15] Cronstein et al[8] and others[16] have shown that adenosine inhibits superoxide radical generation by neutrophils activated in vitro by chemotactic agents. Neither metabolism nor uptake of adenosine into PMNs were required for this inhibition, suggesting an interaction on the PMN membrane, i.e. by receptors. Subsequent studies[17] suggested that an A_2 receptor-mediated mechanism was involved. Adenosine was also found to inhibit adherence of PMNs with subsequent damage to the vascular endothelium.[18] This interaction is dependent on the well-choreographed interaction between adhesion molecules on both cell types. An initial loose adherence is mediated by the glycoprotein, p-selectin, on the endothelium, and L-selectin on the PMN. After stimulation with superoxide, H_2O_2, histamine or thrombin, P-selectin is rapidly translocated from the cytoplasmic Weibel-Palade bodies to the surface of endothelial cells. A firm adherence follows this rolling phenomenon, involving the β_2-integrins CD11a/CD18 and CD11b/CD18 complexes on PMNs and ICAM-1 on the endothelium. Adenosine directly inhibits the expression of CD11/CD18 on PMNs stimulated by FMLP, and this inhibitory effect is blocked by an adenosine receptor antagonist.[19] Furthermore, CD11/CD18 expression is inhibited by an A_2 agonist (5'N-ethlycarboxamido-adenosine), but not by an A_1-selective agonist (N^6-cyclopentyl-adenosine).[19] The adenosine regulating agent, acadesine (5 amino-4 imidazole carboxamide riboside), which purportedly increases the endogenous production of adenosine,[20]inhibited CD11b/CD18 expression on neutrophils, ostensibly by augmenting release of adenosine from neutrophils themselves.

Studies from our laboratory[21] using canine coronary artery segments have confirmed that adenosine directly inhibits superoxide generation by canine PMN suspensions activated by platelet activating factor (PAF) (Fig. 5-1A). This inhibitory effect was reversed by 8-SPT, suggesting a receptor-mediated effect. Adenosine (100 µM) in the presence of the A_1-selective antagonist KW-3902 retained its inhibitory effects, implying an A_2-mediated mechanism. An A_2-subtype mechanism was further supported by similar inhibition with the specific A_2-agonist CGS-21680. In addition, adenosine inhibited adherence of PMNs to the endothelium in an in vitro system where PAF was used to activate both cell types. Similar to the effects on superoxide anion production by PMNs, adenosine-induced inhibition of PMN adherence was not attenuated by A_1 antagonism, and was mimicked by the A_2-agonist CGS-21680 (Fig. 5-1B), again implying activation of A_2-receptors in this neutrophil-inhibitory effect. Superoxide anions generated by direct activation of PMNs by PAF, and cytotoxic mediators resulting from the interaction between PMNs and endothelium, injures the coronary vascular endothelium, quantified as a reduction in vasodilator responses to agonist stimulators of nitric oxide synthase in a bioassay system (Fig. 5-1C). Adenosine partially inhibited this endothelial injury, again by A_2-receptor mechanisms. The residual endothelial injury not inhibited by adenosine may have been related to PMN-derived proteases (elastase, collagenase) the release of which (by degranulation) adenosine does not seem to inhibit.

Direct Inhibitory Effects on the Endothelium

The endothelium plays an active and important role in initiating and promulgating the cell-cell interactions ultimately leading to PMN-induced damage to the myocardium. The observation by Nolte et al[22,23] that adenosine and A_2-selective

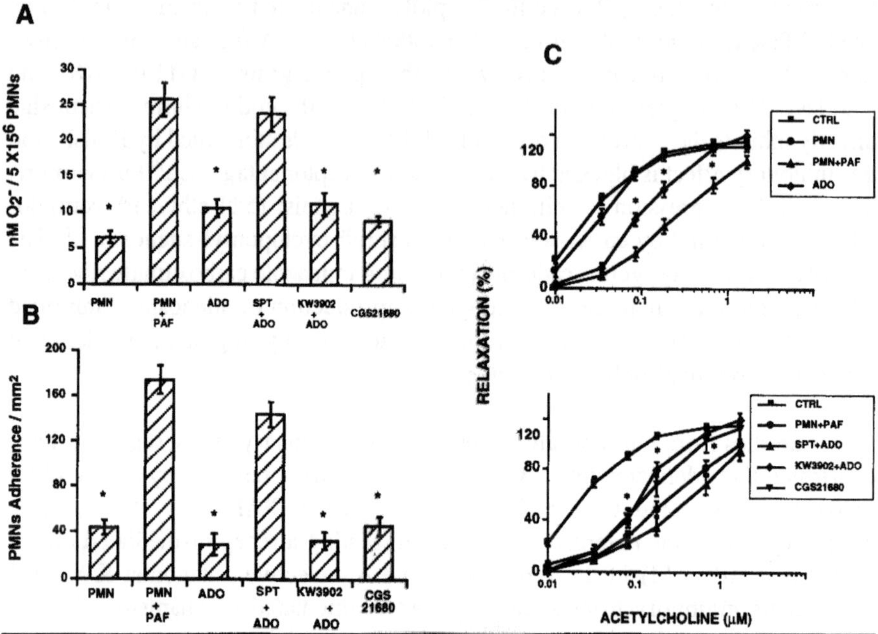

FIGURE 5-1. Graphs of superoxide radical generation (cytochrome C reduction) from platelet activating factor (PAF)-stimulated neutrophils (PMN) (Panel A), PMN adherence to coronary artery endothelium (Panel B), and PMN-mediated damage to endothelium-dependent and -independent relaxation in coronary artery rings (Panel C). Adenosine (ADO) significantly inhibited superoxide radical generation and adherence by PAF-stimulated PMNs, and blunted relaxation responses, which were reversed with the ADO antagonist 8-SPT. ADO plus the A_1-antagonist KW-3902 did not alter ADO's inhibition; the ADO A_2-receptor analog mimicked ADO inhibition. Mean ± standard error. *P<0.05 vs PAF-stimulated PMN group. From Zhao et al.[21]

agonists reduced leukocyte "rolling" on and firm adherence to the endothelium in dorsal subcutaneous muscle during reperfusion suggested to us that adenosine may inhibit this initial stage by acting directly on the endothelium, rather than on the PMNs. Accordingly, Williams et al[24] tested the hypothesis that adenosine directly inhibits the thrombin activated coronary vascular endothelium to attenuate adherence of *unstimulated* neutrophils. The endothelium of coronary arteries was activate with thrombin (100nM) and exposed to unstimulated neutrophils, which increased adherence six-fold over unstimulated endothelium. Adenosine attenuated PMN adherence to thrombin stimulated endothelium in a concentration-dependent manner, with 100 μM showing complete inhibition to baseline levels of adherence (Fig. 5-2). This was reversed by the adenosine receptor antagonist 8-SPT back to thrombin-stimulated levels. Interestingly, pretreatment and subsequent washout of the endothelium with adenosine did not alter PMN adherence to stimulated endothelium from that seen with adenosine alone. Subsequently, Fernandez et al[25] demonstrated that the inhibitory actions exerted by adenosine were reversed by an A_2-selective antagonist (KF-21326), but not by the A_1-selective antagonist (KW-3902). There was a tendency for KF-21326 to inhibit adherence in the absence of exogenous adenosine, suggesting inhibition of endogenous adenosine A_2-receptor effects. Furthermore, the selective A_2 agonist CGS21680 mimicked adenosine's inhibition of adherence, suggesting that adenosine's actions on activated endothelium were mediated by A_2-receptor mechanisms but not by A_1-receptor mechanisms. Therefore, adenosine directly inhibits both cellular components involved in neutrophil-endothelial cell interactions, i.e. the neutrophil and the endothelium. However, Zahler et al.[26] showed that A_1 receptor activation actually stimulated PMN adherence to thrombin-stimulated endothelium at lower adenosine concentrations (<1 μM). However, A_2 receptor mediated inhibition predominated at higher concentrations of adenosine. Therefore, direct actions of the A_1 and A_2 receptors on PMNs and

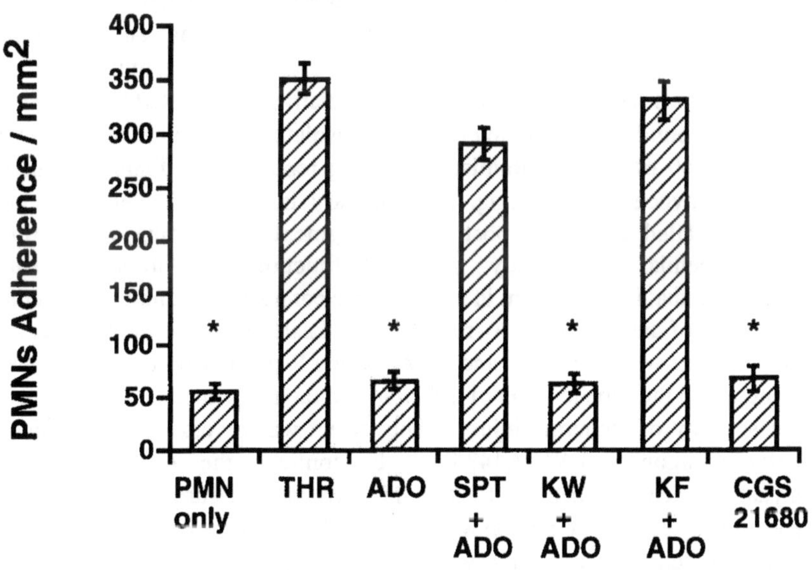

FIGURE 5-2. Graphs showing adherence of *unstimulated* neutrophils (PMNs) to coronary artery endothelium. Thrombin (THR), which stimulates translocation of p-selectin on endothelium, significantly increased PMN adherence. Inhibition of neutrophil adherence by adenosine (ADO) was blocked by the ADO antagonist 8-SPT, but was not altered by the A_1-receptor antagonist KW-3902 (KW). KF21326 (KF), a selective A_2 receptor antagonist, completely reversed the inhibitory effect of ADO. The A_2 receptor agonist, CGS-21680, mimicked the inhibitory effect of ADO, suggesting that PMN adherence is inhibited by A_2 receptor mechanisms. Mean ± standard error. $P<0.05$ vs THR-stimulated PMN group. From taken Williams et al[24] and Fernandez et al.[25]

endothelium seem to be bimodal, with the A_1 receptor increasing adherence and the A_2 receptor inhibiting adherence. Whether this bimodal action occurs in vivo is not clear. These bimodal actions may have important implications for the actions of endogenously released adenosine on postischemic contractile dysfunction[27] and viability, depending upon the periendothelial concentrations achieved. If endogenously released adenosine inhibits PMN adherence, as suggested by Gunther and Herring,[28] then inhibitory concentrations of periendothelial adenosine may be achieved in the unstirred vascular interface. If, however, lower concentrations of adenosine are achieved at the vascular interface during early reperfusion, then activation of PMN will prevail. Consequently, adenosine has the potential of being both a protagonist and an antagonist of reperfusion injury.[26,27]

Exogenous Adenosine Administered During Reperfusion
Non-Lethal Injury (Myocardial Stunning)

Postischemic contractile dysfunction in the absence of myocardial necrosis has been defined as "stunning". Hoffmeister et al[29] found that an intracoronary infusion of adenosine during reperfusion failed to improve stunning, although tissue ATP levels were significantly increased relative to untreated hearts. Similar results were found by Ambrosio et al[30] in the isolated perfused rabbit heart when adenosine (100 μM) was administered during reperfusion. Finally, in in vivo models of myocardial stunning, intracoronary infusion of adenosine during reperfusion failed to improve postischemic segmental shortening, while infusion before ischemia significantly improved function.[31,32] Subsequent studies demonstrated that improvement in postischemic contractile stunning was mediated by activation of the adenosine A_1-receptor.[33,34] Lasley et al[34] found that treatment before ischemia with adenosine and the A_1 analog R-phenylisopropy adenosine (R-PIA) increased the time to onset of ischemic contracture, which is used as a marker of the severity of ischemic injury. This effect was reversed by an adenosine receptor antagonist, BW A1433U. In contrast, the A_2-receptor analog phenylaminoadenosine had no effect on this surrogate measure of ischemic injury. Adenosine A_1-receptor activation was also found to improve postischemic function of globally ischemic rat hearts, while an A_2-receptor analog had no protective effect.[35] It is important to note that in this latter study using buffer-perfused hearts,[35] the agonists were used in a pretreatment modality only, and were washed out at the time of reperfusion. Therefore, the A_1 and A_2 agonists would not be present in the myocardium during reperfusion. Secondly, the perfusate was PMN-free, and the benefit of the A_2 agonist may depend on the presence of PMNs.

The consensus from available data would suggest that exogenous adenosine and adenosine analogs must be administered as a pretreatment before ischemia, and not during reperfusion, in order to inhibit postischemic contractile dysfunction in models of non-lethal injury (i.e. stunning).[32,36,37] The mechanisms involved in this inhibition of stunning include reducing the severity of ischemia by hyperpolarizing the cell, augmenting anaerobic glycolysis,[38] and improving energy status. The failure of adenosine or A_2 agonists to improve contractile stunning when given during reperfusion is still unclear, but may relate to the involvement of the therapeutic target to the pathophysiology of stunning, and to the compartment in which adenosine is present versus the location of the target. A major participant in reperfusion injury is the neutrophil. However, neutrophils may not be important in the pathogenesis of myocardial stunning, since neutrophil inhibition fails to modify stunning,[39,40] and stunning still occurs in neutrophil-free models.[35,38] Although adenosine is a potent inhibitor of PMNs and related events, inhibition of PMNs during reperfusion would have little effect on contractile dysfunction in view of their limited role in its pathogenesis. Likewise, models which preclude neutrophils (i.e. buffer-perfused hearts) would avoid this component of injury and hence adenosine would fail to demonstrate a protective effect. Consequently, adenosine may exert its cardioprotective effects on non-lethal injury (i.e. stunning) during ischemia, rather than during reperfusion because of its therapeutic targets and the time course of those targets in ischemic-reperfusion events.

Lethal Injury

Prolonged coronary occlusion followed by reperfusion produces necrosis within the area at risk, beginning in the subendocardium and extending with occlusion time toward the subepicardium in a wavefront pattern.[41] In a landmark study, Olafsson et al[5] first reported that intracoronary adenosine, transiently infused into the LAD at 3.75 mg/min at the onset of reperfusion, reduced infarct size by 75% and improved regional contractile function 24 hours after the start of reflow. Histology demonstrated preservation of endothelial morphology with decreased neutrophil infiltration and plugging in the central necrotic zone. This study[5] is important because it demonstrated that adenosine could 1) reduce infarct size on a long term basis (inhibition versus delay), 2) inhibit neutrophil accumulation in the area at risk, or at least attenuate plugging of the capillaries, 3) reduce endothelial damage, and 4) attenuate the complex processes of reperfusion injury leading to contractile dysfunction. These data strongly suggested an interaction between neutrophils, endothelium and infarction which has since emerged as a key triad in the pathogenesis of reperfusion injury.[11-13,15,42-45] Similar results were subsequently found by others using intravenous administration of adenosine[46] or adenosine receptor-specific analogues.[47] The attenuation of endothelial injury with intracoronary adenosine was reinforced by a subsequent study from the same group.[48] Using in vivo determination of endothelial-dependent (acetylcholine) and independent (papaverine) vasodilator reserve as a surrogate measure of endothelial function, both components of vasodilator responses were attenuated after reperfusion, consistent with the in vitro studies by Cronstein et al[18] and Zhao et al[21] and regional myocardial blood flow was impaired, both manifestations consistent with microvascular injury. Adenosine attenuated the loss of vasodilator reserve, and also reduced neutrophil infiltration and morphologic injury to the endothelium. This study[48] therefore confirmed the conclusions raised by Olafsson et al[5] that adenosine reduced necrosis, possibly by preventing neutrophil accumulation and microvascular injury.

Although numerous studies have reported a reduction in infarct size by adenosine, several studies have nonetheless failed to show any infarct sparing with adenosine administered only at reperfusion.[49,50] In the study by Homeister et al,[49] intracoronary adenosine was infused at doses similar to that used by Pitarys et al[46] (0.15 mg/kg/min) failed to reduce infarct size. However, the combination of adenosine and lidocaine did significantly reduce infarct size, suggesting a cooperative effect between the two agents. Lidocaine may attenuate infarct extension by reducing adherence, lysosomal enzyme release and superoxide anion generation by PMNs. However, Goto et al[50] failed to show infarct sparing with adenosine, even in combination with lidocaine. Differences in preparation may be one reason cited for this discrepancy since studies performed by both Pitarys et al[46] and Babbitt et al[48] were in closed-chest preparations, while that of Homeister et al[49] was performed in open-chest dogs. However, other studies demonstrated cardioprotective effects of pretreatment adenosine[51] and endogenous adenosine[52,53] without the concomitant use of lidocaine. Therefore, the issue remains unresolved.

Since adenosine has potent anti-neutrophil properties, it was hypothesized that adenosine would reduce reperfusion injury in part by inhibiting neutrophil events, including accumulation in the area at risk, through an A_2 receptor mechanism. Jordan et al[54] used a canine model of LAD occlusion with reperfusion via a carotid to LAD shunt used to introduce pharmacologic agents intracoronarily. After 60 minutes of collateral-deficient (LAD arteriotomy) occlusion, reperfusion was initiated with an infusion of either saline (control) or the A_2 receptor-specific analogue CGS-23680 for the first hour of reperfusion. Similar to the study by Schlack et al[55], Jordan et al found that the adenosine A_2-receptor analogue CGS-21680 significantly reduced infarct size from 29.8 ± 2.3 % of the area at risk in a saline vehicle group to $15.4 \pm 2.9\%$ of the area at risk. However, there was no improvement in wall motion, in contrast to that reported by Schlack et al.[55] CGS-21680 significantly reduced neutrophil accumulation in the area at risk, as well as inhibiting in vitro neutrophil superoxide radical production and neutrophil adherence to the endothelium of isolated coronary artery segments. These data provide an association between adenosine's antineutrophil effects and its infarct-sparing effect.

If the cardioprotective effects of adenosine specifically administered during reperfusion are related to its inhibitory actions on PMNs and endothelium, then the vascular compartment is a primary site of action. Adenosine A_2 receptors are present and functional on both neutrophils[56] and the vascular endothelium.[57,58] To test the hypothesis that the vascular compartment is a primary site of adenosine actions against reperfusion injury, Todd et al[59] used a large molecular weight adenosine congener (polyadenylic acid, PolyA) that contains only one adenosine moiety at its 3' end, and is retained in the vascular compartment. A nearly subvasodilator dose of PolyA administered at repersusion in a rabbit model of coronary occlusion-reperfusion reduced infarct size by 50% (Figure 5-3A). Furthermore, the effects of PolyA were reversed by 8-SPT, confirming an adenosine receptor-mediated mechanism. However, infarct size was not altered by the highly A_1-selective antagonist 8-(3-noradamantyl)-1,3-dipropylxanthine (KW-3902, 1 mg/kg i.v.), implicating an A_2 receptor mechanism. In addition, PolyA significantly inhibited PMN superoxide generation and adherence to coronary endothelium. This study strongly suggested that the intravascular compartment, by inhibiting PMN-endothelial cell interactions, is important site for the cardioprotective actions of adenosine during reperfusion. Activation (and inhibition) of adenosine receptors has been linked to the release of other endothelial-derived factors,[60] and interactions exist between nitric oxide and adenosine that impact on infarct size[61] and postischemic function.[62] To what extent the co-release of other anti-neutrophil factors contributes to the inhibitory effcts of adenosine in the vascular compartment is not known.

Inherent Cardioprotection by Endogenous Adenosine

It has been established that adenosine is tonically released by the endothelium and myocytes. Ischemia and hypoxia significantly augment the release of adenosine from both cell sources into the interstitium and into the vascular compartments. Therefore, endogenously released adenosine could act in either compartment, based on the concentrations achieved, the time when sufficient concentrations are achieved in a given compartment, and the targets in each of the compartments. The question arises whether *endogenous* adenosine exerts cardioprotective effects, and if so, are these effects exerted during ischemia, reperfusion or both "windows"? In 1990, Lasley et al[34] made the important observation that the adenosine antagonist BW A1433U alone increased the time to onset of ischemic contracture, suggesting that endogenously released adenosine played an inherent cardioprotective role in the heart. A preliminary report by Khatchician et al[63] suggested that the protective

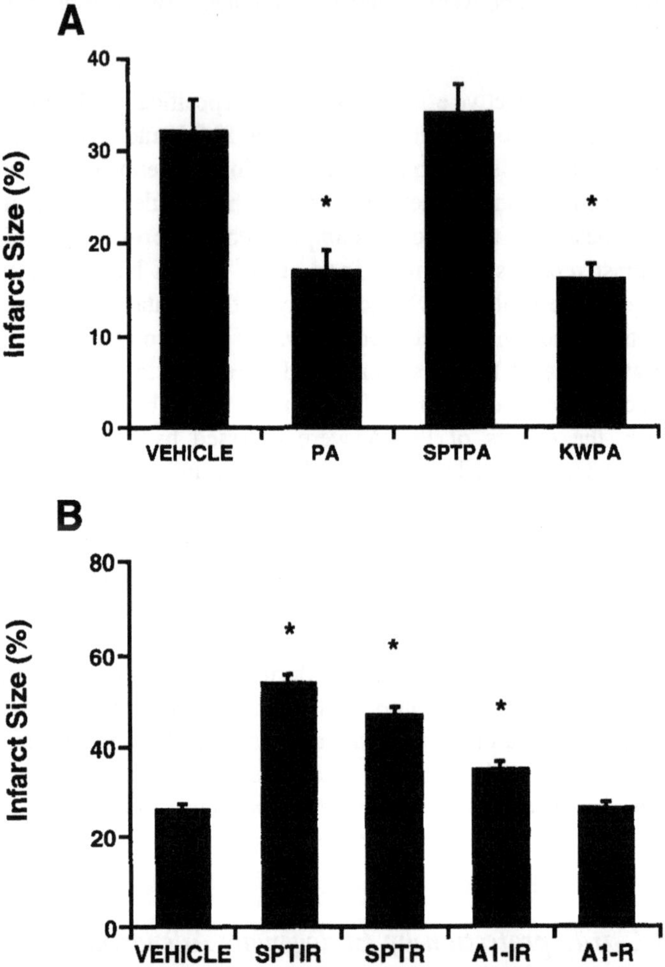

FIGURE 5-3. A. Infarct size, expressed as the area of necrosis/area of left ventricle at risk (%) in rabbits undergoing 30 minutes left coronary occlusion and 2 hours reperfusion. Vehicle-treated group (VEHICLE) received saline, PA received 1mg/kg bolus followed by 0.5 mg/kg/h Polyadenylic acid (PolyA), the SPTPA group received PolyA plus SPT (20 mg/kg), and KWPA group received Polyadenylic acid plus the A_1-receptor antagonist KW3902 (1 mg/kg). Data taken from Todd et al.[59] B. Infarct size data in rabbits exposed to 30 minutes left coronary occlusion and 2 hours reperfusion. SPTIR, SPT (10 mg/kg) was given throughout ischemic and reperfusion; SPTR, SPT was given 2 minutes before reperfusion only; A1-IR, the A_1-receptor antagonist KW-3902 (1 mg/kg) was given throughout ischemia-reperfusion, A1-R, KW-3902 was given 2 minutes before reperfusion.

effects of endogenous adenosine may reduce the extent of postischemic dysfunction (i.e. stunning) in a model of global ischemia-reperfusion. In contrast, studies by Liu et al[64] and Tsuchida et al [65] demonstrated a failure of the antagonists 8-*p*-sulfophenyl theophylline (8-SPT) or PD 115,199 to augment infarct size when infused before ischemia to block the effects of endogenously released adenosine. Therefore, whether tonic and ischemia-induced adenosine conferred an inherent cardioprotection was indeed controversial. Toombs et al[66] and Zhao et al,[67] using a rabbit model of 30 minutes left coronary artery occlusion (blood flow reduction 96% by microspheres) and 2 hours reperfusion showed that 8-SPT significantly increased infarct size by 60% to 100%, respectively, over a vehicle group, suggesting that endogenously released adenosine did participate in inherent modulation of infarct development. Zhao et al[67] then infused 8-SPT before ischemia and continuing into reperfusion , or only during reperfusion. As shown in Figure 5-3B, infarct size was increased by 100% over the vehicle group when 8-SPT was administered during ischemia and reperfusion, and was increased by 75% when given only during reperfusion. However, when 8-SPT was infused 30 minutes after reperfusion, there was no effect on infarct size. These data suggested that cardioprotection exerted specifically by endogenous adenosine 1) was receptor-mediated, 2) was expressed largely during reperfusion, with a smaller (25%) fraction exerted during the ischemic period, and 3) the injury processes acted on by endogenous adenosine were acutely complete within 30 minutes of reperfusion. In addition to reducing infarct size, adenosine reduced the severity in blood flow defects and improved postischemic blood flow in both the ischemic non-necrotic zone and the necrotic zone. The observation that adenosine exerts cardioprotection in this model of lethal injury during reperfusion is consistent with the protective effects of *exogenous* adenosine,[54,55] and is intriguing in that adenosine concentrations are augmented during ischemia, and reduced in concentration either by washout, rephosphorylation to AMP, or deaminated to inosine during reperfusion.

The important role of neutrophils in mediating the inflammatory-like component of reperfusion injury, combined with inhibition of neutrophil functions by predominantly A_2-receptor mechanisms led to the hypothesis that adenosine's cardioprotective effects during reperfusion were primarily A_2-mediated. Using the previously described[67] rabbit infarct model, Zhao et al used a potent, highly selective A_1-receptor antagonist 8-(3-noradamantyl)-1,3-dipropylxanthine (KW-3902, 1 mg/kg i.v.) administered throughout ischemia and reperfusion or during reperfusion only. As shown in Figure 5-3B, the A_1-receptor antagonist increased infarct size 25% above that in the vehicle group; this infarct increase was similar to the difference between SPT given during combined ischemia-reperfusion and reperfusion only, i.e. 25%. In contrast, when the A_1 antagonist was given during reperfusion only, there was no increase in infarct size over vehicle. These data suggested that 1) A_1-receptor mediated effects of endogenous adenosine predominate during ischemia, but 2) A_1-receptor effects are not exerted during reperfusion, implicating A_2-mediated effects. At the time of these studies, no water soluble A_2-receptor antagonists were available. The role of the A_3 receptor in this setting is very unclear at this time.

These results differ somewhat from those reported by Norton et al[47] that the 700-fold A_1-selective agonist N^6-cyclopentyladenosine (CPA) given intravenously before reperfusuion significantly reduced infarct size in a similar rabbit model of ischemia-reperfusion. It is possible that the A_1-mediated effects leading to infarct reduction are expressed during later (>4 hours) phases of reperfusion. This point emphasizes the need to perform definitive studies in long-term models of reperfusion to determine whether adenosine permanently reduces infarct size, or simply delays the development of a predetermined extent of infarction.

Taken together, adenosine exerts protection against lethal injury primarily by A_2-mediated mechanisms targeting PMN-related injury during reperfusion. Although the severity of ischemia may be a target by A_1 receptor mechanisms as it is in non-lethal injury, the impact of this effect on subsequent infarct size is most likely modest in lethal injury. However, this explanation needs further investigation.

The endothelium may play an important part in the endogenous cardioprotection mediated by adenosine. Adenosine is rapidly taken up by vascular endothelial cells via simple diffusion and via transport mechanisms,[68] and stored in the endothelium , primarily as nucleotides.[69] Therefore, the vascular endothelium acts as a metabolic barrier for adenosine that participates in the regulation of bidirectional movement of adenosine into the interstitial and vascular compartments. Adenosine is tonically released by the endothelium,[69] to which extracellular ecto-5'-nucleotidase activity adds a significant additional amount.[69,70] However, the release of adenosine from the endothelium is dramatically increased by hypoxia[71] and ischemia.[72]

The adenosine released by the PMNs and endothelial cells may play an important role in inhibiting neutrophil-induced damage. Unstimulated PMNs continuously produce and release adenosine from intracellular sources and in part by extracellular dephosphorylation of AMP by ecto-5'-nucleotidase activity.[73,74] Using co-incubated and co-stimulated PMNs and endothelium, Cronstein et al.[18] reported that tonically released adenosine attenuated neutrophil superoxide radical generation and endothelial damage. However, the source of this endogenous adenosine PMN or endothelium) was not identified. Gunther et al[28] found that adenosine tonically released from endothelial cell monolayers inhibited superoxide anion production from human neutrophils by 49%, which could be reversed by addition of adenosine deaminase to metabolize adenosine. Therefore, the endothelium may release adenosine, as well as other factors, that participate in normal homeostatic regulation of PMN-endothelial cell interactions and their sequelae.

Should Adenosine Join the Surgical Cardioprotective Armamentarium?

Many of the mechanisms involved in non-surgical ischemic-reperfusion injury are involved also in reperfusion following cardiac surgery. However, the situation in cardiac surgery is more complex than nonsurgical reperfusion[75,76] because aortic cross-clamping a vented heart interposes an additional interval of ischemia in a heart with reduced oxygen demands, which differs in time course of pathology to working hearts with coronary occlusion (for example) in which the oxygen demands in the ischemic segment are paradoxically high.[77,78] Furthermore, the infusion of a cardioplegic solution adds several opportunities for (re)perfusion injury, but also presents opportunities for protection, viz-a-viz modification of the *conditions* of cardioplegia infusion and *composition* of the perfusate (hypothermia, hypocalcemia, hyperkalemia, hyperglycemia, alkalosis, and additives).[79] However, since the surgical team exercises control over the conduct of cardiopulmonary bypass and the delivery of cardioplegia, cardiac surgery allows the unique opportunity for the cardioprotective potential of adenosine to be exerted in all three windows of opportunity: pretreatment, ischemia and reperfusion. Alas, despite the preliminary studies showing great promise as a potent cardioprotective agent, and a resounding call for studies on the use of adenosine as a surgical adjunct,[80] primary studies exploring adenosine and its mechanisms of protection in surgical models of ischemia, cardioplegia and reperfusion are woefully and disappointingly lacking.

Pretreatment

The plasma half-life of adenosine is very short, on the order of seconds in humans. Nonetheless, numerous studies have shown that a brief pretreatment with adenosine reduces infarct size in isolated-perfused (no circulating PMNs, platelets, etc)[81] and in vivo[66,82] models, improves postischemic contractile function[37] and preserves metabolic or energy status of the ischemic-reperfused myocardium.[37] These pretreatment cardioprotective effects may be mediated by a number of mechanisms including activation of A_1-receptors,[83] ATP-sensitive potassium (K_{ATP}) channels and reducing calcium overload, while favorably altering calcium transients involved in excitation-contraction coupling.[84] The effect of pretreatment adenosine on PMN function in vivo is not clear, although in vitro studies indicate no direct inhibitory effect on either PMNs[26] or on endothelium.[24] Lee et al[85] first reported favorable results with pretreatment adenosine given preoperatively to patients with poor left ventricular performance (ejection fraction approximately 30%) and three vessel disease. Adenosine was infused at a hemodynamically benign dose of 250 to 350 μg/kg for 10 minutes prior to cardiopulmonary bypass. Cardiac index was improved over nontreated patients (by 42% of prebypass vs 10% of prebypass, respectively) immediately after discontinuation of bypass and 40 hours postoperatively, and creatine kinase levels 24 hours post-operatively were significantly lower in adenosine treated patients. Obviously, these data are extremely promising since the question of unwanted complications (hypotension, bradycardia) or other side effects do not enter into the evaluation process at this dose and regimen.

Ischemia (Cardioplegic Arrest)

In 1976, Hearse et al[86] reported that adenosine, either used alone during ischemia or as an adjunct to hyperkalemic cardioplegia was cardioprotective. Subsequently, other studies demonstrated that adenosine, either alone[87,88] or in combintion with crystalloid potassium cardioplegia,[87,89] could be useful to accelerate cardiac arrest through membrane hyperpolarization and increased potassium permeability,[89] and improved indices of postischemic contractile performance as well. Other studies have shown that adenosine improved postischemic performance variables after long-term storage of hearts.[90,91] The beneficial effects of adenosine applied during ischemia (during cardioplegia) have been attributed to a number of mechanisms, including improvement in the rate of anaerobic glycolysis and energy status, as well as reduction in calcium accumulation secondary to cell hyperpolarization. Although some studies report that adenosine repletes tissue ATP content during reperfusion, but not during arrest,[92,93] others show no correlation between tissue ATP content after reperfusion and functional recovery.[30,88,94-96]

Few studies have tested adenosine as an adjunct to blood cardioplegia, perhaps because there is concern that the nucleoside will be too rapidly degraded by adenosine deaminase and thereby not achieve therapeutic levels, or the generation of superoxide radicals metabolite xanthine by xanthine oxidase will induce severe injury. However, catabolism of adenosine in blood cardioplegia can be attenuated by hypothermia, mixing the adenosine as close as possible to the aortic root, and co-infusion of a short acting deaminase inhibitor. Alternatively, degradation can be compensated for by judisciously increasing the concentration of adenosine delivered at the aortic root. Hudspeth et al[97] investigated adenosine as an adjunct to a standard hypothermic, hyperkalemic blood cardioplegic solution in ischemically injured (30 minutes normothermic global ischemia) hearts. Adenosine-supplemented (400 µmole/L final concentration) blood cardioplegia reversed the postischemic systolic dysfunction (left ventricular pressure-volume analysis) observed with unsupplemented blood cardioplegia. This protection was inhibited with 8-SPT, suggesting a receptor-mediated mechanism rather than a purely biochemical mechanism. Interestingly, adenosine did not increase the total volume of blood cardioplegia delivered, probably because the myocardium was maximally dilated by antecedant ischemia or intermittent ischemia. The study by Hudspeth et al[97] did not determine the mechanisms by which adenosine reduced postcardioplegia dysfunction in these injured hearts, a topic which would provide some interesting science. However, based on the known mechanisms summarized above, it can be speculated that these mechanisms include 1) increasing the tolerance to ischemia between infusions of cardioplegia related to improved glycolysis and phosphorylation potential, K_{ATP} channel activation, calcium accumulation, anti-adrenergic effect (all possibly A_1-receptor mediated events during ischemia) and , 2) attenuating neutrophil events and endothelial injury by direct inhibition of PMNs, endothelium or their interactions (purportedly A_2-mediated events occurring during infusion of blood cardioplegia and during reperfusion).

As in non-surgical models of regional ischemia-reperfusion, coronary endothelial injury is not manifest until reperfusion with normal blood after clinically relevant short-term global ischemia or cardioplegic arrest,[98]. The coronary vascular endothelium is injured during global normothermic ischemia that is significantly prolonged (>1 hour).[99] However, Sellke et al[100] have shown that adenosine-enhanced crystalloid cardioplegia improves postischemic contractile function, but fails to inhibit endothelial dysfunction seen after one hour of chemical arrest. This observation is in conflict with the known effects of adenosine to inhibit PMN-endotheoial cell interactions and endothelial injury in non-cardioplegia models, and the observation that other antineutrophil agents improve postischemic function in association with better endothelial function.[101,102] The interactions between ischemia, cardioplegia solutions and reperfusion creates a more complex situation than presented in non-surgical studies, and requires further study.

Reperfusion

Because adenosine has potent antineutrophil effects which reduce lethal postischemic injury when given only at the onset of reperfusion, infusion of the nucleside at reperfusion (declamping) may be beneficial. Indeed, this has been shown by Ledingham et al[94] and Thelin et al[88] in which transient adenosine infusion only at the start of reperfusion was associated with improved functional recovery.

Although a beneficial effect exerted during reperfusion would be in keeping with adenosine's antineutrophil effects listed above, this benefit would apply to lethal injury, and not necessarily to non-lethal injury (postcardioplegia or postischemic contractile dysfunction). The use of adenosine as a post-cardioplegia treatment has been virtually ignored in other models of surgical ischemic-reperfusion injury, and well-controlled studies of mechanisms are lacking.

Conclusions

Adenosine has a broad spectrum of physiological effects which make it suitable as a cardioprotective agent with effectiveness in all three windows of opportunity. It has potential for reducing ischemic injury by largely A_1-receptor mediated mechanisms involving effectors or targets in the myocyte or interstitial compartment, including K_{ATP} channel activation, improved anaerobic metabolism, improved energy status and attenuated PMN-myocyte interactions. Such effects can be instigated by treatment remote from or adjacent to the ischemic interval. The duration of the physiological actions seem to extend well beyond its plasma half-life. In addition, adenosine reduces reperfusion injury by inhibiting the neutrophil and the endothelium directly, and their interactions by largely A_2-receptor mechanisms largely in the vascular space. Exogenous as well as endogenous adenosine can be exploited for their therapeutic potential. Since adenosine's cardioprotection is dose-dependent,[81,103] the optimal dose needs to be identified, taking full advantage of beneficial effects while avoiding unwanted side effects. Further research is required to elucidate the role of adenosine in potentially modulating "late" reperfusion injury, and its role in modulating signals involved in the neutrophil-mediated response to ischemia-reperfusion, and its potential role in modulating the apoptotic component of post-ischemic cell death.[104] Other effects of adenosine which may attract the surgeon's interest are termination of supraventricular tachyarrhythmias, negative chronotropy, and negative inotropic effects. The latter is effective only against adrenergically augmented inotropic state, and may have mixed blessings in the postbypass patient.

To echo a previous editorial,[80] there has been a hesitation to investigate and incorporate adenosine into the surgical strategy of cardioprotection. This reticence may be related to concern over vasodilation resulting in hypotension and potential cardioplegia "overload" with delivery of high volumes of solution, or to pain and discomfort. However, these adverse effects may be related to the dose of adenosine used in previous studies; the vasodilatory effects of adenosine, if present, may be counterbalanced with short acting vasoconstrictors delivered in synchrony with adenosine-enhanced cardioplegia. These untoward effects may be overcome by identifying a subvasodilatory dose of adenosine, and appropriate analogues that do

not induce vasodilate at therapeutic doses. Also, it is not known whether the PMN inhibitory effects of adenosine are short-term effects, or whether they persist for days and may interfere with the patient's defense mechanisms against infection.

References

1. Drury AN, Szent-Györgyi A. The physiological activity of adenine compounds with especial reference to their action upon the mammalian heart. J Physiol (Lond) 1929;68:213-237.
2. Berne RM, Knabb RM, Ely SW, et al. Adenosine in the local regulation of blood flow: a brief overview. Fed Proc 1983;42:3136-3142.
3. Belardinelli L, West A, Crampton R, et al. Chronotropic and dromotropic actions of adenosine. In: Berne RM, Rall TW, Rubio R, eds. The regulatory function of adenosine. The Hague: Martinus Nijhoff, 1983:378-398.
4. Froldi G, Belardinelli L. Species-dependent effects of adenosine on heart rate and atrioventricular nodal conduction. Mechanism and physiological implications. Circ Res 1990;67:960-978.
5. Olafsson B, Forman MB, Puett DW, et al. Reduction of reperfusion injury in the canine preparation by intracoronary adenosine: importance of the endothelium and the no-reflow phenomenon. Circulation 1987;76:1135-1145.
6. Vinten-Johansen J, Hammon JW, Jr. Cardioprotection by adenosine: Is it a question of effective dose, timing, or the target compartment? Letters to the editor. J Thorac Cardiovasc Surg 1996;112:202-204.
7. Van Wylen DGL. Relationship between intracoronary adenosine, interstitial fluid purine metabolites, and coronary blood flow. Drug Devel Res 1994;31:330
8. Cronstein BN, Kramer SB, Weissmann G, et al. Adenosine: a physiological modulator of superoxide anion generation by human neutrophils. J Exp Med 1983;158:1160-1177.
9. Kitakaze M, Hori M, Sato H, et al. Endogenous adenosine inhibits platelet aggregation during myocardial ischemia in dogs. Circ Res 1991;69:1402-1408.
10. Colli S, Tremoli E. Multiple effects of dipyridamole on neutrophils and mononuclear leukocytes: adenosine-dependent and adenosine-independent mechanisms. J Lab Clin Med 1991;118:136-145.
11. Mullane K. Neutrophil and endothelial changes in reperfusion injury. Trends Cardiovasc Med 1991;1:282-289.
12. Dreyer WJ, Michael LH, West MW, et al. Neutrophil accumulation in ischemic canine myocardium: Insights into time course, distribution, and mechanism of localization during early reperfusion. Circulation 1991;84:400-411.
13. Lucchesi BR, Werns SW, Fantone JC. The role of neutrophils and free radicals in ischemic myocardial injury. J Mol Cell Cardiol 1989;21:1241-1251.
14. Mullane KM. Myocardial ischemia-reperfusion injury: Role of neutrophils and neutrophil-derived mediators. In: Marone G, Lichtestein L, Condorelly M, Fauci AS, eds. Human Inflammatory Disease: Clinical Immunology. 1st ed. Toronto: Decker, Inc. 1988:143
15. Mehta JL, Nichols WW, Mehta P. Neutrophils as potential participants in acute myocardial ischemia: Relevance to reperfusion. J Am Coll Cardiol 1988;11:1309-1316.
16. Roberts PA, Newby AC, Hallett MB, et al. Inhibition by adenosine of reactive oxygen metabolite production by human polymorphonuclear leucocytes. Biochem J 1985;227:669-674.
17. Cronstein BN, Rosenstein ED, Kramer SB, et al. Adenosine: a physiologic modulator of superoxide anion generation by human neutrophils. Adenosine acts via an A_2 receptor on human neutrophils. J Immunol 1985;135:1366-1371.

18. Cronstein BN, Levin RI, Belanoff J, et al. Adenosine: an endogenous inhibitor of neutrophil-mediated injury to endothelial cells. J Clin Invest 1986;78:760-770.
19. Wollner A, Wollner S, Smith JB. Acting via A2 receptors, adenosine inhibits the upregulation of Mac-1 (CD11b/CD18) expression on FMLP-stimulated neutrophils. Am J Resp Cell & Mol Biol 1993;9:179-185.
20. Gruber HE, Hoffer ME, McAllister DR, et al. Increased adenosine concentration in blood from ischemic myocardium by AICA Riboside. Effects on flow, granulocytes, and injury. Circulation 1989;80:1400-1411.
21. Zhao Z-Q, Sato H, Williams MW, et al. Adenosine A_2-Receptor Activation Inhibits Neutrophil-Mediated Injury to Coronary Endothelium. Am J Physiol 1996;271;H1456-1464.
22. Nolte D, Lorenzen A, Lehr HA, et al. Reduction of postischemic leukocyte-endothelium interaction by adenosine via A2 receptor. Naunyn-Schmiedebergs Archives of Pharmacology 1992;346.234-237.
23. Nolte D, Lehr HA, Messmer K. Adenosine inhibits postischemic leukocyte-endothelium interaction in postcapillary venules of the hamster. Am J Physiol 1991;261:H651-5.
24. Williams MW, Jordan JE, Fernandez AZ, et al. Adenosine (ADO) inhibits unactivated neutrophil (PMN) adherence to thrombin stimulated coronary vascular endothelium (EC) by a p-selectin mechanism. FASEB J 1996;10:A280(Abstract)
25. Fernandez AZ, Williams MW, Jordan JE, et al. Neutrophil (PMN) adherence to thrombin stimulated coronary vascular endothelium is inhibited by an adenosine (ADO) A_2-receptor mechanism. FASEB J 1996;10:A611(Abstract)
26. Zahler S, Becker BF, Raschke P, et al. Stimulation of endothelial adenosine A_1 receptors enhances adhesion of neutrophils in the intact guinea pig coronary system. Cardiovasc Res 1994;28:1366-1372.
27. Raschke P, Becker BF. Adenosine and PAF dependent mechanisms lead to myocardial reperfusion injury by neutrophils after brief ischaemia. Cardiovasc Res 1995;29:569-576.
28. Gunther GR, Herring MB. Inhibition of neutrophil superoxide production by adenosine released from vascular endothelial cells. Ann Vasc Surg 1991;5:325-330.
29. Hoffmeister HM, Mauser M, Schaper W. Effect of adenosine and AICAR on ATP content and regional contractile function in reperfused canine myocardium. Bas Res Cardiol 1985;80:445-458.
30. Ambrosio G, Jacobus WE, Mitchell MC, et al. Effects of ATP precursors on ATP and free ADP content and functional recovery of postischemic hearts. Am J Physiol 1989;256:H560-H566.
31. Sekili S, Jeroudi MO, Tang X, et al. Effect of adenosine on myocardial 'stunning' in the dog. Circ Res 1995;76:82-94.
32. Randhawa MPS, Jr., Lasley RD, Mentzer RM, Jr. Salutary effects of exogenous adenosine administration on in vivo myocardial stunning. J Thorac Cardiovasc Surg 1995;110:63-74.
33. Jeroudi MO, Tang X-L, Abd-Elfattah AS, et al. Effect of adenosine A_1-receptor activation on myocardial stunning in intact dogs. Circulation 1994;90 (No 4, Part 2):I-479(Abstract)
34. Lasley RD, Rhee JW, Van Wylen DGL, et al. Adenosine A_1 receptor mediated protection of the globally ischemic isolated rat heart. J Mol Cell Cardiol 1990;22:39-47.
35. Lasley RD, Mentzer RM. Adenosine improves recovery of postischemic myocardial function via an adenosine A_1 receptor mechanism. Am J Physiol 1992;263:H1460-H1465.
36. Lasley RD, Mentzer RM, Jr. Protective effects of adenosine in the reversibly injured heart. Ann Thorac Surg 1995;60:843-846.
37. Zhou Z, Bunger R, Lasley RD, et al. Adenosine pretreatment increases cytosolic phosphorylation potential and attenuates postischemic cardiac dysfunction in swine. Surg Forum 1993;249-251.
38. Janier MF, Vanoverschelde JJ, Bergmann SR. Adenosine protects ischemic and reperfused myocardium by receptor-mediated mechanisms. Am J Physiol 1993;264:H163-H170.
39. Bolli R. Role of neutrophils in myocardial stunning after brief ischaemia: the end of a six year old controversy (1987-1993) [comment]. Cardiovasc Res 1993;27:728-730.

40. Juneau CF, Ito BR, del Balzo U, et al. Severe neutrophil depletion by leucocyte filters or cytotoxic drug does not improve recovery of contractile function in stunned porcine myocardium [see comments]. Cardiovasc Res 1993;27:720-727.
41. Reimer KA, Jennings RB. The "wavefront phenomenon" of myocardial ischemic cell death. II. Transmural progression of necrosis within the framework of ischemic bed size (myocardial at risk) and collateral flow. Lab Invest 1979;40:633-644.
42. Ma X, Tsao PS, Viehman GE, et al. Neutrophil-mediated vasoconstriction and endothelial dysfunction in low-flow perfusion-reperfused cat coronary artery. Circ Res 1991;69:95-106.
43. Ma X, Weyrich AS, Lefer DJ, et al. Diminished basal nitric oxide release after myocardial ischemia and reperfusion promotes neutrophil adherence to coronary endothelium. Circ Res 1993;72:403-412.
44. Lefer AM, Tsao PS, Lefer DJ, et al. Role of endothelial dysfunction in the pathogenesis of reperfusion injury after myocardial ischemia. FASEB J 1991;5:2029-2034.
45. Siminiak T, Ozawa T. Neutrophil mediated myocardial injury. [Review]. International Journal of Biochemistry 1993;25:147-156.
46. Pitarys CJ, Virmani R, Vildibill HD, Jr., et al. Reduction of myocardial reperfusion injury by intravenous adenosine administered during the early reperfusion period. Circulation 1991;83:237-247.
47. Norton ED, Jackson EK, Turner MB, et al. The effects of intravenous infusions of selective adenosine A_1-receptor and A_2-receptor agonists on myocardial reperfusion injury. Am Heart J 1992;123:332-338.
48. Babbitt DG, Virmani R, Forman MB. Intracoronary adenosine administered after reperfusion limits vascular injury after prolonged ischemia in the canine model. Circulation 1989;80:1388-1399.
49. Homeister JW, Hoff PT, Fletcher DD, et al. Combined adenosine and lidocaine administration limits myocardial reperfusion injury. Circulation 1990;82:595-608.
50. Goto M, Miura T, Iliodoromitis EK, et al. Adenosine infusion during early reperfusion failed to limit myocardial infarct size in a collateral deficient species. Cardiovasc Res 1991;25:943-949.
51. Toombs CF, McGee DS, Johnston WE, et al. Protection from ischaemic-reperfusion injury with adenosine pretreatment is reversed by inhibition of ATP-sensitive potassium channels. Cardiovasc Res 1993;27:623-629.
52. Vinten-Johansen J, Lefer DJ, Nakanishi K, et al. Controlled coronary hydrodynamics at the time of reperfusion reduces postischemic injury. Cor Art Dis 1992;3:1081-1093.
53. Zhao Z-Q, Nakanishi K, McGee DS, et al. A_1-receptor mediated myocardial infarct size reduction by endogenous adenosine is exerted primarily during ischemia. Cardiovasc Res 1994;28:270-279.
54. Jordan JE, Zhao Z-Q, Sato H, et al. Adenosine A_2 activation attenuates reperfusion injury by inhibiting neutrophil accumulation, superoxide generation and coronary endothelial adherence. J Pharmacol Exp Ther 1996;
55. Schlack W, Schäfer M, Uebing A, et al. Adenosine A_2-receptor activation at reperfusion reduces infarct size and improves myocardial wall function in dog heart. J Cardiovasc Pharmacol 1993;22:89-96.
56. Cronstein BN, Daguma L, Nichols D, et al. The adenosine/neutrophil paradox resolved: human neutrophils possess both A_1 and A_2 receptors that promote chemotaxis and inhibit O_2 generation, respectively. J Clin Invest 1990;85:1150-1157.
57. Nees S. Coronary flow increases induced by adenosine and adenine nucleotides are mediated by the coronary endothelium: a new principle of the regulation of coronary flow. Eur Heart J 1989;10:28-35.
58. Balcells E, Suarez J, Rubio R. Functional role of intravascular coronary endothelial adenosine receptors. Eur J Pharmacol 1992;210:1-9.
59. Todd JC, Zhao Z-Q, Williams MW, et al. Intravascular adenosine at reperfusion reduces infarct size and neutrophil adherence. Ann Thorac Surg 1996;62;1364-1372.

60. Headrick JP, Berne RM. Endothelium-dependent and -independent relaxations to adenosine in guinea pig aorta. Am J Physiol 1990;259:H62-H67.
61. Woolfson RG, Patel VC, Neild GH, et al. Inhibition of nitric oxide synthesis reduces infarct size by an adenosine-dependent mechanism. Circulation 1995;91:1545-1551.
62. Hasebe N, Shen Y-T, Vatner SF. Inhibition of endothelium-derived relaxing factor enhances myocardial stunning in conscious dogs. Circulation 1993;88:2862-2871.
63. Khatchikian GS, Mikhail EA, Zweier JL, et al. Role of endogenous adenosine in protecting against neutrophil-mediated injury in postischemic hearts. Circulation 1996;92:I-712(Abstract)
64. Liu GS, Thornton J, Van Winkle DM, et al. Protection against infarction afforded by preconditioning is mediated by A_1 adenosine receptors in rabbit hearts. Circulation 1991;84:350-356.
65. Tsuchida A, Miura T, Miki T, et al. Role of adenosine receptor activation in myocardial infarct size limitation by ischaemic preconditioning. Cardiovasc Res 1992;26:456-461.
66. Toombs CF, McGee DS, Johnston WE, et al. Myocardial protective effects of adenosine: Infarct size reduction with pretreatment and continued receptor stimulation during ischemia. Circulation 1992;86:986-994.
67. Zhao Z-Q, McGee DS, Nakanishi K, et al. Receptor-mediated cardioprotective effects of endogenous adenosine are exerted primarily during reperfusion after coronary occlusion in the rabbit. Circulation 1993;88:709-719.
68. Pearson JD, Carleton JS, Hutchings A, et al. Uptake and metabolism of adenosine by pig aortic endothelial and smooth-muscle cells in culture. Biochem J 1978;170:265-271.
69. Deussen A, Bading B, Kelm M, et al. Formation and salvage of adenosine by macrovascular endothelial cells. Am J Physiol 1993;264:H692-H700.
70. Smolenski RT, Kochan Z, McDouall R, et al. Endothelial nucleotide catabolism and adenosine production. Cardiovasc Res 1994;28:100-104.
71. Deussen A, Möser G, Schrader J. Contribution of coronary endothelial cells to cardiac adenosine production. Pflug Archiv 1986;406:608-614.
72. Borst MM, Schrader J. Adenine nucleotide release from isolated perfused guinea pig hearts and extracellular formation of adenosine. Circ Res 1991;68:797-806.
73. van Waeg G, Van den Berghe G. Purine Catabolism in Polymorphonuclear Neutrophils: Phorbol myristate acetate-induced accumulation of adenosine owing to inactivation of extracellularly released adenosine deaminase. J Clin Invest 1991;87:305-312.
74. Kitakaze M, Hori M, Morioka T, et al. Attenuation of ecto-5'-nucleotidase activity and adenosine release in activated human polymorphonuclear leukocytes. Circ Res 1993;73:524-533.
75. Vinten-Johansen J, Hammon JW, Jr. Myocardial Protection During Cardiac Surgery. In: Utley J, Gravlee GP, eds. Cardiopulmonary Bypass: Principles and Practice. New York: Williams & Wilkins, 1993:155-206.
76. Vinten-Johansen J, Nakanishi K. Postcardioplegia acute cardiac dysfunction and reperfusion injury. [Review]. J Cardiothorac Vasc Anesth 1993;7:6-18.
77. Gayheart PA, Vinten-Johansen J, Johnston WE, et al. Oxygen requirements of the dyskinetic myocardial segment. Am J Physiol 1989;257:H1184-H1191.
78. Allen BS, Rosenkranz ER, Buckberg GD, et al. Studies of controlled reperfusion after ischemia. VII. High oxygen requirements of dyskinetic cardiac muscle. J Thorac Cardiovasc Surg 1986;92:543-552.
79. Buckberg GD. Myocardial protection: An overview. Semin Thorac Cardiovasc Surg 1993;5:98-106.
80. Galiñanes M, Chambers DJ, Hearse DJ. Should adenosine continue to be ignored as a cardioprotective agent in cardiac operations? J Thorac Cardiovasc Surg 1993;105:180-183.
81. Woolfson RG, Patel VC, Yellon DM. Pre-conditioning with adenosine leads to concentration-dependent infarct size reduction in the isolated rabbit heart. Cardiovasc Res 1996;31:148-151.
82. Jennings RB. Myocardial ischemia-observation, definitions, and speculations. J Mol Cell Cardiol 1970;1:345-349.

83. Thornton JD, Liu GS, Olsson RA, et al. Intravenous pretreatment with A_1-selective adenosine analogues protects the heart against infarction. Circulation 1992;85:659-665.
84. Randhawa MPS, Jr., Lasley RD, Mentzer, Jr. Adenosine and the stunned heart. J Card Surg 1993;8 (Suppl):332-337.
85. Friedrichs GS, Kilgore KS, Manley PJ, et al. Effects of heparin and *N*-Acetyl heparin on ischemia/reperfusion-induced alterations in myocardial function in the rabbit isolated heart. Circ Res 1994;75:701-710.
86. Hearse DJ, Stewart DA, Braimbridge MV. Cellular protection during myocardial ischemia. The development and characterization of a procedure for the induction of reversible ischemic arrest. Circulation 1976;54:193-202.
87. Schubert T, Vetter H, Owen P, et al. Adenosine cardioplegia: Adenosine versus potassium cardioplegia: Effects on cardiac arrest and postischemic recovery in the isolated rat heart. J Thorac Cardiovasc Surg 1989;98:1057-1065.
88. Thelin S, Hultman J, Ronquist G. Effects of adenosine infusion on the pig heart during normothermic ischemia and reperfusion. Scand J Thorac Cardiovasc Surg 1991;25:207-213.
89. de Jong JW, van der Meer P, van Loon H, et al. Adenosine as adjunct to potassium cardioplegia: Effect on function, energy metabolism, and electrophysiology. J Thorac Cardiovasc Surg 1990;100:445-454.
90. Galiñanes M, Hearse DJ. Exogenous adenosine accelerates recovery of cardiac function and improves coronary flow after long-term hypothermic storage and transplantation. J Thorac Cardiovasc Surg 1992;104:151-158.
91. Fremes SE, Zhang J, Furukawa RD, et al. Cardiopulmonary bypass, myocardial management, and support techniques. *Adenosine pretreatment for prolonged cardiac storage.* An evaluation with St. Thomas' Hospital and University of Wisconsin solutions. J Thorac Cardiovasc Surg 1995;110:293-301.
92. Bolling SF, Bies LE, Bove EL, et al. Augmenting intracellular adenosine improves myocardial recovery. J Thorac Cardiovasc Surg 1990;99:469-474.
93. Bolling SF, Bies LE, Bove EL. Effect of ATP synthesis promoters on postischemic myocardial recovery. J Surg Res 1990;49:205-211.
94. Ledingham S, Katayama O, Lachno D, et al. Beneficial effect of adenosine during reperfusion following prolonged cardioplegic arrest. Cardiovasc Res 1990;24:247-253.
95. Rosenkranz ER, Okamoto F, Buckberg GD, et al. Studies of controlled reperfusion after ischemia. II. Biochemical studies: failure of tissue adenosine triphosphate levels to predict recovery of contractile function after controlled reperfusion. J Thorac Cardiovasc Surg 1986;92:488-501.
96. Hohlfeld T, Hearse DJ, Yellon DM, et al. Adenosine-induced increase in myocardial ATP: Are there beneficial effects for the ischaemic myocardial? Bas Res Cardiol 1989;84:499-509.
97. Hudspeth DA, Nakanishi K, Vinten-Johansen J, et al. Adenosine in blood cardioplegia prevents postischemic dysfunction in ischemically injured hearts. Ann Thorac Surg 1994;58:1637-1644.
98. Nakanishi K, Zhao Z-Q, Vinten-Johansen J, et al. Coronary artery endothelial dysfunction after ischemia, blood cardioplegia, and reperfusion. Ann Thorac Surg 1994;58:191-199.
99. Dignan RJ, Dyke CM, Abd-Elfattah AS, et al. Coronary artery endothelial cell and smooth muscle dysfunction after global myocardial ischemia. Ann Thorac Surg 1992;53:311-317.
100. Sellke FW, Friedman M, Wang SY, et al. Adenosine and AICA-riboside fail to enhance microvascular endothelial preservation. Ann Thorac Surg 1994;58:200-206.
101. Nakanishi K, Zhao Z-Q, Vinten-Johansen J, et al. Blood cardioplegia enhanced with nitric oxide donor SPM-5185 counteracts postischemic endothelial and ventricular dysfunction. J Thorac Cardiovasc Surg 1995;109:1146-1154.
102. Sato H, Zhao Z-Q, McGee DS, et al. Supplemental L-arginine during cardioplegic arrest and reperfusion avoids regional postischemic injury. J Thorac Cardiovasc Surg 1995;110:302-314.
103. Bolling SF, Bies LE, Gallagher KP, et al. Enhanced myocardial protection with adenosine. Ann Thorac Surg 1989;47:809-815.

104. Gottlieb RA, Burleson KO, Kloner RA, et al. Reperfusion injury induces apoptosis in rabbit cardiomyocytes. J Clin Invest 1994;94:1621-1628.

In: Mentzer, R.M., Jr., Kitakaze, M., Downey, J.M., Hori, M, eds. Adenosine, Cardioprotection and Clinical Application. Kluwer Academic Publishers, Norwell, MA, USA, 1997.

III. CELLULAR MECHANISMS OF CARDIOPROTECTION IN ISCHEMIC PRECONDITIONING

6. Protein Kinase C - the Key-Enzyme in Ischemic Preconditioning?

Christof Weinbrenner
James M. Downey

Introduction

Ischemic preconditioning of the heart is a phenomenon whereby one or more brief episodes of ischemia render the heart more resistant to injury from a subsequent longer ischemic insult. Preconditioning was originally described a decade ago as a protective intervention that reduced the area of necrosis from a standardized ischemic insult.[1] Subsequently numerous studies have shown that preconditioning can also provide protection against other detrimental effects of ischemia, such as arrhythmia and possibly even postischemic contractile dysfunction as occurs in the stunned myocardium.[2,3] There is of course no proof that the mechanisms responsible for the protective effects against necrosis, recovery of function and arrhythmias are all the same. In fact current evidence would suggest that the anti-arrhythmic and the anti-infarct effects are accomplished by quite different pathways. Ischemic preconditioning against infarction has been confirmed in every animal model that has been studied and there is considerable evidence, albeit indirect, that ischemic preconditioning also occurs in man.[4] The actual mechanism of ischemic preconditioning has not yet been determined although considerable light has been shed on the signal transduction systems that are involved. Investigations in ischemic preconditioning have revealed that protection against infarction, at least in some species, is mediated through activation of protein kinase C (PKC), but it is not yet known how PKC is being activated nor what the final effector might be.[5,6]

The PKC-family

The phospholipid-dependent PKC family is a group of protein serine/threonine kinases originally identified in the brain.[7] Comparison of the amino acid sequence of these proteins has revealed that up to five regions of variable sequence (V1-V5) alternate with four highly conserved regions (C1-C4 as shown in Fig. 6-1). The amino-terminal regulatory domain of PKC is linked through the V3 hinge region to the carboxyl-terminal catalytic domain which effects the actual phosphorylation of a substrate.[8] The C1 region contains what is called the pseudosubstrate site because its sequence is similar to the unique amino acid sequence that the enzyme recognizes as substrate for phosphorylation. The catalytic domain binds tightly to this region and activity is thus inhibited. In addition the enzyme also has one or two Zn^{2+}-finger-like cysteine rich motifs which bind the physiological activators of PKC diacylglycerol (DAG) or their analogues e.g. the phorbol ester 12-myristate 13-acetate (PMA). The binding of an activator to the regulatory domain is thought to cause an allosteric change so that the pseudosubstrate region is displaced from the active site of the kinase, rendering the PKC catalytically active and allowing true substrate access to the catalytic domain.[9] The C2 region contains acidic amino acids residues that bind calcium (Ca^{2+}). Binding of Ca^{2+} to PKC is thought to expose a binding site for phosphatidylserine (PtdSer), a component of the inner leaflet of the plasma membrane. The C3 and C4 regions contain the catalytic domain, that transfers a phosphate from ATP to the protein substrate. Upon activation, PKC undergoes autophosphorylation at three separate sites.[10] The role of these autophosphorylation events in the activation and function

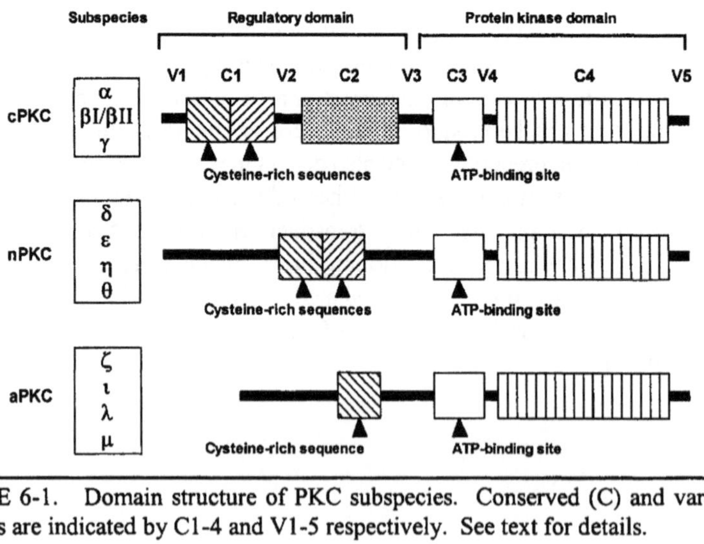

FIGURE 6-1. Domain structure of PKC subspecies. Conserved (C) and variable (V) domains are indicated by C1-4 and V1-5 respectively. See text for details.

of PKC has not been established, but they are thought to be required for PKC activity.[11,12] On the basis of their structures and biochemical properties the PKC family can be divided into three major subfamilies. The conventional PKCs (cPKC) comprising the α, β_I, β_{II} and γ isoforms are activated by PtdSer, Ca^{2+} and DAG (or PMA).[13-15] The members of the novel PKC subfamily (nPKC) comprising the δ, ϵ, η and θ isoforms lack the C2 region which is responsible for the Ca^{2+} binding of the enzyme.[16-18] Therefore the nPKCs require PtdSer and DAG (or PMA) for activation, but the requirement for Ca^{2+} as an activator has been lost. The atypical group (aPKC) comprising the ζ, ι, λ and μ isoforms, lack the C2 region and one of the two Zn^{2+}-finger-like Cysteine rich motifs in the C1 region.[19-22] Therefore aPKCs require only PtdSer for activation, they can neither be activated by Ca^{2+} nor by DAG (or PMA). Unsaturated fatty acids (especially arachidonic acid) are possible physiological activators for this third group.

Protein kinase C isoform diversity in the heart

PKC is present in the heart although concentrations of most isoforms are much lower than in the brain. Using immunoblot technique cPKCα, nPKCδ, nPKCϵ and aPKCζ can be detected in the rat heart (for references see Table 1). cPKCβ_I/β_{II} seems only to be present in the neonatal rat heart. cPKCγ cannot be found in the rat heart. The newly characterized PKC isoforms nPKCη, nPKCθ, aPKCι, aPKCλ and aPKCμ have yet to be demonstrated in the heart. This pattern of PKC expression in the heart that was found by immunoblotting and immunohistochemistry is in good agreement with that found by examining gene expression with northern blotting techniques.[23] The amounts of all expressed PKC isoforms dramatically decline postnatally.[24] Translocation of PKC from a cytosolic compartment to the membranes is thought to be a necessary step in activation[25] and has provided an important tool for monitoring in vivo activity of PKC. Cardiac substrates that can be phosphorylated by activated PKC in vitro may include troponin I and T,[26] myosin light chain 2,[27] adenylyl cyclase,[28] inhibitory G-protein,[29,30] the muscarinic receptor,[31] Ca^{2+}-pumps[32] and glycogen synthase.[33] In vivo phosphorylation of troponin[34] and the ATP dependent K^+-channel (causing it to open) may be induced by activation of PKC.[35] A highly specific substrate for PKC is the 80 kDa myristoylated alanine-rich C kinase substrate (MARCKS)[36] which has been used as an in vivo marker of PKC activation. But the physiological function of MARCKS in phosphorylation remains poorly understood. MARCKS can be phosphorylated by the members of the subfamilies cPKC and nPKC. aPKCζ however does not appear to phosphorylate the intact MARCKS protein.[37,38]

TABLE 6-1. Studies in the rat heart on the expression of PKC isoforms

Study	Preparation	Method	PKCα	PKCβ	PKCγ	PKCδ	PKCε	PKCζ	Other PKCs
Wetsel[101]	adult whole heart	IB	+	+	ND	+	ND	+	ND
		IF	+	+	-	+	+	+	ND
Gu[102]	postnatal whole heart	IB	+	+	-	+	+	+	ND
Bogoyevitch[84]	adult whole heart	IB	-	-	-	-	+	+	η
	adult myocytes		-	-	-	-	+	+	no η
Weinbrenner[85]	adult whole heart	IB	+	-	-	+	+	+	ND
Kohout[23]	neonatal myocytes adult myocytes	NB	+	-	-	+	+	+	η
Pucéat[103]	neonatal myocytes	IB	+	-	-	+	+	+	ND
	adult myocytes		+	-	-	+	+	(+)	ND
Disatnik[104]	neonatal myocytes	IF	+	+	ND	+	+	+	ND
Rybin[24]	neonatal whole heart		+	+	ND	+	+	+	ND
	adult whole heart	IB	(+)	+	ND	+	+	(+)	ND
	neonatal myocytes		+	(+)	ND	+	+	+	ND
	adult myocytes		-	-	ND	+	+	-	ND
Clerk[105]	postnatal ventricle	IB	(+)	(+)	ND	+	+	+	ND
	adult ventricle		(+)	-	ND	+	+	+	ND
Mitchell[80]	adult whole heart	IB	-	(+)	ND	+	+	+	ND

IF: immunofluorescence, IB: immunoblotting, NB: northern blotting

Activation of protein kinase C

PKC is activated upon external stimulation of the myocyte by various ligands including hormones, neurotransmitters and growth factors. These external signals activate phospholipases which induce the hydrolysis of membrane phospholipids, particularly the inositol containing species. Hydrolysis of phospholipids by removing the base and phosphate from position 3 produces sn-1,2diacylglycerol (Fig. 6-2). One isoform of phospholipase C (PLC-β) is coupled to some receptors through G-proteins[39] and generates DAG and inositol-1,4,5-triphosphate (IP_3) when its preferred substrate phosphatidylinositol 4,5 bisphosphate (PtdIns-4,$5P_2$) is hydrolyzed.[40,41] IP_3 mobilizes Ca^{2+} from intracellular stores[42] and along with the liberated DAG causes activation of both c and nPKCs. DAG can also be derived from phosphatidylcholine (PtdCho) by two pathways - a distinct isoform of PLC which can hydrolyze PtdCho and an indirect pathway involving sequential actions of phospholipase D (PLD). PLD produces phosphatidic acid (PtdOH) rather than DAG. The PtdOH is subsequently dephosporylated to DAG by a phospho-hydrolase (PPH). Thus PLD action generates not only PtdOH, a molecule with potential second messenger functions, but also the second messenger DAG which activates PKC. As PLD does not produce IP_3 and its subsequent calcium release PLD would be expected to more strongly activate the nPKCs while cPKCs would be better activated by PLC. PLD also appears to be a substrate for PKC. PMA causes activation of both PKC and PLD.[41] This PLD activation is inhibited by PKC inhibitors suggesting that PKC may be involved in PLD activation. The physiological significance of this regulation of PLD by PKC is not completely understood but the potential for an interesting positive-feedback control appears to

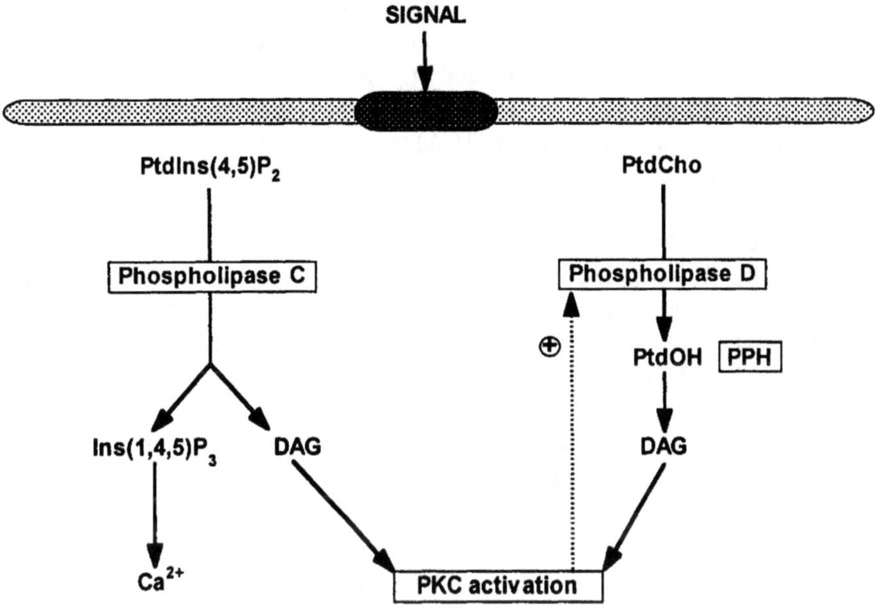

FIGURE 6-2. Potential pathway for the signal-induced degradation of membrane phospholipids by phospholipase C and phospholipase D. PtdIns(4,5)P_2: phosphatidylinositol 4,5-biphosphate, PtdCho: phosphatidylcholine, Ins(1,4,5)P_3: inositol 1,4,5-trisphosphate, DAG: diacylglycerol, Ca^{2+}: calcium, PtdOH: phosphatidic acid, PPH: phosphatidic acid phosphohydrolase, PKC: protein kinase C. Dashed line indicates the positive feedback effect of PKC on the activity of phospholipase D.

exist.[43] Recent evidence suggests that adenosine receptors couple to PKC via PLD and that this is an important pathway in preconditioning, at least in rabbit heart.[44]

Ischemic preconditioning

The basis for the phenomenon of ischemic preconditioning in the heart is that a short period of ischemia that does not lead to irreversible cell injury can paradoxically trigger an adaptive mechanism within the heart causing the heart to become resistant to infarction from a subsequent period of ischemia. The prerequisite for transition to a preconditioned state is a period of ischemia of at least 3 to 5 minutes followed by a minimum of at least one minute of reperfusion.[45] Protection wanes if the reflow is extended beyond one hour.[46] However in the rabbit protection can be renewed after 2 hours by a second cycle of brief coronary occlusion and reperfusion.[47] It appears that the threshold for protection is species dependent. In rabbits a single cycle of 5 minutes of ischemia appears to be as effective as multiple cycles[46,48] whereas in rats we found that three cycles of 5 minutes of ischemia were required to induce an anti-infarct effect.[49] Preconditioning appears to be induced in humans undergoing percutaneous transluminal coronary angioplasty (PTCA) with coronary occlusions only lasting 2 minutes.[50] Protection does not appear to be limited to the vascular bed subjected to a brief coronary occlusion. Przyklenk[51] found that myocardium was protected against infarction by a brief episode of ischemia in a distant vascular bed in the canine model. This implies, that humoral or mechanical factors act throughout the heart during a brief occlusion.Factors besides ischemia can put the heart into a preconditioned state. Ovize[52] showed in dogs that stretching the heart fibers with a volume overload mimicked preconditioning against infarction. He postulated the involvement of stretch-activated membrane channels because he could block protection by Gd^{3+}, a documented blocker of stretch-activated channels. But it is also known, that stretch of myocytes activates PKC.[53]

Non-ischemic or pharmacological preconditioning

The first indication that preconditioning utilizes signal transduction occurred when Liu et al.[54] showed that pretreatment of rabbits with an A_1-agonist or Adenosine can substitute for the preconditioning ischemia in the rabbit model. Conversely the ischemic preconditioning effect could be abolished by the non-selective adenosine antagonist 8-p-sulphophenyl theophylline. Since then a number of receptor agonists have been shown to mimic preconditioning. Tsuchida[55] preconditioned the rabbit heart with α_1-adrenergic agonists. Banerjee[56] simultaneously made the same observation in rat heart. Activation of Bradykinin B_2-receptors in both rabbits[57] and rats[58] also preconditioned as did activation of angiotensin II receptors in rabbits[59] and muscarinic receptors in dogs,[60] rabbits and rats.[61] The common factor of these receptor systems is that all activate PKC in the heart. Since a number of receptor systems converge on PKC in the heart it appears that the pathway for triggering protection is highly redundant as agonists for most of the above receptors are released to some degree during ischemia. There are, however, some species differences. Protection does not seem to involve Adenosine or A_1-agonists in the rat heart.[49,62,63] It has been proposed that protection in rats is mediated by an adrenergic mechanism,[56] but that conclusion is controversial as several investigators have failed to confirm an adrenergic role in the rat.[64,65] More recently Gross has found that opiate receptors may be the primary stimulus for preconditioning in rat heart.[66] Some cardiac opiate receptors are also PKC-coupled. Many of these receptors are coupled to PKC via an inhibitory G-protein. Therefore the hypothesis is that the inhibitory G-protein may be involved in ischemic preconditioning. Furthermore an increased responsiveness of the G_i protein after a brief period of ischemia and reperfusion was found.[67] However there is conflicting evidence as to wether treatment with pertussis toxin prevents preconditioning.[61,68-70] This is probably a result of species differences.

Preconditioning - involvement of protein kinase C?

In 1994 Ytrehus[5] found that either staurosporine, a non-specific inhibitor of PKC which blocks ATP-binding to the enzyme, or polymyxin B, an inhibitor which inhibits membrane-binding of PKC, could abolish the protection of ischemic preconditioning in the rabbit heart. Non-preconditioned hearts without drug or treated with staurosporine or polymyxin B all resulted in about 40% infarction of the risk zone after 30 minutes of regional ischemia. Preconditioning reduced infarct size to below 10% in the same model. Figure 6-3 reveals that staurosporine completely blocked preconditioning's protection. On the other hand, activation of PKC with PMA or with 1-oleyl-2acetyl glycerol (OAG) mimicked preconditioning in buffer perfused hearts subjected to 30 minutes regional ischemia. Infarct size in the PMA and OAG groups was only 6.4±1.4 and 11.7±3.3% (Fig. 6-3). Speechly-Dick[71] confirmed the results of Ytrehus in the rat heart. She could completely inhibit preconditioning by the PKC-inhibitor chelerythrine, a more specific PKC inhibitor than staurosporine. Also she could mimic preconditioning with 1,2-dioctanoyl-sn-glycerol (DOG), a DAG analogue. Hu[72] inhibited PKC activation by the PKC-inhibitors 1-(5-isoquinolinesulfonyl)-2-methylpiperazine and bisindolylmaleimide in rat hearts. Li[6] tested the more specific PKC-inhibitor calphostin C, an inhibitor which inhibits translocation of PKC in *in situ* rat hearts. He gave two doses of calphostin C as an intravenous bolus. One was given 5 minutes before preconditioning, another dose between preconditioning and the sustained 90 minutes of ischemia. Calphostin C completely blocked the effect of preconditioning on infarct size. Calphostin C also attenuated preconditioning's protection against ventricular tachycardia (VT) but did not completely block it. Simkhovich[73] showed, that acidotic preincubation of isolated perfused rabbit hearts improves the cardiac recovery of function after 30 minutes of global ischemia. Strasser[74] found that acidotic perfusion activated PKC in isolated rat hearts. The observation that acidosis can mimic preconditioning could therefore again be explained on the basis of activation of cardiac PKC. Acidotic activation of PKC could have a physiologic significance in preconditioning since transient acidosis occurs during a brief coronary occlusion.

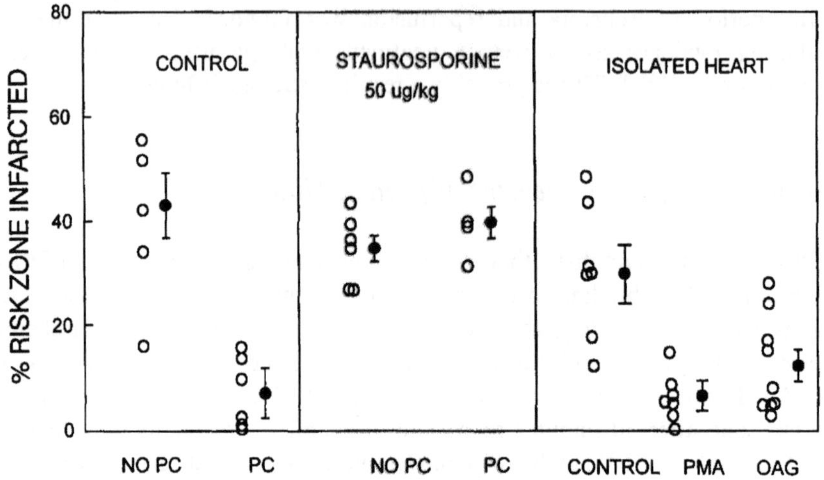

FIGURE 6-3. Percentage infarction of the risk zone for 4 in vivo experimental groups. Control hearts did not receive any drug. Staurosporine (50 mg/kg) was given 5 min before the prolonged regional ischemia. There was no significant difference between PC and no PC hearts with staurosporine indicating that protection from preconditioning had been blocked. Isolated perfused control hearts were subjected to 30 min regional ischemia without treatment. Preconditioned hearts experienced 5 min global ischemia followed by 10 min reperfusion. Treatment hearts received a 5 min exposer of OAG (50 nM) or PMA (0.05 nM) followed by a 10 min washout period before the onset of regional ischemia[5].

The translocation hypothesis of preconditioning

One of the most vexing questions concerning preconditioning is: What is preconditioning's memory? The simplest mechanism would be for PKC to phosphorylate a substrate during the preconditioning period and as long as that protein was phosphorylated the heart would be in a protected state. Unfortunately laboratory observations strongly argue against that phosphorylation theory. When staurosporine was introduced after the 5 minute preconditioning ischemia but before the 30 minutes of sustained ischemia protection was blocked.[5] Conversely, when staurosporine was only present during the preconditioning ischemia hearts continued to be protected.[75] These results indicate that kinase activity is not required during the preconditioning period in order to realize protection. But rather, PKC's kinase activity is essential only during the prolonged ischemia for the protective effect. Liu and Downey[75] proposed that translocation of PKC might account for this interesting behavior. In their theory they proposed that the delay associated with translocation prevents a virgin heart from being protected by its own PKC. If the PKC had been translocated to the membranes by a previous

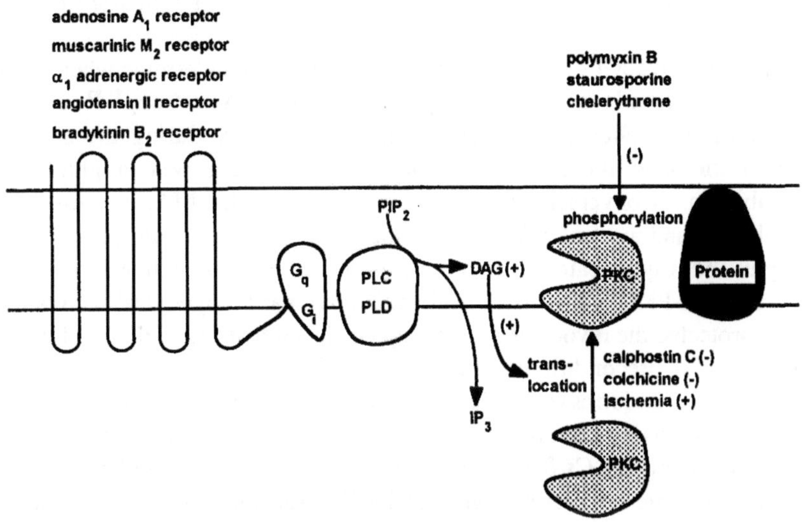

FIGURE 6-4. Activation of phospholipase C (PLC) (via a G protein) or phospholipase D results in the formation of sn-1,2-diacylglycerol (DAG) and the translocation of protein kinase C (PKC) to the membrane where it is subsequently activated. PKC then phosphorylates a membrane protein that may be linked to the ATP-dependent K^+-channel. IP_3: inositol 1,4,5-trisphosphate, PIP_2: phosphatidylinositol 4,5-bisphosphate.

ischemic event, however, then PKC could be quickly reactivated on a subsequent ischemia and protect the heart. Liu et al.[75] could also block preconditioning's protection with colchicine in rabbits. Colchicine disrupts microtubules and thereby inhibits translocation of PKC, a necessary step in its activation. The colchicine data therefore supported the translocation hypothesis. The translocation hypothesis states that the only difference between a preconditioned and non-preconditioned heart is that the former has PKC translocated into the membranes (Fig. 6-4). When the PKC reverts to the cytosol, protection will have waned. The evidence for the translocation hypothesis is, at present, only circumstantial. Furthermore attempts to directly test it to date have been controversial.[76-80] The translocation theory could not be supported by the findings of Armstrong et al.[78] Using western blot analysis they found no translocation of the PKC-isozymes a, ϵ and ζ after preconditioning either with 100 μM adenosine or with 10 minutes of ischemia. Contrary to this finding Henry et al.[79] reported a significant translocation of PKC-δ in rat myocytes after incubation with 100 μM adenosine. Mitchell et al.[80] (see below) also found, that preconditioning stimuli caused translocation of δ- and ϵ-isoforms.

Which isoforms are responsible for preconditioning's protection?

Isolated rabbit myocytes can also be preconditioned. To determine whether PKC in the myocyte plays a role in preconditioning, Armstrong[81,82] used the PKC-inhibitor calphostin C. Calphostin C added only during the simulated ischemia inhibited the protection from preconditioning with a glucose-free preincubation. Conversely direct PKC activation with PMA, a non-selective phorbol ester, and ingenol, a δ-, ϵ-PKC isozyme selective activator, protected the myocytes, but thymeleatoxin, an α-, β-, γ-PKC isozyme selective activator, did not.[83] Since ϵ-PKC is the major isoform in adult cardiomyocytes[84] and because ingenol protected the myocytes Armstrong concluded that the ϵ-PKC isoform was responsible for preconditioning the isolated rabbit cardiomyocytes. Mitchell[80] monitored PKC-isoforms (α, β_I, β_{II}, γ, δ, ϵ, ζ, η) during ischemic preconditioning in rat hearts by using immunofluorescent microscopy. He demonstrated that the Ca^{2+}-independent nPKCs δ and ϵ translocate with ischemic stimulation. PKC-δ translocated to the sarcolemma whereas PKC-ϵ translocated mostly into cardiac myocyte nuclei. Similarly, direct α_1-adrenergic receptor stimulation by phenylephrine which could mimic ischemic preconditioning in rat hearts also translocated PKC-δ to the sarcolemma and sporadically translocated the aPKC isoform ζ into cardiac myocyte nuclei. In contrast phenylephrine did not mobilize perinuclear ϵ-PKC. He also detected the cPKCs α and β_I as well as the nPKC-η, however, these isoforms did not show translocation either with ischemic preconditioning or with phenylephrine. Therefore he concluded that the PKC-δ, rather than the ϵ isoform, was responsible for preconditioning in the heart. Brew from the same group as Mitchell[58] addressed the role of PKC activation in bradykinin-mediated cardioprotection in isolated rat hearts. Recovery of the developed pressure after global ischemia-reperfusion was improved in hearts treated with bradykinin by an amount similar to that with ischemic preconditioning. Bradykinin-mediated preconditioning was eliminated with either the B_2-receptor antagonist (D-Arg[Hyp^3-Thi^{5,8}-D-Phe^7]Bk) or the PKC-inhibitor chelerythrine. Immunofluorescence staining again revealed translocation of the PKC-δ isoform into both cellular and perinuclear membranes of bradykinin treated hearts. PKC-ϵ also showed some sarcolemmal translocation, and the PKC-ζ isoform was predominantly concentrated in the intranuclear region in those hearts. These data are consistent with the observation that after only 2.5 minutes of acute myocardial ischemia the α, δ, ϵ and ζ-isoforms of PKC translocate to the particulate fraction as shown by immunoblotting.[85] Taken together activation of PKC appears to be a critical step in the process of ischemic preconditioning and the δ- or/and ϵ-PKC seem to be the major isoforms involved.

The PKC hypothesis has not been confirmed in all species

There is also some evidence that in the canine or the porcine models PKC may not be involved in ischemic preconditioning. Przyklenk et al.[76] showed that H-7 and polymyxin B, both PKC inhibitors fail to blunt the reduction in infarct size achieved with ischemic preconditioning. Also neither fluorescence staining with a bisindolylmaleimide PKC inhibitor (fim) nor biochemical quantification with a PKC enzyme assay system (Amersham) revealed evidence of preconditioning-induced translocation of PKC to the cell membrane. There are some limitations in the Przyklenk et al. study as mentioned by the author herself. First H-7 and polymyxin B are both non-selective inhibitors of PKC. For inhibition of PKC in vivo higher concentrations of the inhibitors than were used may have been required. Due to side effects like reduced mean arterial pressure and bradycardia the doses had to be limited. Because polymyxin B decreased coronary blood flow, hemodynamic alterations could have masked any direct effect of these PKC inhibitors to abolish the effect of ischemic preconditioning. It is quite possible that a single PKC isoform is responsible for the protection. The assay systems that were used were not selective for the different PKC isoforms. Furthermore, most activity assays can easily detect the cPKCs. However, they are not very sensitive for n and aPKCs. As mentioned before, it is likely that one or more of the PKC-isoforms δ, ϵ and ζ are the important ones. Thus it is not resolved whether PKC is simply not important in the dog or whether technical problems have prevented a clear demonstration of its involvement. Finally one group has recently reported that PKC inhibitors can block preconditioning's protection against infarction in the dog model.[86] Vogt[77] used a model of intramyocardial microinfusion in pigs. The infusion of the specific A_1-receptor agonist cyclohexyladenosine (CHA) achieved a local protection of the ischemic myocardium against ischemic damage. Biopsies taken from this tissue showed no PKC-translocation from the cytosol to the membranous fraction. So he concluded that preconditioning induced by A_1-receptor stimulation does not involve an activation of PKC in the porcine heart in vivo. However, the same group[87] reported in isolated pig myocytes a preconditioning effect at 30 and 60 minutes anoxia after PMA treatment. Therefore it cannot be excluded that in pigs, too, preconditioning is mediated through PKC. There are also practical difficulties with PKC activation studies. Activation of PKC in coronary arteries causes constriction and in leukocytes and mast cells it causes degranulation, all of which tend to exacerbate ischemia and could easily mask the protective effect of PKC activation in the cardiomyocyte. PKC activation of the whole heart is profoundly proarrhythmic rather than antiarrhythmic.[88] In the myocyte activation of PKC results in sensitization of adenylyl cyclase[89] which could increase cAMP and the promotion of ventricular arrhythmias, stimulate the Na^+H^+-exchanger which would lead to activation of the sodium-calcium-exchanger and to calcium overload. However, phorbol esters result in the translocation and activation of a wide variety of PKC isoenzymes. If PKC activation is a key step in ischemic preconditioning, then it probably involves the selective activation of one particular isoenzyme and only in the cardiomyocyte.

K_{ATP}-channels as the end-effectors of preconditioning - is it compatible with the PKC-hypothesis?

Kirsch[90] found that occupancy of A_1 adenosine receptors caused ATP-sensitive potassium-channels (K_{ATP}) to open in rat myocytes. Therefore it was proposed that K_{ATP}-channels might be involved in ischemic preconditioning because preconditioning appears to be triggered by activation of adenosine receptors. Gross and Auchampach[91] found that the K_{ATP}-channel blocker glibenclamide completely abolished the protective effect of ischemic preconditioning. Inversely RP 52891, a selective K_{ATP}-channel opener, produced a significant reduction in infarct size. Again, however, species differences were seen. Thornton[92] found that glibenclamide did not block the protection afforded by preconditioning nor did the K_{ATP}-opener pinacidil mimic preconditioning in the pentobarbital anaesthetized rabbit. But in the ketamine-xylazine anaesthetized rabbit these agents did perform as in the dog.[93,94] Armstrong et al.[95] showed in isolated rabbit cardiomyocytes that glibenclamide abolished the protective effect of ischemic preconditioning. Moreover the protection mimicked by preincubation with the K_{ATP}-channel opener pinacidil could be completely abolished by the PKC inhibitors chelerythrine and calphostin C. Interestingly pinacidil added only into the ischemic pellet resulted in no protection. The conclusion of the authors was that ischemically preconditioned cells do not require opened K_{ATP}-channels for protection although they appear to only be important during initiation of the preconditioned state. In the rat K_{ATP}-channels are clearly not involved in the protection.[96] Today there is certainly convincing evidence that these channels are involved in the protection of preconditioning, but their exact role is not clear. It is not proven yet if K_{ATP}-channels are the end-effector of preconditioning nor if the channels are phosphorylated following the activation of PKC. One possible scenario that we find attractive is that adenosine receptor activation opens K_{ATP}-channels by a direct coupling mechanism but only if the channel or one of ist associated control proteins has first been phosphorylated by PKC. Liu et al.[97] recently found evidence in support of this hypothesis.

Preconditioning in man - involvement of protein kinase C?

Deutsch et al.[50] showed that during PTCA a second occlusion was characterized by less subjective anginal discomfort, less ST-segment shift and lower mean pulmonary artery pressure. They concluded that these changes reflected preconditioning during the first inflation. Tomai[98] found during PTCA in humans that the preconditioning-effect described by Deutsch is completely abolished by pretreatment with glibenclamide. Therefore K_{ATP}-channels may also be involved in the process of ischemic preconditioning in humans. Yellon[99] found during coronary artery bypass surgery that ventricular ATP concentrations were preserved in preconditioned hearts during aortic cross clamping. In human right atrial trabeculae, Speechly-Dick from the same group[35] found that several minutes of hypoxia plus pacing caused improved recovery of contractile function following a prolonged hypoxic insult. This preconditioning-effect could be blocked by the K_{ATP}-blocker glibenclamide and also by the PKC antagonist chelerythrine. The K_{ATP}-channel opener cromakalim and the PKC activator DOG could mimic the protective effect of ischemic preconditioning. This was the first study in human heart tissue that showed the involvement of PKC in ischemic preconditioning. Ikonimedis et al. also showed a similar involvement of PKC in isolated human ventriculocytes.[100] Thus it would appear that the animal models are representative of the human heart with regards to preconditioning and its mechanism.

Concluding comments

Many lines of evidence indicate that PKC is involved in ischemic preconditioning of the heart. The exact role played by PKC has yet to be elucidated. There is also controversy about the different PKC-coupled receptor systems which might be involved in ischemic preconditioning. Much of this discrepancy can now be explained by species differences. Because the pathway for triggering preconditioning appears to be very redundant at the receptor level it is not surprising that differing pathways will be predominant in different species. Another intriguing question is which membrane-bound protein is phosphorylated by PKC during the preconditioning and why is it so protective in its phosphorylated state. The best candidate for this end-effector seems to be the K_{ATP}-channel, but other mechanisms cannot be ruled out at this time. Before we can learn much more about how PKC acts to control the protective state of the myocyte it will probably be necessary to develop PKC isoform-specific activators and inhibitors since it is likely that only one PKC isoform is involved in the process.

Acknowledgment

Christof Weinbrenner is sponsored by a grant of the Deutsche Forschungsgemeinschaft (We 1955/1-1).

References

1. Murry CE, Jennings RB, Reimer KA. Preconditioning with ischemia: a delay of lethal cell injury in ischemic myocardium. Circulation 1986;74:1124-1136.
2. Lasley RD, Anderson GM, Mentzer RM. Ischemic and hypoxic preconditioning enhance postischemic recovery of function in the rat heart. Cardiovasc Res 1993;27:565-570.
3. Lawson CS, Coltart DJ, Hearse DJ. "Dose"-dependency and temporal characteristics of protection by ischaemic preconditioning against ischaemia-induced arrhythmias in rat hearts. J Mol Cell Cardiol 1993;25:1391-1402.
4. Lawson CS. Does ischemic preconditioning occur in the human heart. Cardiovasc Res 1994;28:1461-1466.
5. Ytrehus K, Liu Y, Downey JM. Preconditioning protects ischemic rabbit heart by protein kinase C activation. Am J Physiol 1994;266:H1145-H1152.
6. Li Y, Kloner RA. Does protein kinase C play a role in ischemic preconditioning in rat heart? Am J Physiol 1995;268:H426-H431.
7. Nishizuka Y. Studies and perspectives of protein kinase C. Science 1986;233:305-312.
8. Stabel S, Parker PJ. Protein kinase C. Pharmac Ther 1991;51:71-95.
9. Pears C, Parker PJ. Domain interactions in protein kinase C. J Cell Sci 1992;100:683-686.
10. Flint AJ, Paladini RD, Koshland DEJ. Autophosphorylation of protein kinase C at three separated regions of its primary sequence. Science 1990;249:408-411.
11. Mitchell FE, Marais RM, Parker PJ. The phosphorylation of protein kinase C as a potential measure of activation. Biochem J 1989;261:131-136.
12. Cazaubon SM, Parker PJ. Identification of the phosphorylated region responsible for the permissive activation of protein kinase C. J Biol Chem 1993;268:17559-17563.
13. Marais RM, Parker PJ. Purification and characterisation of bovine brain protein kinase C isotypes alpha, beta and gamma. Eur J Biochem 1989;182:129-137.
14. Ono Y, Fujii T, Igarashi K, et al. Nucleotide sequences of cDNAs for alpha and gamma subspecies of rat protein kinase C. Nucl Acids Res 1988;16:5199-5200.
15. Blobe GC, Khan WA, Halpern AE, et al. Selective regulation of expression of protein kinase C b isoenzymes occurs via alternative splicing. J Biol Chem 1993;268:10627-10635.
16. Ono Y, Fujii T, Ogita K, et al. Identification of three additional members of rat protein kinase C family: delta, epsilon and zeta subspecies. FEBS Lett 1987;226:125-128.
17. Bacher N, Zisman Y, Berent E, et al. Isolation and characterization of PKC-L, a new member of the protein kinase C-related gene family specifically expressed in lung, skin, and heart. Mol Cell Biol 1991;11:126-133.
18. Osada S, Mizuno K, Saido TC, et al. A new member of the protein kinase C family, nPKC-teta, predominantly expressed in skeletal muscle. Mol Cell Biol 1992;12:3930-3938.
19. Ono Y, Fujii T, Ogita K,et al. Protein kinase C-zeta subspecies from rat brain: Its structure, expression and properties. Proc Natl Acad Sci U S A 1989;86:3099-3103.
20. Johannes FJ, Prestle J, Eis S,et al. PKC-m is a novel, atypical member of the protein kinase C family. J Biol Chem 1994;269:6140-6148.
21. Selbie LA, Schmitz Peiffer C, Sheng Y,et al. Molecular cloning and characterization of PKC-iota, an atypical isoform of protein kinase C derived from insulin-secreting cells. J Biol Chem 1993;268:24296-24302.

22. Akimoto K, Mizuno K, Osada S, et al. A new member of the third class in the protein kinase C family, PKC lambda, expressed dominantly in an undifferentiated mouse embryonal carcinoma cell line and also in many tissues and cells. J Biol Chem 1994;269:12677-12683.
23. Kohout TA, Rogers TB. Use of a PCR-based method to characterize protein kinase C isoform expression in cardiac cells. Am J Physiol 1993;264:C1350-C1359.
24. Rybin VO, Steinberg SF. Protein kinase C isoform expression and regulation in the developing rat heart. Circ Res 1994;74:299-309.
25. Kraft AS, Anderson WB. Phorbol esters increase the amount of Ca^{2+}, phospholipid-dependent protein kinase associated with plasma membrane. Nature 1983;301:621-623.
26. Noland TAJ, Kuo JF. Protein kinase C phosphorylation of cardiac troponin I and troponin T inhibits Ca^{2+}-stimulated MgATPase activity in reconstituted actomyosin and isolated myofibrils, and decreases actin-myosin interactions. J Mol Cell Cardiol 1993;25:53-65.
27. Noland TAJ, Kuo JF. Phosphorylation of cardiac myosin light chain 2 by protein kinase C and myosin light chain kinase increases Ca^{2+}- stimulated actomyosin MgATPase activity. Biochem Biophys Res Commun 1993;193:254-260.
28. Kawabe J, Iwami G, Ebina T, et al. Differential activation of adenylyl cyclase by protein kinase C isoenzymes. J Biol Chem 1994;269:16554-16558.
29. Katada T, Gilman AG, Watanabe Y, et al. Protein kinase C phosphorylates the inhibitory guanine-nucleotide-binding regulatory component and apparently suppresses its function in hormonal inhibition of adenylate cyclase. Eur J Biochem 1985;151:431-437.
30. Yatomi Y, Arata Y, Tada S, et al. Phosphorylation of the inhibitory guanine-nucleotide-binding protein as a possible mechanism of inhibition by protein kinase C of agonist-induced Ca^{2+} mobilization in human platelet. Eur J Biochem 1992;205:1003-1009.
31. Richardson RM, Ptasienski J, Hosey MM. Functional effects of protein kinase C-mediated phosphorylation of chick heart muscarinic cholinergic receptors. J Biol Chem 1992;267:10127-10132.
32. Qu Y, Torchia J, Sen AK. Protein kinase C mediated activation and phosphorylation of Ca^{2+}-pump in cardiac sarcolemma. Can J Physiol Pharmacol 1992;70:1230-1235.
33. Grekinis D, Reimann EM, Schlender KK. Phosphorylation and inactivation of rat heart glycogen synthase by cAMP-dependent and cAMP-independent protein kinases. Int J Biochem Cell Biol 1995;27:565-573.
34. Liu JD, Wood JG, Raynor RL, et al. Subcellular distribution and immunocytochemical localization of protein kinase C in myocardium, and phosphorylation of troponin in isolated myocytes stimulated by isoproterenol or phorbol ester. Biochem Biophys Res Commun 1989;162:1105-1110.
35. Speechly-Dick ME, Grover GJ, Yellon DM. Does ischemic preconditioning in the human involve protein kinase C and the ATP-dependent K^+ channel? Studies of contractile function after simulated ischemia in an atrial in vitro model. Circ Res 1995;77:1030-1035.
36. Stumpo DJ, Graff JM, Albert KA, et al. Molecular cloning, characterization, and expression of cDNA encoding the "80- to 87-kDa" myristoylated alanine-rich kinase substrate: a major cellular substrate for protein kinase C. Proc Natl Acad Sci U S A 1989;86:4012-4016.
37. Herget T, Oehrlein SA, Pappin DJC, et al. The myristoylated alanine-rich C-kinase substrate (MARCKS) is sequentially phosphorylated by conventional, novel and atypical isotypes of protein kinase C. Eur J Biochem 1995;233:448-457.
38. Nishizuka Y. The molecular heterogeneity of protein kinase C and its implications for cellular regulation. Nature 1988;334:661-665.
39. Cockcroft S, Geny B, Thomas GM. Regulation of cytosolic phosphoinositide-phospholipase C by G- protein, G_p. Biochem Soc Trans 1991;19:299-302.
40. Lamers JM, Dekkers DH, Bezstarosti K, Meij JT, van Heugten HA. Occurrence and functions of the phosphatidylinositol cycle in the myocardium. Mol Cell Biochem 1992;116:59-67.
41. Billah MM, Anthes JC. The regulation and cellular functions of phosphatidylcholine hydrolysis. Biochem J 1990;269:281-291.
42. Berridge MJ. Inositol triphosphate and calcium signalling. Nature 1993;361:315-325.

43. Conricode KM, Smith JL, Burns DJ, Exton JH. Phospholipase D activation in fibroblast membranes by the alpha and beta isoforms of protein kinase C. FEBS Lett 1994;342:149-153.
44. Liu Y, Cordis GA, Das DK, Downey JM, Cohen MV. Protein kinase C may be activated by phospholipase D rather than C in ischemic preconditioning. J Mol Cell Cardiol 1995;27:A41 (abstract).
45. Alkhulaifi AM, Pugsley WB, Yellon DM. The influence of the time period between preconditioning ischemia and prolonged ischemia on myocardial protection. Cardioscience 1993;4:163-169.
46. Lawson CS, Downey JM. Preconditioning: state of the art myocardial protection. Cardiovasc Res 1993;27:542-550.
47. Yang XM, Arnoult S, Tsuchida A, Cope D, Thornton JD, Daly JF, Cohen MV, Downey JM. The protection of ischemic preconditioning can be reinstated in the rabbit heart after the initial protection has waned. Cardiovasc Res 1993;27:556-558.
48. Miura T, Iimura O. Infarct size limitation by preconditioning: it's phenomenological features and the key role of adenosine. Cardiovasc Res 1993;27:36-42.
49. Liu Y, Downey JM. Ischemic preconditioning protects against infarction in rat heart. Am J Physiol 1992;263:H1107-H1112.
50. Deutsch E, Berger M, Kussmaul WG, et al. Adaption to ischemia during percutaneous transluminal coronary angioplasty. Clinical, hemodynamic, and metabolic features. Circulation 1990;82:2044-2051.
51. Przyklenk K, Bauer B, Ovize M, et al. Regional ischemic 'preconditioning' protects remote virgin myocardium from subsequent sustained coronary occlusion. Circulation 1993;87:893-899.
52. Ovize M, Kloner RA, Przyklenk K. Stretch preconditions canine myocardium. Am J Physiol 1994;266:H137-H146.
53. Yazaki Y, Komuro I, Yamazaki T, et al. Role of protein kinase system in the signal transduction of stretch-mediated protooncogene expression and hypertrophy of cardiac myocytes. Mol Cell Biochem 1993;119:11-16.
54. Liu GS, Thornton JD, Van-Winkle DM, et al. Protection against infarction afforded by preconditioning is mediated by A_1 adenosine receptors in rabbit heart. Circulation 1991;84:350-356.
55. Tsuchida A, Liu Y, Liu GS, et al. α_1-adrenergic agonists precondition rabbit ischemic myocardium independent of Adenosine by direct activation of protein kinase C. Circ Res 1994;75:576-585.
56. Banerjee A, Locke-Winter C, Rogers KB, et al. Preconditioning against myocardial dysfunction after ischemia and reperfusion by an α_1-adrenergic mechanism. Circ Res 1993;73:656-670.
57. Goto M, Liu YG, Yang XM, et al. Role of Bradykinin in protection of ischemic preconditioning in rabbit hearts. Circ Res 1995;77:611-621.
58. Brew EC, Mitchell MB, Rehring TF, et al. Role of bradykinin in cardiac functional protection after global ischemia-reperfusion in rat heart. Am J Physiol 1995;269:H1370-H1378.
59. Liu Y, Tsuchida A, Cohen MV, et al. Pretreatment with angiotensin II activates protein kinase C and limits myocardial infarction in isolated rabbit hearts. J Mol Cell Cardiol 1995;27:883-892.
60. Yao Z, Gross GJ. Acetylcholine mimics ischemic preconditioning via a glibenclamide-sensitive mechanism in dogs. Am J Physiol 1993;264:H2221-H2225.
61. Thornton JD, Liu GS, Downey JM. Pretreatment with pertussis toxin blocks the protective effects of preconditioning: evidence for a G-protein mechanism. J Mol Cell Cardiol 1993;25:311-320.
62. Ganote CE, Armstrong S, Downey JM. Adenosine and A_1 selective agonists offer minimal protection against ischaemic injury to isolated rat cardiomyocytes. Cardiovasc Res 1993;27:1670-1676.

63. Cave AC, Collis CS, Downey JM, et al. Improved functional recovery by ischaemic preconditioning is not mediated by adenosine in the globally ischaemic isolated rat heart. Cardiovasc Res 1993;27:663-668.
64. Asimakis GK, Inners-McBride K, Conti VR, et al. Transient beta adrenergic stimulation can precondition the rat heart against postischaemic contractile dysfunction. Cardiovasc Res 1994;28:1726-1734.
65. Weselcouch EO, Baird AJ, Sleph PG, et al. Endogenous catecholamines are not necessary for ischemic preconditioning in the isolated perfused rat heart. Cardiovasc Res 1995;29:126-132.
66. Schultz JEJ, Rose E, Yao Z, et al. Evidence for the involvement of opioid receptors in ischemic preconditioning in the rat heart. Am J Physiol 1995;268:H2157-H2161.
67. Niroomand F, Weinbrenner C, Weis A, et al. Impaired function of inhibitory G proteins during acute myocardial ischemia of canine hearts and its reversal during reperfusion and a second period of ischemia. Possible implications for the protective mechanism of ischemic preconditioning. Circ Res 1995;76:861-870.
68. Piacentini L, Wainwright CL, Parratt JR. The antiarrhythmic effect of ischaemic preconditioning in isolated rat heart involves a pertussis toxin sensitive mechanism. Cardiovasc Res 1993;27:674-680.
69. Lawson CS, Coltart DJ, Hearse DJ. The antiarrhythmic action of ischemic preconditioning in rat hearts does not involve functional G_i proteins. Cardiovasc Res 1993;27:681-687.
70. Liu Y, Downey JM. Preconditioning against infarction in the rat heart does not involve a pertussis toxin sensitive G protein. Cardiovasc Res 1993;27:608-611.
71. Speechly-Dick ME, Mocanu MM, Yellon DM. Protein kinase C: its role in ischemic preconditioning in the rat. Circ Res 1994;75:586-590.
72. Hu KL, Nattel S. Mechanisms of ischemic preconditioning in rat hearts. Involvement of a_{1b}-adrenoceptors, pertussis toxin-sensitive G proteins, and protein kinase C. Circulation 1995;92:2259-2265.
73. Simkhovich BZ, Whittaker P, Przyklenk K, et al. Transient pre-ischemic acidosis protects the isolated heart subjected to 30 minutes, but not 60 minutes, of global ischemia. Basic Res Cardiol 1995;90:397-403.
74. Strasser RH, Simonis G, Weinbrenner C, et al. Ischemia-induced activation of protein kinase C: Evidence for an acidose-dependent, but energy-independent mechanism. Circulation 1994;90:I-208 (abstract).
75. Liu Y, Ytrehus K, Downey JM. Evidence that translocation of protein kinase C is a key event during ischemic preconditioning of rabbit myocardium. J Mol Cell Cardiol 1994;26:661-668.
76. Przyklenk K, Sussman MA, Simkhovich BZ, et al. Does ischemic preconditioning trigger translocation of protein kinase C in the canine model? Circulation 1995;92:1546-1557.
77. Vogt A, Barancik M, Weihrauch D, et al. Protection of ischemic porcine myocardium from infarction by an A_1-receptor agonist is not mediated by protein kinase C. Circulation 1994;90:I-371 (abstract).
78. Armstrong SC, Hoover DB, DeLacey MH, et al. Translocation of PKC, protein phosphatase inhibition and in vitro preconditioning of rabbit myocytes. J Mol Cell Cardiol 1996; (abstract).
79. Henry P, Demolombe S, Puceat M, et al. Adenosine A_1 stimulation activates δ-protein kinase C in rat ventricular myocytes. Circ Res 1996;78:161-165.
80. Mitchell MB, Meng X, Ao L, et al. Preconditioning of isolated rat heart is mediated by protein kinase C. Circ Res 1995;76:73-81.
81. Armstrong S, Downey JM, Ganote CE. Preconditioning of isolated rabbit cardiomyocytes: induction by metabolic stress and blockade by the adenosine antagonist SPT and calphostin C, a protein kinase C inhibitor. Cardiovasc Res 1994;28:72-77.
82. Armstrong S, Ganote CE. In vitro ischaemic preconditioning of isolated rabbit cardiomyocytes: effects of selective adenosine receptor blockade and calphostin C. Cardiovasc Res 1995;29:647-652.
83. Armstrong S, Ganote CE. Preconditioning of isolated rabbit cardiomyocytes: effects of glycolytic blockade, phorbol esters, and ischaemia. Cardiovasc Res 1994;28:1700-1706.

84. Bogoyevitch MA, Parker PJ, Sugden PH. Characterization of protein kinase C isotype expression in adult rat heart. Protein kinase C-epsilon is a major isotype present, and it is activated by phorbol esters, epinephrine, and endothelin. Circ Res 1993;72:757-767.
85. Weinbrenner C, Simonis G, Marquetant R, et al. Selective regulation of calcium-dependent and calcium- independent subtypes of protein kinase C in acute and prolonged ischemia. Circulation 1993;88:I-101 (abstract).
86. Kitakaze M, Node K, Minamino T, et al. Role of activation of protein kinase C in the infarct size-limiting effect of ischemic preconditioning through activation of ecto-5'-nucleotidase. Circulation 1996;93:781-791.
87. Rennollet H, Barancik M, Westernacher D, et al. The preconditioning-effect of PKC-stimulation is dose-, time-, and species-dependent. Circulation 1994;90:I-371 (abstract).
88. Black SC, Fagbemi SO, Chi L, et al. Phorbol-ester-induced ventricular fibrillation in the Langendorff-perfused rabbit heart: antagonism by staurosporine and glibenclamide. J Mol Cell Cardiol 1993;25:1427-1438.
89. Strasser RH, Braun Dullaeus R, Walendzik H, et al. α_1-receptor-independent activation of protein kinase C in acute myocardial ischemia. Circ Res 1992;70:1304-1312.
90. Kirsch GE, Codina J, Birnbaumer L, et al. Coupling of ATP-sensitive K^+ channels to A_1-receptors by G-proteins in rat ventricular myocytes. Am J Physiol 1990;259:H820-H826.
91. Gross GJ, Auchampach JA. Blockade of ATP-sensitive potassium channels prevents myocardial preconditioning in dogs. Circ Res 1992;70:223-233.
92. Thornton JD, Thornton CS, Sterling DL, et al. Blockade of ATP-sensitive potassium channels increases infarct size but does not prevent preconditioning in rabbit hearts. Circ Res 1993;72:44-49.
93. Walsh RS, Tsuchida A, Daly JJF, et al. Ketamine-xylazine anaesthesia permits a K_{ATP} channel antagonist to attenuate preconditioning in rabbit myoardium. Cardiovasc Res 1994;28:1337-1341.
94. Toombs CF, McGee DS, Johnston WE, et al. Protection from ischemic-reperfusion injury with adenosine pretreatment is reversed by inhibition of ATP sensitive potassium channels. Cardiovasc Res 1993;27:623-629.
95. Armstrong SC, Liu GS, Downey JM, et al. Potassium channels and preconditioning of isolated rabbit cardiomyocytes: effects of glyburide and pinacidil. J Mol Cell Cardiol 1995;27:1765-1774.
96. Grover GJ, Dzwonczyk S, Sleph PG. ATP-sensitive K^+-channel activation does not mediate preconditioning in isolated rat hearts. Circulation 1992;86:I-341 (abstract).
97. Liu Y, Gao WD, O'Rourke B, et al. Synergistic modulation of ATP-sensitive K^+ currents by protein kinase C and adenosine. Implications for ischemic preconditioning. Circ Res 1996;78:443-454.
98. Tomai F, Crea F, Gaspardone A, et al. Ischemic preconditioning during coronary angioplasty is prevented by glibenclamide, a selective ATP-sensitive K^+ channel blocker. Circulation 1994;90:700-705.
99. Yellon DM, Alkhulaifi AM, Pugsley WB. Preconditioning the human myocardium. Lancet 1993;342:276-277.
100. Ikonomidis JS, Shirai T, Weisel RD, et al. "Ischemic" or adenosine preconditioning of human ventricular cardiomyocytes is protein kinase C dependent. Circulation 1995;92:I-12 (abstract).
101. Wetsel WC, Khan WA, Merchenthaler I, et al. Tissue and cellular distribution of the extended family of protein kinase C isoenzymes. J Cell Biol 1992;117:121-133.
102. Gu X, Bishop SP. Protein kinase isoenzyme expression in the developing rat heart and changes in expression in response to pressure overload hypertrophy. J Mol Cell Cardiol 1994;27:CLXVI (65) (abstract).
103. Puceat M, Hilal Dandan R, Strulovici B, et al. Differential regulation of protein kinase C isoforms in isolated neonatal and adult rat cardiomyocytes. J Biol Chem 1994;269:16938-16944.
104. Disatnik MH, Buraggi G, Mochly Rosen D. Localization of protein kinase C isoenzymes in cardiac myocytes. Exp Cell Res 1994;210:287-297.

105. Clerk A, Bogoyevitch MA, Fuller SJ, et al. Expression of protein kinase C isoforms during cardiac ventricular development. Am J Physiol 1995;269:H1087-H1097.

In: Mentzer, R.M., Jr., Kitakaze, M., Downey, J.M., Hori, M, eds. Adenosine, Cardioprotection and Clinical Application. Kluwer Academic Publishers, Norwell, MA, USA, 1997.

7. Adenosine Cardioprotection and Potential Mechanisms

Robert D. Lasley

Introduction

The purine nucleoside adenosine exerts numerous physiological effects in normal mammalian myocardium, including modulation of coronary blood flow and negative chronotropic, dromotropic, and anti-adrenergic properties. The cellular mechanisms of these effects have, for the most part, been well delineated.[1] In the last several years it has been established that adenosine also exerts effects in ischemic and reperfused myocardium. Infusion of adenosine prior to ischemia enhances postischemic ventricular function and reduces infarct size. Endogenous adenosine also appears to modulate myocardial ischemic and reperfusion injury. This review will summarize the beneficial effects of adenosine in reversibly and irreversibly injured myocardium and address potential mechanisms of action.

The administration of adenosine prior to ischemia delays the onset of ischemic contracture, improves postischemic left ventricular function and reduces infarct size.[2-4] These beneficial effects of adenosine have been observed in rats, rabbits, dogs, and pigs. Adenosine treatment is also associated with effects on metabolism during ischemia. Adenosine pretreatment reduces the rate of ATP decline during the initial minutes of ischemia, but this effect wanes after approximately 10 minutes of ischemia.[2,3] Exogenous adenosine increases postischemic myocardial phosphorylation potential in isolated guinea pig hearts[5] and in vivo porcine myocardium.[6] Phosphorylation potential determines the energy available from ATP hydrolysis that drives cellular energy-dependent processes, such as the sarcoplasmic reticulum (SR) Ca^{2+}-Mg^{2+} ATPase, the sarcolemmal Ca^{2+} ATPase, and the myofibrillar contractile apparatus (actomyosin ATPase). Adenosine induced increases in myocardial phosphorylation potential may reduce alterations in Ca^{2+} homeostasis and contractile proteins that are thought to play a role in myocardial stunning. The role of the adenosine-induced increase in phosphorylation potential in adenosine-mediated attenuation of myocardial stunning however remains to be determined.

Adenosine Receptors and Cardioprotection

Although the exact mechanism of adenosine-induced attenuation of post-ischemic ventricular dysfunction is not known, there is extensive evidence that it involves activation of cardiac myocyte membrane-bound adenosine A_1 receptors. This conclusion is based on observations that adenosine's cardioprotective effects are: 1) mimicked by relatively selective adenosine A_1 receptor agonists but not by A_2 receptor agonists,[2,7,8] 2) blocked by selective adenosine A_1 antagonists,[2,7,8] and 3) blocked by pertussis toxin, which ADP-ribosylates and inactivates inhibitory guanine nucleotide binding (G_i) proteins which couple to adenosine A_1 receptors.[9] The anti-stunning effect of adenosine appears to be mediated during ischemia since adenosine infusion during reperfusion does not attenuate myocardial stunning.[10,11]

Results obtained in isolated heart and in vivo preparations indicate that exogenous adenosine must be delivered in high doses to exert a cardioprotective effect. This is most likely due to the rapid metabolism of adenosine by red blood cells and endothelial cells which produces a large concentration gradient between intravascular and interstitial fluid (ISF) adenosine concentrations. Since cardiac myocyte adenosine A_1 receptors are bathed by ISF, elevations in ISF adenosine provide indirect evidence of increased adenosine A_1 receptor activation. Our laboratory modified the brain microdialysis technique to measure cardiac ISF adenosine and its metabolites.[12] Results obtained in the isolated rat heart with this technique support the hypothesis that exogenous adenosine must accumulate in the ISF prior to ischemia to exert its cardioprotective effect (Figure 7-1).

Preischemic treatment with 1 μM adenosine increased coronary effluent adenosine concentrations almost 10-fold (from 0.034 ± 0.005 to 0.31 ± 0.06 μM), but did not alter dialysate adenosine levels. Infusion of 10 μM adenosine increased effluent adenosine concentration to 7.2 ± 0.4 μM and dialysate adenosine levels from 0.22 ± 0.06 μM to 2.4 ± 0.3 μM. Consistent with these metabolic findings 1 and 10 μM adenosine exhibited similar increases in coronary flow (A_2 receptor activation), but only the 10 μM dose reduced spontaneous heart rate (A_1 receptor activation). After 30 minutes global ischemia and 30 minutes reperfusion hearts pretreated with 1 μM adenosine exhibited a similar recovery of preischemic function ($46 \pm 7\%$) as control hearts ($48 \pm 4\%$). In contrast hearts treated with 10 μM adenosine showed significantly improved postischemic function ($80 \pm 5\%$).

Exogenous adenosine also reduces irreversible ischemic injury, i.e. myocardial infarction.[4,13] This effect appears to be mediated via the activation of adenosine A_1 receptors, since it is mimicked by adenosine A_1, but not A_2 receptor

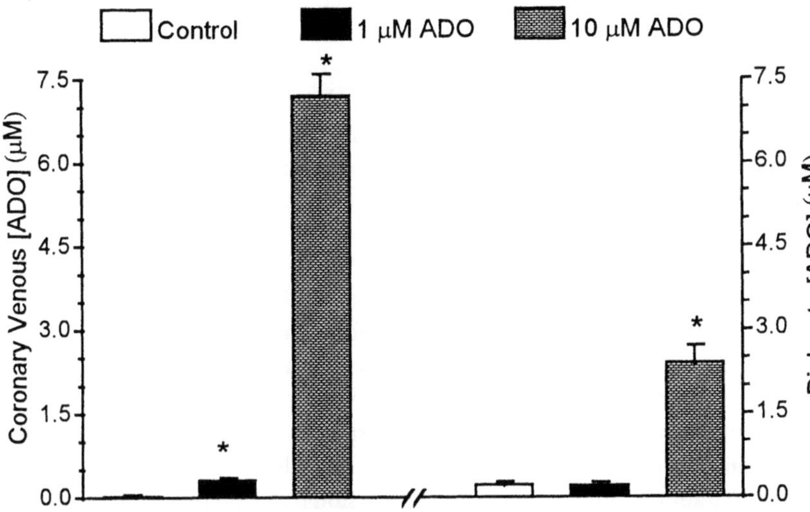

FIGURE 7-1. Effects of exogenous adenosine on coronary venous and dialysate adenosine concentrations in isolated rat hearts. Dialysis samples were collected from 8.0 mm fibers perfused at 0.75 μl/min. Samples were collected during a 10 minute treatment with either 1 or 10 μM adenosine immediately prior to 30 minutes global normothermic ischemia. * $p < 0.05$ vs. Control.

analogues[14,15] and blocked by DPCPX.[15] As with adenosine's anti-stunning effect, this protection appears to occur during ischemia, since the infusion of adenosine alone during reperfusion does not reduce infarct size.[16] There is however one major difference between the effects of adenosine in reversibly and irreversibly injured myocardium. A transient adenosine infusion that is terminated prior to ischemia (adenosine preconditioning) reduces infarct size[4,13] but does not attenuate postischemic dysfunction.[11,15] There is no clear explanation for these dissimilar effects of adenosine preconditioning on postischemic function and infarct size, but it may indicate that adenosine A_1 receptor activation reduces reversible and irreversible injury via different mechanisms.

Endogenous adenosine, which accumulates rapidly during ischemia-induced adenylate metabolism, also exerts beneficial effects in both stunned and irreversibly injured myocardium. Since adenosine itself is rapidly metabolized, these effects have been documented primarily by using agents which reduce adenosine metabolism directly or by blocking the nucleoside transporter. Treatment with adenosine deaminase inhibitors (erythro-9-[2-hydroxy-3-nonyl] adenine HCl (EHNA) or pentostatin) increases endogenous ISF adenosine and attenuates postischemic ventricular dysfunction.[17,18] Pretreatment with the nucleoside transport inhibitor draflazine (R75231) has also been reported to attenuate in vivo myocardial stunning.[19] Although it has been reported that pentostatin does not decrease infarct size in the dog,[20] recent findings in our laboratory indicate that R75231 decreases infarct size in the pig.[21] The cardioprotective effects of adenosine metabolism inhibitors have been presumed to be due to the augmentation of endogenous myocardial adenosine levels during ischemia. However since these agents also increase preischemic ISF adenosine, their beneficial effects may be due in part to activation of adenosine A_1 receptors prior to occlusion.

The exact role of endogenous adenosine during reperfusion in the irreversibly injured heart is not clear. In the aforementioned experiments in our laboratory, administration of the nucleoside transport inhibitor R75231 prior to reperfusion after a 60 minute occlusion in the pig increased both ISF and plasma adenosine but did not reduce infarct size.[21] Disparate results have been obtained with adenosine receptor antagonists, such as 8-p-sulfophenyl theophylline (8-SPT), as the administration of this agent during reperfusion has been reported to increase infarct size in some studies[22] but not in others.[23] The hypothesis that endogenous vascular adenosine may modulate infarct size during reperfusion is based on observations that adenosine A_2 receptors are located on coronary endothelial cells and neutrophils, and adenosine both inhibits neutrophil adherence to endothelium and neutrophil production of superoxide radicals.[24] Despite this solid theoretical basis for protection by vascular adenosine, the conflicting results on infarct size with reperfusion infusions of adenosine and adenosine antagonists indicate that the role of vascular adenosine and thus adenosine A_2 receptors in altering myocardial infarct size remains equivocal.

Adenosine and Ischemic Preconditioning

In addition to the well-documented beneficial effects of exogenous adenosine and adenosine A_1 receptor analogs in the ischemic reperfused heart, adenosine is thought to play a role in the cardioprotection induced by ischemic preconditioning. Ischemic preconditioning is the phenomenon whereby a brief period of myocardial ischemia and reperfusion reduces ischemic injury produced by a subsequent period of prolonged occlusion.[25] The hypothesis that adenosine plays a role in the infarct size reducing effect of ischemic preconditioning is supported by the observations that: 1) the brief preconditioning ischemia is associated with increased ISF adenosine accumulation, [4] suggesting that there is transient activation of adenosine A_1 receptors, 2) a transient infusion of adenosine and adenosine A receptor agonists can reduce infarct size,[4,13-15] and 3) adenosine receptor antagonists block the infarct size reducing effect of ischemic preconditioning.[14,26] Thus the evidence that adenosine participates in ischemic preconditioning is compelling.

The exact role of adenosine in this phenomenon however remains to be determined, since there are several differences between adenosine cardioprotection and ischemic preconditioning. A key difference between the two is that the selective adenosine A_1 receptor antagonist DPCPX blocks the cardioprotective effects of adenosine in rat and rabbit myocardium[3,15] but does not block ischemic preconditioning in either species.[15,27] It has been reported that DPCPX blocks ischemic preconditioning in the dog,[26] however it has also been shown that in the dog the window of protection (and the extent of infarct size reduction) are greater with ischemic preconditioning than with adenosine preconditioning.[13] In general, the extent of infarct size reduction with ischemic preconditioning is greater than that achieved with adenosine and long-acting adenosine A_1 receptor analogs. As shown in Figure 7-2, adenosine preconditioning and ischemic preconditioning in the rabbit are associated with similar increases in ISF adenosine (measured by microdialysis), but ischemic preconditioning produces a 40% smaller infarct size.[4] These results suggest that adenosine may play a modulatory role in ischemic preconditioning but other factors are also involved. For instance adenosine may potentiate the effect of some other metabolite or transmitter released during a brief occlusion.

Mechanism(s) of Adenosine Cardioprotection

As detailed above it appears that the cardioprotective effects of adenosine pretreatment and adenosine preconditioning are due to adenosine A_1 receptor activation. Adenosine also appears to play some role in ischemic preconditioning. However, other than the apparent involvement of a pertussis toxin-sensitive G_i protein[9] there is no consensus on adenosine's mechanism of action. The difficulty in determining the mechanism of adenosine cardioprotection is that in normal ventricular myocytes adenosine exerts no significant direct effects. Even under simulated ischemia conditions in cardiac myocytes adenosine does not exert the same degree of protection as it does in the whole heart or intact animal.[28] These observations suggest that adenosine cardioprotection may be mediated via adenosine receptor modulation of responses to other autocrine or paracrine factors that are released during ischemia and reperfusion.

Two signal transduction pathways that have been proposed to play a role in adenosine cardioprotection and ischemic preconditioning are the activation of ATP dependent K^+ (K_{ATP}) channels and stimulation of protein kinase C. Cellular studies indicate that adenosine can facilitate activation of ATP dependent K^+ channels in rat[29] and guinea pig ventricular myocytes[30] under conditions of low ATP and GTP. There are also reports that adenosine cardioprotection and ischemic preconditioning can be blocked with ATP dependent K^+ channel blockers such as

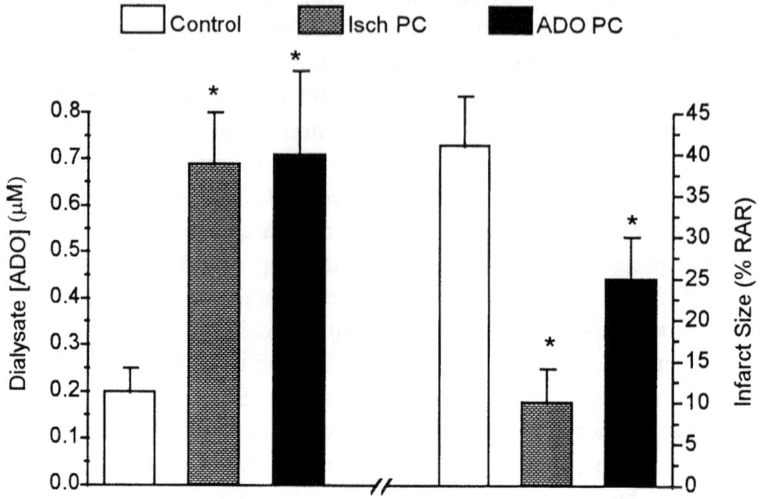

FIGURE 7-2. Comparison of the effects of adenosine preconditioning and ischemic preconditioning on dialysate (ISF) adenosine concentration and infarct size in the in situ rabbit. Hearts were preconditioned with 5 minutes intravenous adenosine (140 μg/kg/min) or 5 minutes ischemia followed by 10 minutes washout/reperfusion prior to 45 minutes coronary artery occlusion. Infarct size was determined by triphenyl tetrazolium chloride (TTC) staining after two hours reperfusion. * $p < 0.05$ vs. Control hearts.

glibenclamide.[7,26,31] However, there are several discrepancies between the documented effects of adenosine on K_{ATP} channel activity and the results of adenosine cardioprotection studies that need to be reconciled. The first report of adenosine A_1 receptor activation of K_{ATP} channels was in rat ventricular myocytes,[29] but it is thought that adenosine does not play a role in ischemic preconditioning in this species. Furthermore, Grover et al[8] recently reported that DPCPX, but not glibenclamide, blocked adenosine A_1 receptor-mediated cardioprotection in the rat. Xu et al[32] also reported that endogenous adenosine did not activate ventricular K_{ATP} channels during hypoxia in the intact guinea pig. Finally, the K_{ATP} channel blocker glibenclamide blocks ischemic preconditioning in ketamine/xylazine anesthetized rabbits, but not in pentobarbital anesthetized rabbits.[33]

Another signal transduction pathway that has been proposed to mediate adenosine cardioprotection is protein kinase C (PKC). Since adenosine appears to play some role in ischemic preconditioning, and there is pharmacological evidence that transient PKC activation prior to prolonged ischemia may mediate the infarct size reducing effect of ischemic preconditioning,[34,35] it has been proposed that adenosine A_1 receptor stimulation activates PKC. Although ischemic preconditioning can be mimicked by numerous agents that couple to phospholipase C and subsequently activate PKC, there is no evidence in mammalian myocardium that adenosine A_1 receptor effects are mediated by PKC activation. Henry et al[36] reported that treatment of rat ventricular myocytes with adenosine and the adenosine A_1 receptor analog phenylisopropyladenosine (PIA) was associated with a transient cytosol to membrane translocation of the δ-PKC isoform. The membrane translocation, however, peaked at 1 minute and then decreased back to basal levels within 5-10 minutes, despite the continued presence of adenosine or PIA. Since Mitchell et al[35] have reported that ischemic preconditioning in the isolated rat heart is also associated with the translocation of the δ-PKC isoform, these results would seem to indicate a role for adenosine activation of PKC in ischemic preconditioning.

Despite the above evidence suggesting a link between adenosine and PKC, there are several inconsistencies between these results and adenosine/ischemic preconditioning cardioprotection. First, the observations of Henry et al[36] were obtained in the rat, and there is widespread agreement that adenosine does not mediate ischemic preconditioning in the rat. Second, in the Henry et al.[36] study adenosine and PIA-induced PKC translocation were blocked by the selective adenosine A_1 receptor blocker DPCPX, but DPCPX does not block ischemic preconditioning in the rat or rabbit.[15,27] Third, although adenosine appears to play a role in ischemic preconditioning in the dog,[13,26] Przyklenk et al.[37] reported that ischemic preconditioning in the dog was not associated with PKC membrane translocation and could not be blocked by PKC inhibitors. Finally, we have reported that adenosine and the adenosine A_1 receptor agonist chlorocyclopentyladenosine (CCPA) significantly blunt the PKC dependent negative inotropic effects of phorbol esters and diacylglycerol analogs in the isolated rat heart.[38] As shown in Figure 7-3, CCPA also antagonizes the negative inotropic effect of PKC activation in the isolated rabbit heart.

Conclusion

In conclusion, there is significant experimental data that adenosine exerts a cardioprotective effect in reversibly and irreversibly injured myocardium. It appears that this effect is mediated with activation of adenosine A_1 receptors located on the cardiac myocytes resulting in a decrease in ischemic injury. Since the cardioprotective effect of adenosine is species-independent, one might expect its mechanism of action to also be species-independent. At the present time however there is no definitive information on adenosine receptor modulation of signal transduction in the ischemic reperfused heart. Therefore, it is obvious that

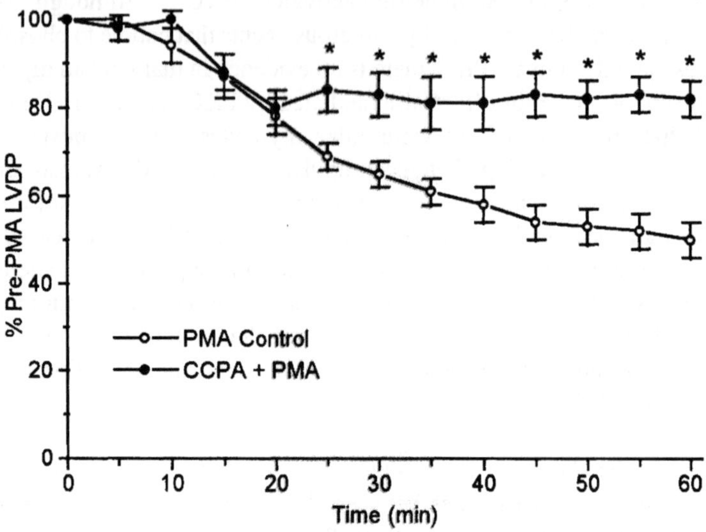

FIGURE 7-3. Adenosine A_1 receptor agonist blockade of the negative inotropic effect of the phorbol ester phorbol 12-myristate 13-acetate (PMA) in isolated rabbit hearts. Results are expressed (mean ± SEM) as percent of pre-PMA left ventricular developed pressure (LVDP). Paced and constant flow perfused hearts were exposed to 5 nM PMA for 30 minutes and then monitored for an additional 30 minutes. A second group was treated prior to and during the PMA infusion with the adenosine A_1 agonist 2-chlorocyclopentyladenosine (CCPA, 0.1 μM). * $p < 0.05$ vs Control PMA.

much work remains to be done in elucidating the mechanism of adenosine's cardioprotective effect.

References

1. Belardinelli L, Shryock JC, Song Y, Wang D, Srinivas M (1995) Ionic basis of the electrophysiological actions of adenosine on cardiomyocytes. FASEB Journal 9:359-365.
2. Lasley RD, Rhee JW, Van Wylen DGL, Mentzer RM (1990) Adenosine A_1 receptor mediated protection of the globally ischemic isolated rat heart. J Mol Cell Cardiol 22:39-47.
3. Lasley RD, Mentzer RM Jr (1992) Adenosine improves the recovery of postischemic myocardial function via an adenosine A_1 receptor mechanism. Am J Physiol 263:H1460-H1465.
4. Lasley RD, Konyn PJ, Hegge JO, Mentzer RM Jr (1995) The effects of ischemic and adenosine preconditioning on interstitial fluid adenosine and myocardial infarct size. Am J Physiol 269:H1460-H1466.
5. Mentzer RM Jr, Bünger R, Lasley RD (1993) Adenosine enhanced preservation of myocardial function and energetics. Possible involvement of the adenosine A_1 receptor system. Cardiovasc Res 27:28-35.

6. Zhou Z, Bünger R, Lasley RD, Hegge JO, Mentzer RM Jr (1993) Adenosine pretreatment increases cytosolic phosphorylation potential and attenuates postischemic cardiac dysfunction in swine. Surg Forum 44:249-252.
7. Yao Z, Gross GJ (1993) Glibenclamide antagonizes adenosine A1 receptor-mediated cardioprotection in stunned canine myocardium. Circulation 88:235-244.
8. Grover GJ, Baird AJ, Sleph PG (1996). Lack of a pharmacologic interaction between ATP-sensitive potassium channels and adenosine A(1) receptors in ischemic rat hearts. Cardiovasc Res 31:511-517.
9. Lasley RD, Mentzer RM Jr (1993): Pertussis toxin blocks adenosine A_1 receptor mediated protection of the ischemic rat heart. J Mol Cell Cardiol 25:815-821.
10. Randhawa MPS Jr, Lasley RD, Mentzer RM Jr (1995): Salutary effects of exogenous adenosine on canine myocardial stunning in vivo. J Thorac Cardiovasc Surg 110:63-74.
11. Sekili S, Jeroudi MO, Tang XL, Zughaib M, Sun JZ, Bolli R (1995) Effect of adenosine on myocardial 'stunning' in the dog. Circ Res 76:82-94.
12. Van Wylen DGL, Willis J, Sodhi J, Weiss RJ, Lasley RD, Mentzer RM (1990) Cardiac microdialysis to estimate interstitial adenosine and coronary blood flow. Am J Physiol 258:H1642-H1649.
13. Yao Z, Gross GJ (1994) A comparison of adenosine-induced cardioprotection and ischemic preconditioning in dogs. Efficacy, time course, and role of KATP channels. Circulation 89:1229-1236.
14. Liu GS, Thornton J, Van Winkle D, Stanley AWH, Olsson RA, Downey JM (1991) Protection against infarction afforded by preconditioning is mediated by A_1 adenosine receptors in rabbit heart. Circulation 84:350-356.
15. Lasley RD, Noble MA, Konyn PJ, Mentzer RM Jr (1995) Different effects of an adenosine A_1 analogue and ischemic preconditioning in isolated rabbit hearts. Ann Thorac Surg 60:1698-1703.
16. Homeister JW, Hoff PT, Fletcher DD, Lucchesi BR (1990): Combined adenosine and lidocaine administration limits myocardial reperfusion injury. Circulation 82:595-608.
17. Dorheim TA, Hoffman A, Van Wylen DGL, Mentzer RM Jr (1991) Enhanced interstitial fluid adenosine attenuates myocardial stunning. Surgery 110: 136-145.
18. Hudspeth DA, Williams MW, Zhao ZQ, Sato H, Nakanishi K, McGee DS, Hammon JW Jr, Vinten-Johansen J, Van Wylen DGL (1994) Pentostatin-augmented interstitial adenosine prevents postcardioplegia injury in damaged hearts. Ann Thorac Surg 58:719-727.
19. Kirkeboen KA, Ilebekk A, Tonnessen T, Leistad E, Naess PA, Christensen G, Aksnes G (1994) Cardiac contractile function following repetitive brief ischemia: effects of nucleoside transport inhibition. Am J Physiol 267:H57-H65.
20. Silva PH, Dillon D, Van Wylen DG (1995) Adenosine deaminase inhibition augments interstitial adenosine but does not attenuate myocardial infarction. Cardiovasc Res 29:616-623.
21. Martin BJ, Lasley RD, Mentzer RM Jr (1996): Infarct size reduction with the nucleoside transport inhibitor R75231 in swine. Am J Physiol In Press.
22. Zhao ZQ, McGee S, Nakanishi K, Toombs CF, Johnston WE, Ashar MS, Vinten-Johansen J (1993) Receptor-mediated cardioprotective effects of endogenous adenosine are exerted primarily during reperfusion after coronary occlusion in the rabbit. Circulation 88:709-719.
23. Hoshida S, Kuzuya T, Nishida M, Yamashita N, Oe H, Hori M, Kamada T, Tada M (1994) Adenosine blockade during reperfusion reverses the infarct limiting effect in preconditioned canine hearts. Cardiovasc Res 28:1083-1088.
24. Cronstein BN, Levin RI, Belanoff J, Weissmann G, Hirschhorn R (1986) Adenosine: an endogenous inhibitor of neutrophil-mediated injury to endothelial cells. J Clin Invest 78: 760-770.
25. Murry CE, Jennings RB, Reimer KA (1986): Preconditioning with ischemia: a delay of lethal cell injury in ischemic myocardium. Circulation 74:1124-1136.
26. Auchampach JA, Gross GJ (1993): Adenosine A1 receptors, KATP channels, and ischemic preconditioning in dogs. Am J Physiol 264:H1327-H1336.

27. Lasley RD, Anderson GM, Mentzer RM Jr (1993): Ischemic and hypoxic preconditioning enhance postischemic recovery of function in the rat heart. Cardiovasc Res 27:565-570.
28. Ganote CE, Armstrong S, Downey JM (1993) Adenosine and A1 selective agonists offer minimal protection against ischaemic injury to isolated rat cardiomyocytes. Cardiovasc Res 27:1670-1676.
29. Kirsch GE, Codina J, Birnbaumer L, Brown AM (1990) Coupling of ATP-sensitive K+ channels to A1 receptors by G proteins in rat ventricular myocytes. Am J Physiol 259:H820-H826.
30. Ito H, Vereecke J, Carmeliet E (1994) Mode of regulation by G protein of the ATP-sensitive K+ channel in guinea-pig ventricular cell membrane. J Physiol 478:101-107.
31. Toombs CF, McGee DS, Johnston WE, Vinten-Johansen J (1993) Protection from ischaemic-reperfusion injury with adenosine pretreatment is reversed by inhibition of ATP sensitive potassium channels. Cardiovasc Res 27:623-629.
32. Xu J, Wang L, Hurt CM, Pelleg A (1994): Endogenous adenosine does not activate ATP-sensitive potassium channels in the hypoxic guinea pig ventricle in vivo. Circulation 89:1209-1216.
33. Miura T, Goto M, Miki T, Sakamoto J, Shimamoto K, Iimura O (1995) Glibenclamide, a blocker of ATP-sensitive potassium channels, abolishes infarct size limitation by preconditioning in rabbits anesthetized with xylazine/pentobarbital but not with pentobarbital alone. J Cardiovasc Pharmacol 25:531-538.
34. Ytrehus K, Liu Y, Downey JM (1994): Preconditioning protects ischemic rabbit heart by protein kinase C activation. Am J Physiol 266:H1145-H1152.
35. Mitchell MB, Meng X, Ao L, Brown JM, Harken AH, Banerjee A (1995) Preconditioning of isolated rat heart is mediated by protein kinase C. Circ Res 76:73-81.
36. Henry P, Demolombe S, Puceat M, Escande D (1996) Adenosine A(1) stimulation activates delta-protein kinase c in rat ventricular myocytes. Circ Res 78:161-165.
37. Przyklenk K, Sussman MA, Simkhovich BZ, Kloner RA (1995) Does ischemic preconditioning trigger translocation of protein kinase C in the canine model? Circulation 92:1546-1557.
38. Lasley RD, Anderson GM, Mentzer RM Jr (1994) Adenosine attenuates phorbol ester-induced negative inotropic and vasoconstrictive effects in rat hearts. Am J Physiol 266:H2159-H2166.

In: Mentzer, R.M., Jr., Kitakaze, M., Downey, J.M., Hori, M, eds. Adenosine, Cardioprotection and Clinical Application. Kluwer Academic Publishers, Norwell, MA, USA, 1997.

8. Activation of Ecto-5'-nucleotidase Mediates Cardioprotection in Ischemic Preconditioning: Important Role of Protein Kinase C

Masafumi Kitakaze
Tetsuo Minamino
Koichi Node
Hiroharu Funaya
Masatsugu Hori

Introduction

When brief periods of ischemia precede sustained ischemia, infarct size is markedly limited, a phenomenon known as ischemic preconditioning.[1,2] The precise mechanisms underlying this phenomenon have been investigated[3,4] because identification of the primary mediator of ischemic preconditioning may contribute to the development of the potential treatment of acute myocardial infarction. Several lines of evidence suggest that beneficial effects of ischemic preconditioning are observed in the clinical settings.[5,6] Recently, Liu et al[7] experimentally demonstrated that an exposure to 8-sulfophenyltheophylline blunts the infarct size-limiting effect of ischemic preconditioning, and that brief periods of exposures to adenosine, instead of transient ischemia, mimic ischemic preconditioning. Thornton et al.[8] showed that adenosine A_1 receptors activation is responsible for the infarct size-limiting effect of ischemic preconditioning. Indeed, it has been clarified that adenosine contributes to limit infarct size.[9,10] There are two different possibilities by which adenosine links with cardioprotection in ischemic preconditioning. One possibility is that release of adenosine during ischemia and reperfusion is enhanced by ischemic preconditioning, and the other possibility is that released adenosine makes myocardium resistant to ischemia and reperfusion. Here, we will discuss the possibility that ischemic preconditioning activates the enzymes responsible for adenosine release, i.e., ecto-5'-nucleotidase, and test the cause-effect relationship between activation of ecto-5'-nucleotidase and the infarct size-limiting effect in ischemic preconditioning.

Adenosine release and 5'-nucleotidase activity in ischemic preconditioning

First of all, we tested whether the ischemic preconditioning procedure increases ecto-5'-nucleotidase activity and adenosine release during reperfusion.[11] In the anesthetized open chest dogs, after intravenous administration of heparin (500 units/kg), we cannulated and perfused the left anterior descending (LAD) coronary artery with blood from the left carotid artery through an extracorporeal bypass tube. Coronary blood flow and coronary perfusion pressure in the perfused area was measured. A small caliber (1 mm), short (7 cm) collecting tube was introduced into a small coronary vein near the center of the perfused area to sample coronary venous blood for measurements of adenosine. The left atrium was catheterized for microsphere injection to determine the collateral flow during ischemia. After the bypass tube to the LAD coronary artery was occluded 4 times for 5 minutes, both ecto- and cytosolic 5'-nucleotidase activity was increased (Fig. 8-1, lower panel). Ecto- and cytosolic 5'-nucleotidase activity was defined as 5'-nucleotidase activity of membrane and cytosolic fractions.[11,12] The upper panel of Figure 8-1 describes the adenosine concentration of coronary arterial and venous blood during reperfusion following 40 minutes of ischemia. Adenosine concentration in the coronary venous blood was higher in the group of ischemic preconditioning compared with the untreated control group. Does activation of ecto-5'-nucleotidase directly link with the enhanced release of adenosine during ischemia and reperfusion? Adenosine is produced simply by the enzymatic reactions; the dephosphorylation of 5'-AMP by 5'-nucleotidase and the hydrolysis of S-adenosylhomocysteine (SAH) by SAH-hydrolase. Although adenosine is produced through the latter pathway in the normoxic hearts,[13] 5'-nucleotidase is related to adenosine production during ischemia and hypoxia.[14-17] This idea is supported by the fact that α,β-methyleneadenosine 5'-diphosphate (AOPCP, an inhibitor of ecto-5'-nucleotidase, 80 μg/kg/min) potently reduces adenosine production in the ischemic myocardium.[12] Furthermore, the extents of decreases in reactive hyperemic flow following a brief period of coronary occlusion were comparably reduced under the treatment with either AOPCP or 8-sulfophenyltheophylline (an adenosine receptor antagonist), suggesting that adenosine production during ischemia is attributable to the activity of

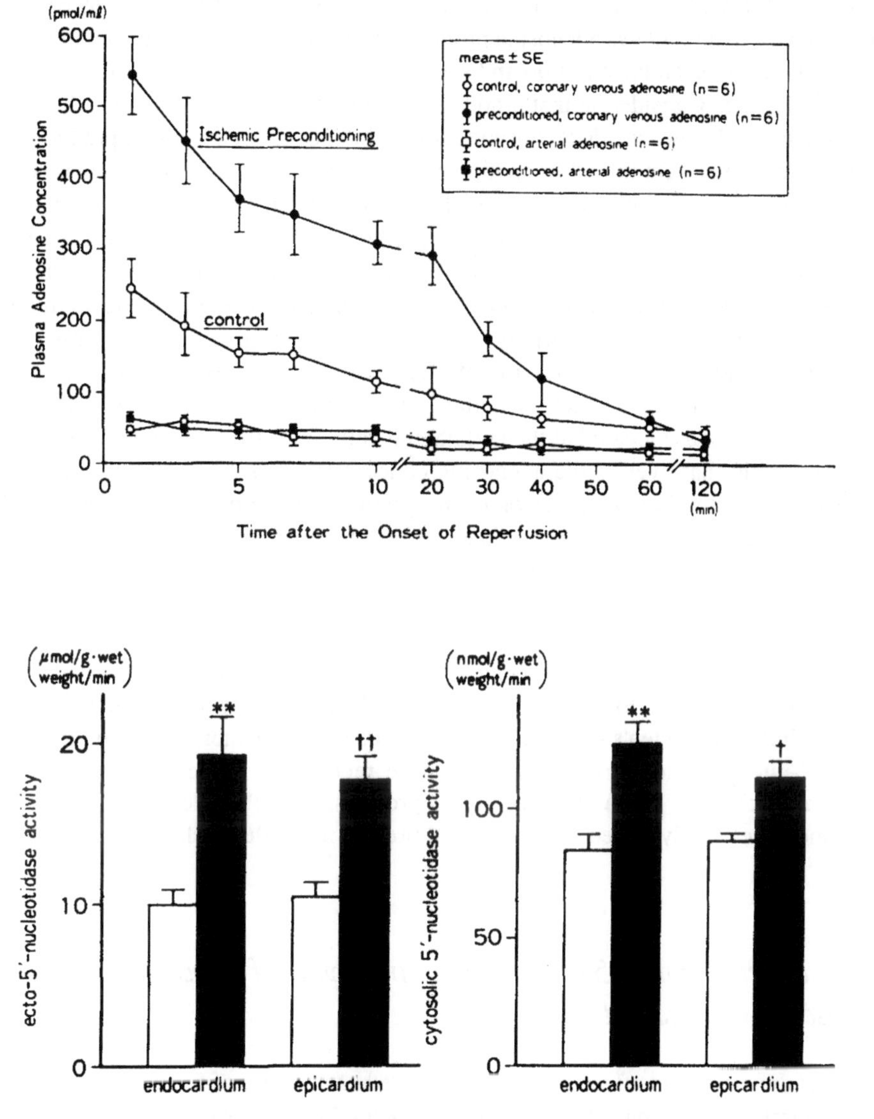

FIGURE 8-1. The upper panel indicates the graph showing adenosine release during reperfusion after 40 minutes of coronary occlusion with and without ischemic preconditioning. Adenosine release in the group that underwent ischemic preconditioning is enhanced (P<0.01) for 40 minutes compared with the untreated control condition. The lower panel indicates bar graphs showing ecto- and cytosolic 5'-nucleotidase activity in the control and ischemic preconditioned myocardium before the 40 minutes coronary occlusion. Both ecto- and cytosolic 5'-nucleotidase activity was augmented by ischemic preconditioning. (Ref. 11).

5'-nucleotidase.[18] On the other hand, accumulation of 5'-AMP seems to be the other factor that regulates adenosine production. Cytosolic 5'-AMP concentration crucially depends on the duration and severity of ischemia and culminates up to 1 x 10^{-2} - 10^{-4} M. Considering that production of adenosine is 1 x 10^{-6} - 10^{-8} M, even considerable changes in AMP concentration would not affect adenosine production during ischemia. On the other hand, there is a report indicating that increases in adenosine concentration in the interstitial space are not augmented during sustained ischemia in the group of ischemic preconditioning,[19] which seems contradict to our findings. One possible explanation for this difference is that we measured adenosine concentration in coronary venous blood, and the adenosine level in the coronary venous blood is largely affected by endothelial cells. In turn, the interstitial adenosine levels might be largely affected by myocardial ecto-5'-nucleotidase. Thus ischemic preconditioning differently activates ecto-5'-nucleotidase located at the endothelial cells and cardiomyocytes. Second, it is possible that even if the adenosine concentration in the microenvironment surrounding ecto-5'-nucleotidase on the myocardial cellular membrane is increased by the activated ecto-5'-nucleotidase, the alteration of interstitial volume determined by myocardial cellular swelling and the rate of washout due to the lymphatic stream may change the interstitial adenosine concentration. In any of these possible situations, the temporal and topical increases in the adenosine concentration surrounding ecto-5'-nucleotidase may be able to directly activate the adenosine receptors located at the same cellular membrane, which may not contradict Van Wylen's observation. This close juxtaposition may explain how ecto-5'-nucleotidase activates the adenosine receptors. Indeed, the regulatory systems including the ATP receptors, G proteins, ecto-5'-nucleotidase and K_{ATP} channels are closely linked each other and present in single patch of no more than 1 μm^2.[20]

Role of activation of 5'-nucleotidase in salvage of myocardial necrosis in ischemic preconditioning

To test the cause and effect relationship between activation of 5'-nucleotidase and the infarct size-limiting effect in ischemic preconditioning, we examined whether AOPCP blunted the infarct size limiting-effect of ischemic preconditioning.[12] We occluded the coronary artery 4 times 5 minutes with intracoronary administration of AOPCP. AOPCP was administered into the LAD coronary artery 5 minutes prior to the ischemic preconditioning (IP) procedures and continued for 60 minutes of reperfusion except for the coronary occlusion period (the AOPCP treatment with IP group). In the other dogs, AOPCP was administered into the LAD coronary artery 40 minutes prior to ischemia and continued for 60 minutes of reperfusion except for the coronary occlusion period (the AOPCP treatment group). To discriminate the role of increases in 5'-nucleotidase activity during the ischemic preconditioning procedure (the AOPCP pretreatment with IP group) or during reperfusion (the AOPCP during reperfusion with IP group) on the infarct size-limiting effect, we infused AOPCP only during the ischemic preconditioning procedure or only during reperfusion up to 60 minutes in the ischemic preconditioned dogs. There are no significant differences in risk area and collateral flow during ischemia between the 6 groups. AOPCP completely abolished the infarct size-limiting effect of ischemic preconditioning. In the AOPCP pretreatment with IP and the AOPCP during reperfusion with IP groups, infarct size was partially attenuated compared with the AOPCP treatment with IP group and the AOPCP treatment group. Infarct size of these two groups were smaller than the control and AOPCP groups and larger than that in the ischemic preconditioning group. These results indicate that increased 5'-nucleotidase activity during ischemic preconditioning procedures and during early reperfusion synergistically contributes to the infarct size-limiting effect of ischemic preconditioning.

Role of activation of protein kinase C via a1-adrenoceptors in salvage of myocardial necrosis in ischemic preconditioning

According to the data of Downey's group,[21] protein kinase C is tightly linked to ischemic preconditioning. We also have reported that activation of protein kinase C increases ecto-5'-nucleotidase activity in the rat cardiomyocytes (Fig. 8-2, Ref.22). Since protein kinase C is activated by ischemic preconditioning,[23] ischemic preconditioning may increase ecto-5'-nucleotidase activity via protein kinase C activation. Figure 8-3 shows that activation of ecto-5'-nucleotidase due to ischemic preconditioning is blunted by GF109203X, an inhibitor of protein kinase C, in the canine hearts. Furthermore, inhibition of protein kinase C by GF109203X blunted the infarct size-limiting effect of ischemic preconditioning (Fig. 8-4). We have also revealed that ecto-5'-nucleotidase is phosphorylated in the preconditioned myocardium. Therefore, we speculate that phosphorylation of ecto-5'-nucleotidase due to protein kinase C may change the characteristics of active site of ecto-5'-nucleotidase or induce a conformational change in the structure of 5'-nucleotidase.

The next question is how protein kinase C is activated during ischemic preconditioning. Since ischemic preconditioning increases release of norepinephrine from the presynaptic vesicles, we tested the role of a1-adrenoceptor activation in cardioprotection in ischemic preconditioning.[24] In the open chest dogs, constant infusion of prazosin (4 μg/kg/min) into the LAD coronary artery was begun 5 minutes prior to ischemic preconditioning, and continued through the first 60 minutes of the reperfusion period, except during coronary occlusion (the

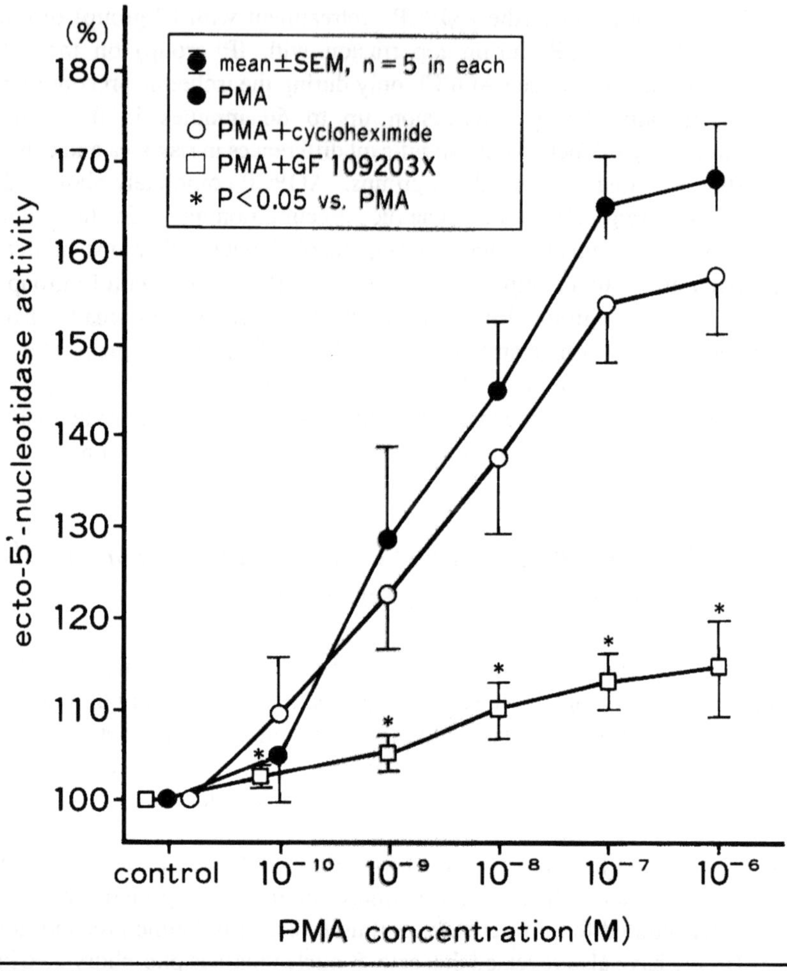

FIGURE 8-2. The dose-response relation between phorbol 12-myristate 13-acetate (PMA) and ecto-5'-nucleotidase activity with and without either GF109203X (an inhibitor of protein kinase C) and cycloheximide (an inhibitor of protein synthesis) in rat cardiomyocytes. Ecto-5'-nucleotidase activity in the control conditions were 6.44 ± 0.89, 5.96 ± 0.78, and 5.81 ± 0.44 nmol/mg protein/min in the PMA, PMA with GF109203X and PMA with cycloheximide groups, respectively. (Ref. 22)

prazosin with IP group). In the other dogs, prazosin was infused into the LAD coronary artery beginning 40 minutes prior to ischemia without ischemic preconditioning and continued for 60 minutes of reperfusion, except during coronary occlusion (the prazosin group). To test whether a1-adrenoceptor stimulation mimics the infarct size-limiting effect of ischemic preconditioning, we

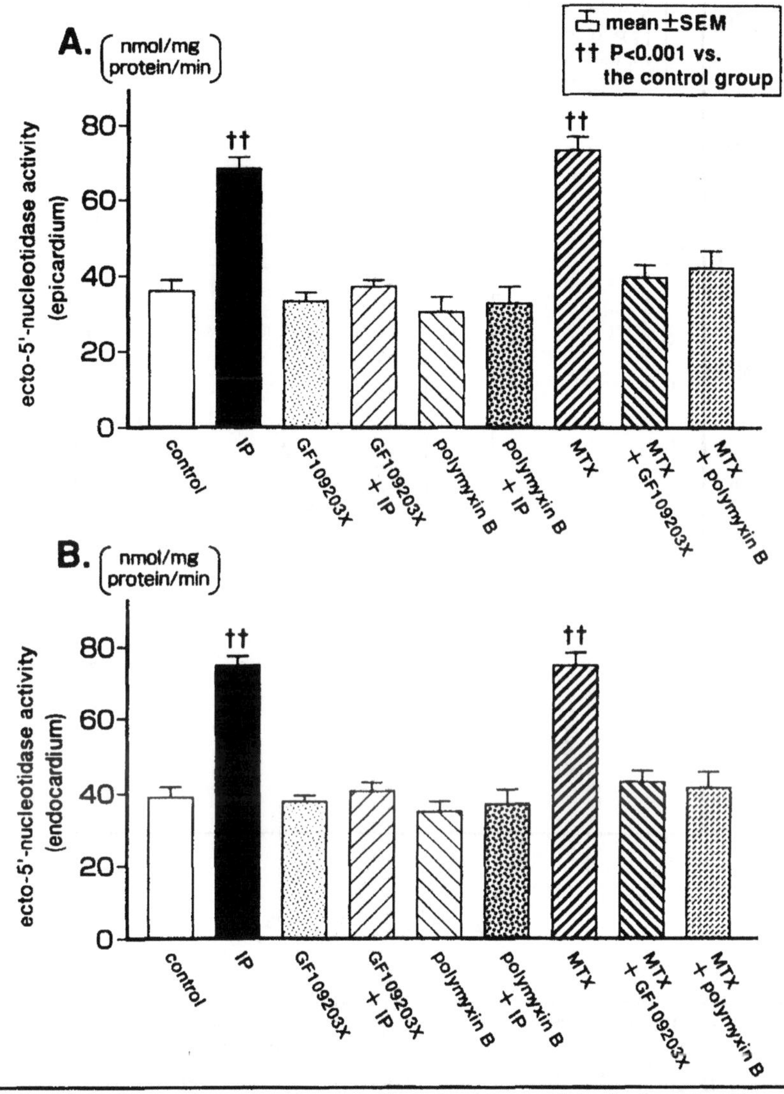

FIGURE 8-3. Comparison of canine ecto-5'-nucleotidase activity in the epicardium (panel A) and endocardium (panel B) following 40 minutes of steady state observation (control group), 40 minutes of either GF109203X or polymyxin B administration, ischemic preconditioning with and without either GF109203X or polymyxin B administration, and intermittent exposure to methoxamine with and without either GF109203X or polymyxin B administration. Ischemic preconditioning increased ecto-5'-nucleotidase activity, which was blunted by both GF109203X and polymyxin B and mimicked by methoxamine. (Ref. 23)

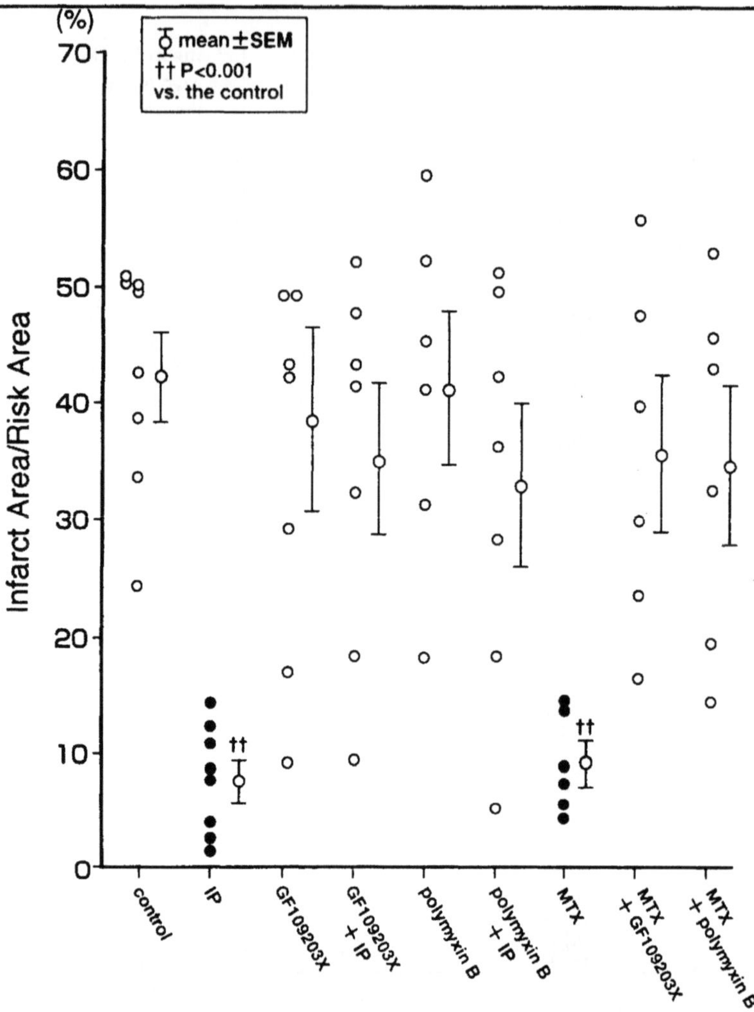

FIGURE 8-4. Infarct size in the control group, the ischemic preconditioning group, the prazosin with IP group, the GF109203X group, the IP with GF109203X group, the polymyxin B group, the IP with polymyxin B group, the methoxamine group, the methoxamine with GF109203X group and the methoxamine with GF109203X group. Infarct size was decreased in the ischemic preconditioning group. The infarct size-limiting effect of ischemic preconditioning was abolished by GF109203X and polymyxin B. On the other hand, methoxamine mimicked the infarct size-limiting effect of ischemic preconditioning, which was blunted by GF109203X and polymyxin B. (Ref. 23)

administered methoxamine into the LAD (40 μg/kg/min, 4 cycles for 5 minutes with 5-minute intervals, the methoxamine group). Following the methoxamine exposure, 90 minutes of coronary occlusion and 6 hours of reperfusion were imposed. Furthermore, to examine the role of increased ecto-5'-nucleotidase activity due to exposures of methoxamine, we concomitantly infused AOPCP 5 minutes prior to ischemic preconditioning and continued 60 minutes of reperfusion, except during 90 minutes of coronary occlusion to animals treated with methoxamine (the methoxamine with AOPCP group). In another group, we determined the effect of AOPCP on infarct size (the AOPCP group). In this group, AOPCP was administered prior to 40 minutes of coronary occlusion and during 1 hour of reperfusion following 90 minutes of coronary occlusion. Ischemic preconditioning increased both ecto- and cytosolic 5'-nucleotidase activity in the myocardium. Prazosin administration without ischemic preconditioning decreased ecto- and cytosolic 5'-nucleotidase activity and blunted the increases in ecto- and cytosolic 5'-nucleotidase activity due to ischemic preconditioning. Methoxamine increased both ecto- and cytosolic 5'-nucleotidase activity to the levels obtained by ischemic preconditioning. Furthermore, prazosin completely abolished the infarct size-limiting effect of ischemic preconditioning. With the methoxamine administration, infarct size was attenuated to the level seen with ischemic preconditioning. However, the infarct size-limiting effect due to exposure of methoxamine was blunted by AOPCP, and no difference in infarct size existed between the methoxamine with AOPCP and the AOPCP groups. We also checked the regression plots of infarct size, as a percentage of the area at risk against collateral flow.[24] This observation is consistent with previous studies. It is reported that α_1-adrenoceptor activation is intimately involved in attenuation of the severity of ischemia and reperfusion[16] and ischemic preconditioning.[25] The present results strongly suggest that α_1-adrenoceptor stimulation mediates cardioprotection seen in ischemic preconditioning, which is attributable to activation of ecto-5'-nucleotidase.

Clinical relevance

The finding in the present study suggests two clinical applications for treatment of acute myocardial infarction. One strategy to limit infarct size is to find a method to increase 5'-nucleotidase activity. As we observed, protein kinase C activation may increase 5'-nucleotidase activity, and may attenuate contractile dysfunction and infarct size. Another possibility is to enhance adenosine release. Administration of adenosine and potentiators of adenosine production, e.g., acadesine, dilazep, or dipyridamole may limit infarct size. Both strategies merit clinical investigation although an enhanced understanding of the basic process involved in ischemic preconditioning is necessary.

References

1. Murry CE, Jennings RB, Reimer KA. Preconditioning with ischemia: A delay of lethal cell injury in ischemic myocardium. Circulation 1986;74:1124-1136.
2. Li GC, Vasquez JA, Gallagher KP et al. Myocardial protection with preconditioning. Circulation 1990;82:609-619.
3. Murry CE, Richard VJ, Reimer KA et al. Ischemic preconditioning slows energy metabolism and delays ultrastructural damage during a sustained ischemic episode. Circ. Res. 1990;66:913-931.
4. Steenbergen CM, Perlman R, London E et al. Mechanism of preconditioning lonic alterations. Circ Res. 1993;72:112-125.
5. Deutsch E, Berger M, Kussmaul WG et al. Adaptation in ischemia during percutaneous transmural coronary angioplasty. Clinical, hemodynamic, and metabolic features. Circulation 1990;82:2044-2051.
6. Okazaki Y, Kodama K, Sato H et al. Attenuation of increased regional oxygen consumption during exercise as a major cause of warm-up phenomenon. J. Am. Coll. Cardiol. 1993;21:1597-1604.
7. Liu GS, Thornton J, Van Winkle DM et al. Protection against infarction afforded by preconditioning is mediated by A1 adenosine receptors in rabbit heart. Circulation 1991;84:350-356.
8. Thornton JD, Liu GS, Olsson RA et al. Intravenous pretreatment with A1-selective adenosine analogue protects the heart against infarction. Circulation 1992;85:659-665.
9. Miura T, Ogawa T, Iwamoto T et al.Dipyridamole potentiates the myocardial infarct size-limiting effect of ischemic preconditioning. Circulation 1992;86:979-985.
10. Olafsson B, Forman MB, Puett DW et al. Reduction of reperfusion injury in the canine preparation by intracoronary adenosine: importance of the endothelium and the no-reflow phenomenon. Circulation 1987;76:1135-1145.
11. Kitakaze M., Hori M, Takashima S et al. Ischemic preconditioning increases adenosine release and 5'-nucleotidase activity during myocardial ischemia and reperfusion in dogs. Implication for myocardial salvage. Circulation 1993;87:208-215.
12. Kitakaze M., Hori M, Morioka T et al. The infarct size-limiting effect of ischemic preconditioning is blunted by inhibition of 5'-nucleotidase activity and attenuation of adenosine release. Circulation. 1994;89:1237-1246.
13. Llyod HGE, Schrader J. The importance of the transmethylation pathway for adenosine metabolism in the hearts. In: Gerlach E, Becker BF (eds) Topics and Perspectives in Adenosine Research. Berlin Heidelberg:Springer-Verlag, 1987:199-207.
14. Sparks NV, Jr., Bardengeuer H. Regulation of adenosine formation by the heart. Circ. Res. 1986;58:193-201.
15. Hori M,. Kitakaze M. Adenosine, the heart, and coronary circulation. Hypertension 1991;18:565-574.
16. Kitakaze M., Hori M, Kamada T. Role of adenosine and its interaction with alpha adrenoceptor activity in ischemic and reperfusion injury of the myocardium. Cardiovasc. Res. 1993;27:18-27.
17. Imai S, Nakazawa M, Imai M et al. 5'-Nucleotidase inhibitors and the myocardial reactive hyperemia and adenosine content. In: Gerlach E, Becker BF (eds) Topics and Perspectives in Adenosine Research. Berlin Heidelberg:Springer-Verlag,1986:416-424.
18. Kitakaze M., Hori M, Takashima S et al. Superoxide dismutase enhances ischemia-induced reactive hyperemic flow and adenosine release in dogs: A role of 5'-nucleotidase activity. Circ Res 1992;71:558-566.
19. Van Wylen DGL. Effects of ischemic preconditioning on interstitial purine metabolite and lactate accumulation during myocardial ischemia Circulation 1994;89:2283-2289.
20. Al-Awqati Q. Regulation of ion channels by ABC transporter that secrete ATP. Science 1995;269:805-806.

21. Tsuchida A., Liu Y, Liu GS et al. Alpha1-adrenergic agonists precondition rabbit ischemic myocardium independent of adenosine by direct activation of protein kinase activation. Circ Res 1994;75:576-585.
22. Kitakaze M., Hori M, Morioka T et al. α_1-Adrenoceptor activation increases ectosolic 5'-nucleotidase activity and adenosine release in rat cardiomyocytes by activing protein kinase C. Circulation 1995;91:2226-2234.
23. Kitakaze M., Node K, Minamino T et al. The role of activation of protein kinase C in the infarct size-limiting effect of ischemic preconditioning through activation of ecto-5'-nucleotidase. Circulation 1995;93:781-791.
24. Kitakaze M., Hori M, Morioka T et al. Alpha$_1$-adrenoceptor activation mediates the infarct size-limiting effect of ischemic preconditioning through augmentation of 5'-nucleotidase activity. J Clin Invest 1994;93:2197-2205.
25. Banerjee A., Locke-Winter C, Rogers KB et al. Preconditioning against myocardial dysfunction after ischemia and reperfusion by α-adrenergic mechanism. Circ Res 1993;73:656-670.

In: Mentzer, R.M., Jr., Kitakaze, M., Downey, J.M., Hori, M, eds. Adenosine, Cardioprotection and Clinical Application. Kluwer Academic Publishers, Norwell, MA, USA, 1997.

9. Role of Mn-SOD Induction in the Second Window Phenomenon of Preconditioning of Ischemic Hearts

Tsunehiko Kuzuya
Masashi Nishida
Shiro Hoshida
Nobushige Yamashita
Michihiko Tada

Introduction

Recently, growing numbers of evidence suggest that the myocardium undergoes adaptation after sub-lethal cellular stresses including ischemia, heat stress and exposure to cytokines.[1-4] The second window, or late phase, of ischemic preconditioning, is one of the adaptation phenomena after non-lethal ischemia, which specifically observed 24 hr after ischemic preconditioning. The mechanism of the acquisition of tolerance to ischemia-reperfusion in the myocardium is still the matter of discussion. However, *de novo* synthesis of rescue proteins, such as heat shock proteins and antioxidants, are strongly implicated in molecular mechanism of the cellular protection. In this review, we will focus on the aspect of oxygen radical metabolism in the heart at ischemia-reperfusion and outline our recent findings on the role of manganese superoxide dismutase, an intrinsic oxygen radical scavenger localized in mitochondria, in the protection of myocardium from ischemia-reperfusion.

Oxygen radical in reperfusion injury

Oxygen radicals, produced at reflow of ischemic myocardium, were proposed to be one of culprits which cause myocardial injury at ischemia-reperfusion. In late

1980s, several groups successfully detected the presence of oxygen radical species in myocardial tissue soon after reperfusion following ischemia by electron paramagnetic resonance (EPR) with or without spin trapping technique.[5,6] We tried to detect continuous production of oxygen-derived free radicals at later phase of reperfusion.[7] Following occlusion of canine left anterior descending coronary artery (LAD) for 90 min, cardiac tissue was freeze clamped at 1 and 3 hr after reperfusion. DMPO adducts of oxygen radicals in tissue sample were detected by EPR. DMPO-OH signal, which represents hydroxyl radical species, was observed at both 1 and 3 hr after reperfusion in much larger quantity than the signal at 15 seconds after reperfusion. These results indicate that oxygen radicals were produced in myocardial tissue after reperfusion and the production of oxygen radicals was augmented during the course of extension of cardiac injury after reperfusion.

Therefore, a lot of studies were designed to scavenge radical species to prevent myocardium from reperfusion injury.[8] In some reports, exogenous radical scavengers such as SOD and catalase successfully reduced reperfusion injury in *in vivo* models. However, the results from other reports were controversial. The controversy might depend on the difference in experimental protocol they used, i.e. species and consciousness of animals, duration of ischemia-reperfusion, and time point of the addition of radical scavengers. One possible reason for this controversy might arise from the diverse mechanism of oxygen radical production in reperfused heart tissue. In the ischemia-reperfused heart, oxygen radicals were generated mainly from three sources. Xanthine - xanthine oxidase system of vascular endothelial cells, NADH oxidase of activated neutrophils in blood stream or in myocardial tissue, and mitochondrial electron transport system of cardiac myocytes. These systems produce superoxide anion, the initial product of oxygen reduction, in coronary circulation, extra-cellular space of cardiac tissue, and inside mitochondria of myocytes. Because exogenous radical scavengers are mainly distributed in blood stream and extra-cellular space, they scavenge oxygen radicals produced by endothelial cells and neutrophils. However, superoxide generated by mitochondrial electron transport system is difficult to be scavenged by exogenous radical scavengers, unless they are modified so as to get into cardiac myocytes like conjugated, lipophylic SODs. Therefore, animal models which emphasize on the production of oxygen radicals outside myocardium could be salvaged by exogenous radical scavengers.

Induction of Mn-SOD after ischemic preconditioning

Recent studies showed, however, that the heart is not merely threatened by oxygen radicals, but also have their own intrinsic radical scavenge system including Mn-

SOD, Cu,Zn-SOD, catalase and glutathione redox system. These enzymes were revealed to be induced by exogenous stimuli, such as endotoxin, cytokines and hyperthermia. Among them, Mn-SOD is located in cardiac mitochondria and is supposed to play a major role in scavenging superoxide generated by electron transport system in the front line. Therefore, we tried to examine whether or not the induction of mitochondrial Mn-SOD is responsible for the acquisition of tolerance to ischemia-reperfusion of the heart by scavenging superoxide generated in mitochondria. Firstly, we examined the relationship between second window protection of ischemic preconditioning and Mn-SOD induction in a canine model of LAD occlusion-reperfusion. Figure 9-1a shows an increase in Mn-SOD content in ischemic myocardium of dog hearts after four 5 min coronary occlusions.[9] Mn-SOD protein was measured by enzyme-linked immuno-sorbent assay soon after, 3 hr, 12 hr and 24 hr after repeated ischemia. Mn-SOD content in the sub-endocardium (open circles) increased gradually with a peak observed 24 hr after sub-lethal ischemia (60 % increase). At this peak point, myocardial Mn-SOD activity, simultaneously measured by nitroblue tetrazolium method, was also increased by about 80% of normal control. We could not see any differences in activity of other antioxidant enzymes, including Cu,Zn-SOD, catalase, and glutathione peroxidase, in this experiment. Nextly, we demonstrated that such an ischemic preconditioning protocol results in a delayed protective response against myocardial necrosis after a subsequent prolonged ischemia in the dog (Fig. 9-1b).[10] Immediately after, or 3, 12 and 24 hr after four 5 min occlusions of LAD, dogs were subjected to 90 min occlusion followed by 5 hr reperfusion. When the second ischemia was applied immediately after the first sub-lethal ischemia, % risk area infarcted was markedly decreased to 14% compared with necrotic area in control animals. However, the reduction of myocardial infarction was disappeared, when the time interval between sub-lethal and sustained ischemia was 3 and 12 hr. Interestingly, the size of myocardial infarction was again reduced, when the prolonged ischemia-reperfusion was applied 24 hr after ischemic preconditioning. Time course of the reappearance of the tolerance to ischemia-reperfusion was identical with that of Mn-SOD induction in the preconditioned myocardium (Fig. 9-1a).

To investigate the role of enhancement of cardiac SOD activity in the protection against ischemia-reperfusion injury, we examined whether the preconditioning phenomenon could be mimicked in cultured rat myocytes by exposing them to hypoxia (7 mmHg) - reoxygenation (143 mmHg) before exposure to sustained hypoxia-reoxygenation (hypoxic preconditioning).[11] In control cells, which were subjected normoxia instead of hypoxia for the first 1 hr, Mn-SOD content and activity showed a slight decrease during the following 36 hr. On the other hand, in the cells exposed to hypoxia, both activity and content of Mn-SOD

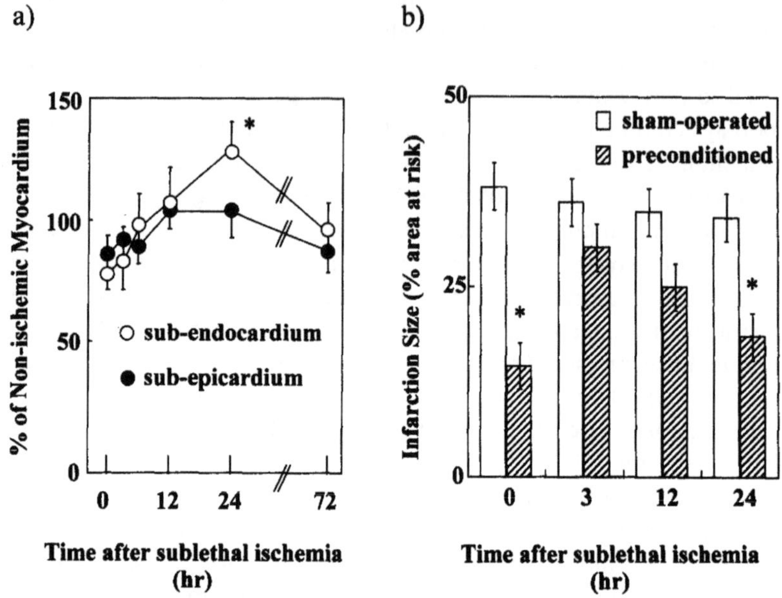

FIGURE 9-1. a) Mn-SOD content in reperfused myocardium was measured at 0, 12, 24, and 36 hr after repeated LAD occlusion. Open circles: Mn-SOD content in sub-endocardium. Closed circles: Mn-SOD content in sub-epicardium. b)LAD was re-occluded for 90 min at 0, 12, 24, and 36 hr after repeated LAD occlusion. Following reperfusion for 5 hr, the size of myocardial infarction was assessed. Animals without repeated LAD occlusion were served as controls.

increased markedly with a peak at 24 hr after reoxygenation from hypoxia. We also examined the expression of Mn-SOD mRNA after hypoxia-reoxygenation by Northern hybridization using a rat Mn-SOD cDNA probe. Mn-SOD mRNA gives two bands at 4.0 kb and 1.0 kb. Basal expression of Mn-SOD mRNA observed before hypoxia, increased after reoxygenation and reached its peak at 30 min after reoxygenation (180% of control level, when it was normalized as to ß-actin signal). Next, we examined myocyte injury by assessing CK release from the cultures after exposure to prolonged hypoxia (3 hr)-reoxygenation (1 hr). When myocyte cultures were pre-exposed to hypoxic preconditioning as above, CK release from myocyte cultures after exposure to prolonged hypoxia was markedly reduced when the second hypoxia was applied 24 hr after the first hypoxia compared with cells without hypoxic preconditioning. The time course of this increase in myocardial tolerance to hypoxia after exposure to brief preceding hypoxia was apparently similar to that of Mn-SOD induction.

Having confirmed that the simulation of ischemia-reperfusion by hypoxia-reoxygenation mimics the second window of protection of ischemic preconditioning in *in vivo*, we examined cause-effect relationship between Mn-SOD induction and tolerance to hypoxia in the culture model using anti-sense oligodeoxyribonucleotides to Mn-SOD mRNA. Induction of Mn-SOD content and activity after exposure to hypoxia were abolished completely when anti-sense oligonucleotides to Mn-SOD mRNA was added to myocyte cultures (Fig. 9-2a). Oligonucleotides having sense sequence did not attenuate the induction of Mn-SOD. Staurosporine, a protein kinase C inhibitor, also attenuated the induction of Mn-SOD in myocyte cultures after exposure to brief hypoxia. As we confirmed that anti-sense oligodeoxyribonucleotides to Mn-SOD mRNA inhibited the induction of Mn-SOD protein, we examined the effect of the oligonucleotides on CK release from myocytes after exposure to prolonged hypoxia-reoxygenation. Cardiac myocytes were exposed to 1 hr hypoxia with or without anti-sense oligonucleotides to Mn-SOD, 24 hr prior to the exposure to prolonged hypoxia (Fig. 9-2b). CK release from myocyte cultures was attenuated by 51 % when the cells were exposed to brief hypoxia compared to the cells without exposure to preceding brief hypoxia. However, anti-sense oligonucleotides to Mn-SOD abolished the expected decrease in CK release from myocytes with hypoxic preconditioning. Sense oligonucleotides did not change CK release from preconditioned myocytes. These results indicate that Mn-SOD induction in cardiac myocytes after exposure to brief hypoxia is the mechanism of the acquisition of tolerance to lethal hypoxia in cardiac myocytes.

Induction of Mn-SOD after heat stress

Heat shock is also known to increase the tolerance of myocardium to ischemic stress by inducing heat shock proteins (HSPs).[4,12] Therefore, a heat shock model of cultured myocytes could be a model to examine the relationship between HSPs and Mn-SOD induction in the acquisition of tolerance to ischemia-reperfusion. We examined the expression of Mn-SOD and HSP72 in rat neonatal cardiac myocytes by exposing them to heat shock at 42 °C for 1 hr. Mn-SOD mRNA exhibited transient expression peaked at 30 min after heat shock. HSP72 mRNA expression probed with PCR fragment of mouse cDNA was also increased dramatically at 30 min after heat shock. As we confirmed that heat shock induces both Mn-SOD and HSP72 in myocardial cells, we used anti-sense oligonucleotides to separate the effect of heat shock protein and Mn-SOD on the acquisition of tolerance to ischemia. Anti-sense oligonucleotides to Mn-SOD was added to myocyte cultures during heat shock and following normo-thermic incubation for 24 hr. Twenty four hr after heat shock at 42 °C for 1 hr, Mn-SOD content increased significantly. This increase in Mn-SOD content was abolished by the addition of 1.5 μM of anti-sense

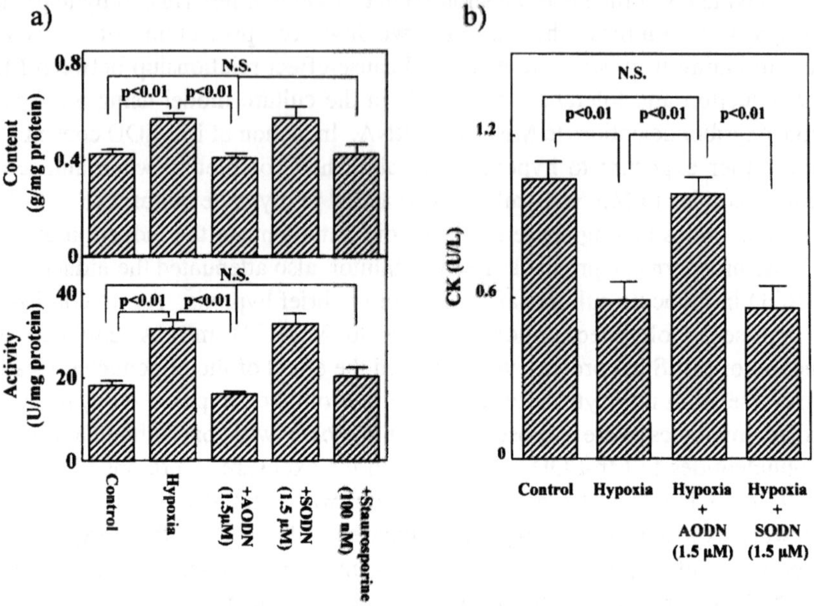

FIGURE 9-2. a) Cardiac myocytes were exposed to hypoxia (1 hr)-reoxygenation (24 hr). Mn-SOD content (upper panel) and activity (lower panel) in the cells were examined. Antisense oligodeoxyribonucleotides (AODN) to Mn-SOD mRNA were applied to some cultures 24 hr before the experiments. b) 24 hr after exposure to hypoxia-reoxygenation, cardiac myocytes were exposed to prolonged hypoxia for 3 hr and reoxygenated for 1 hr. Myocyte injury was assessed by creatine kinase (CK) release into culture medium.

oligonucleotides. HSP72 protein was induced in the myocytes 24 hr after heat shock. The increase in HSP72 was not inhibited by the addition of anti-sense oligonucleotides to Mn-SOD at the dose that abolished Mn-SOD induction. These results indicate anti-sense oligonucleotides used in this experiments inhibited only Mn-SOD induction, but HSP72 was remained to be induced. Although several constructs were examined at a variety of doses, anti-sense oligonucleotides against HSP72 mRNA could not inhibit the induction of HSP72 protein.

Therefore, we used the Mn-SOD anti-sense oligonucleotides to separate the effect of Mn-SOD induction and HSP72 induction. To examine whether Mn-SOD and HSP72 play roles in the acquisition of tolerance to hypoxia after heat stress, we tested the effect of Mn-SOD anti-sense oligonucleotides on CK release from myocytes after hypoxia-reoxygenation. Heat stress for 1 hr at 42°C increased the tolerance of myocytes to hypoxia 24 hr after heat shock, i.e. CK release from myocytes after 3 hr hypoxia followed by 1 hr reoxygenation decreased by 50 % compared with control cells without heat stress. Anti-sense oligonucleotides to

Mn-SOD which inhibited Mn-SOD induction after heat stress, but not HSP72 induction, attenuated significantly the decrease in CK release. Sense oligonucleotides used as control did not alter CK release from heat stressed myocytes. These results indicate that Mn-SOD is induced after heat stress together with HSP72 and plays a pivotal role in the acquisition of the tolerance to ischemia after heat shock. The role of Mn-SOD in cardioprotection might be distinct from that of HSP72, because inhibition of Mn-SOD alone by anti-sense oligonucleotides abolished the tolerance of myocytes to hypoxia-reoxygenation.

Mn-SOD induction after alpha 1 adrenergic stimulation

Finally, we examined the mechanism in which the effect of preconditioning is conducted to the induction of Mn-SOD. Recent studies revealed that cardiac myocytes respond to various stresses such as ischemia, heat shock and adrenergic stimulation and acquire intrinsic cardioprotective capacity in them. In classical preconditioning phenomenon of the heart, the mechanism is well examined as to α1-adrenergic stimulation pathway conducted through adenosine, K-channel or protein kinase C to the final effectors. Therefore, we hypothesized that the induction of Mn-SOD in cardiac myocytes in the second window phenomenon of ischemic preconditioning could be conducted through α1-adrenergic receptor mediated mechanism via protein kinase C.[13] We stimulated cultured rat neonatal cardiac myocytes with norepinephrine in the absence or presence of adrenergic receptor blockades. When norepinephrine was added to myocyte cultures, Mn-SOD activity in culture dish 24 hr after the stimulation increased dose dependently up to 0.2 μM and declined thereafter. Although total protein contents in the cell was also increased after norepinephrine stimulation, the increase in Mn-SOD was shown to be specifically larger than non-specific increase in proteins by dividing Mn-SOD activity with total protein amount. Mn-SOD mRNA expression after the addition of norepinephrine showed that Mn-SOD transcription was augmented at 30 min after stimulation. To confirm the receptor specificity of this phenomenon, we examined the effect of adrenergic receptor antagonists and an agonist on Mn-SOD induction. The augmented Mn-SOD activity in myocytes by the addition of norepinephrine (0.2 μM) was not attenuated by an α2-adrenergic blocker, yohimbine (2 μM), and a ß-adrenergic blocker, propranolol (2 μM). However, an α1-adrenergic blocker, prazosine (2 μM), abolished the increase in Mn-SOD activity induced by norepinephrine. An α1-adrenergic agonist, methoxamine (20 μM), also increased Mn-SOD activity in the myocytes 24 hr after the addition. These results indicate the induction of Mn-SOD after norepinephrine was conducted through α1-adrenergic stimulation. Mn-SOD activity increased by α1-adrenergic stimulation was attenuated by the addition of anti-sense oligonucleotides to Mn-SOD mRNA. A protein kinase C inhibitor, staurosporine (100 nM), also

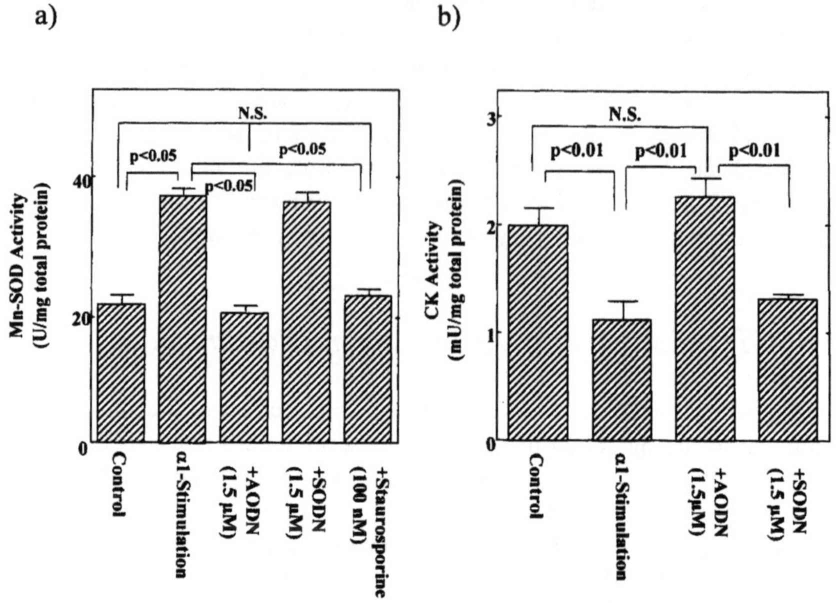

FIGURE 9-3. a) Myocytes were exposed to 0.2 μM norepinephrine in the presence of 2 μM propranolol, and 2 μM yohimbine. 24 hr after stimulation, Mn-SOD activity in cultures were examined. AODN, SODN to Mn-SOD mRNA and staurosporine were added to some cultures. b) Hypoxia (3 hr)-reoxygenation (1 hr) was applied to myocyte cultures 24 hr after α1-adrenergic stimulation. CK release into culture medium was assessed.

attenuated the increase in Mn-SOD activity (Fig. 9-3a). Finally, we examined whether or not Mn-SOD induced by α1-adrenergic stimulation could increase the tolerance of the myocytes to hypoxia-reoxygenation. Cardiac myocytes were exposed to α1-adrenergic stimulation for 24 hr, and then hypoxia (3 hr) followed by reoxygenation (1 hr) was applied to the cells. CK release from the myocytes was significantly attenuated by α1-adrenergic stimulation. However, anti-sense oligonucleotides to Mn-SOD, which inhibited the induction of Mn-SOD by norepinephrine, abolished the expected decrease in CK release from hypoxia-reoxygenated myocytes (Fig. 9-3b).

Conclusion

In this review article, we described our recent findings showing that Mn-SOD induction in cardiac myocytes plays a pivotal role in the acquisition of tolerance to ischemia in the second window of protection in ischemic preconditioning phenomenon. Furthermore, we revealed that:

1) Not only ischemic (hypoxic) preconditioning, heat shock and α1-adrenergic stimulation also induced tolerance of myocytes to hypoxia via Mn-SOD induction.

2) Although HSP72 was also induced in cardiac myocytes, inhibition of the Mn-SOD induction alone abolished the tolerance specifically.

3) A protein kinase C blocker, staurosporine, attenuated the Mn-SOD induction.

Taken these results together, Mn-SOD induction by α1-adrenergic stimulation, heat stress or hypoxia through protein kinase c pathway is one of the key mechanisms by which cardiac myocytes respond to the exogenous stresses and acquire the tolerance to ischemia as an adaptation process.

References

1. Brown JM, White CW, Terada LS et al. Interleukin 1 pretreatment decreases ischemia/reperfusion injury. Proc Natl Acad Sci USA 1990;87: 5026-5030.
2. Eddy LJ, Goeddel DV, Wong GHW. Tumor necrosis factor-a pretreatment is protective in a rat model of myocardial ischemia-reperfusion injury. Biochem Biophys Res Commun 1992;184: 1056-1059.
3. Murry CE, Jennings RB, Reimer KA. Preconditioning with ischemia: a delay of lethal cell injury in ischemic myocardium. Circulation 1986;74: 1124-1136.
4. Yellon DM, Pasini E, Cargnoni A et al. The protective role of heat stress in the ischaemic and reperfused rabbit myocardium. J Mol Cell Cardiol 1992;24: 895-907.
5. Garlick PB, Davies MJ, Hearse DJ et al. Direct detection of free radicals in the reperfused rat heart using electron spin resonance. Circ Res 1987;61: 757-760.
6. Zweier JL, Flaherty JT, Weisfeldt ML. Direct measurement of free radical generation following reperfusion of ischemic myocardium. Proc Natl Acad Sci USA 1987;84:1404-1407.
7. Kuzuya T, Hoshida S, Kim Y et al. Detection of oxygen-derived free radical generation in the canine postischemic heart during late phase of reperfusion. Circ Res 1990;66: 1160-1165.
8. Opie LH. Reperfusion injury and its pharmacologic modification. Circulation 1989;80: 1049-1062.
9. Hoshida S, Kuzuya T, Fuji H et al. Sublethal ischemia alters myocardial antioxidant activity in canine heart. Am J Physiol. 1993;264: H33-H39.
10. Kuzuya T, Hoshida S, Yamashita N et al. Delayed effects of sublethal ischemia on the acquisition of tolerance to ischemia. Circ Res 1993;72: 1293-1299.
11. Yamashita N, Nishida M, Hoshida S et al. Induction of manganese superoxide dismutase in rat cardiac myocytes increases tolerance to hypoxia 24 hours after preconditioning. J Clin Invest 1994;94: 2193-2199.
12. Hutter MM, Sievers RE, Barbosa V et al. Heat-shock protein induction in rat hearts. A direct correlation between the amount of heat-shock protein induced and the degree of myocardial protection. Circulation 1994;89: 355-360.

13. Yamashita N, Nishida M, Hoshida S et al. a1-adrenergic stimulation induced tolerance of cardiac myocytes to hypoxia through induction and activation of manganese superoxide dismutase. Am J Physiol 1996(In Press).

In: Mentzer, R.M., Jr., Kitakaze, M., Downey, J.M., Hori, M, eds. Adenosine, Cardioprotection and Clinical Application. Kluwer Academic Publishers, Norwell, MA, USA, 1997.

10. Opioid Receptors, K_{ATP} Channels and Ischemic Preconditioning

Garrett J. Gross
Jo El Schultz

Introduction

ATP-gated potassium channels (K_{ATP}) were initially identified in the myocardium by Noma[1] using patch clamp methodology in isolated guinea pig ventricular myocytes. Since its discovery, a number of factors and endogenous substances such as the ATP/ADP ratio, certain nucleotide diphosphates, Mg++, lactate, pH, protein kinase C, adenosine and bradykinin have been shown to modulate the gating properties of this channel in the heart.[2] Since K_{ATP} channel activity is regulated by the metabolic state of the myocardial cell, Noma[1] originally proposed that this channel would serve an endogenous cardioprotective function. Subsequently, it was shown that K_{ATP} channel opening produced by ischemia resulted in certain characteristic electrophysiological alterations including a shortening of the ventricular action potential duration (APD) and an attenuation of the rate of membrane depolarization. These changes would be expected to result in a decreased rate of calcium influx via voltage-sensitive calcium channels and sodium-calcium exchange and reduce calcium overload and lethal cell injury if timely reperfusion were to occur. A number of studies support this hypothesis, although several recent reports suggest that APD shortening is not essential in mediating the cardioprotective effect of K_{ATP} channel opening against myocardial infarction or stunning.[3,4] Nevertheless, based upon numerous studies from several laboratories and several species, there is little doubt that the K_{ATP} channel serves an important cardioprotective role during ischemic or hypoxic insults.

Ischemic Preconditioning (PC) - Is the K_{ATP} Channel a Universal Mediator?

Gross and Auchampach[5] were the first investigators to demonstrate a role for the K_{ATP} channel in ischemic PC using myocardial infarct size reduction as the indicator of protection in the canine heart. These investigators found that administration of glibenclamide, a selective K_{ATP} channel antagonist, either prior to or following a 5-minute PC stimulus completely blocked the cardioprotective effects of PC in the dog. Similarly, Auchampach et al.[6] also found that intracoronary administration of glibenclamide or sodium 5-hydroxydecanoate (5-HD) only during PC or following PC also blocked its protective effect. These results suggest that the K_{ATP} channel is both a trigger as well as an end effector of the PC response in the canine heart. Other investigators have also provided evidence that the myocardial K_{ATP} channel mediates the cardioprotective effect of PC in many species including pigs, rabbits and humans. In contrast, Liu and Downey[7] were unable to show that the K_{ATP} channel was involved in ischemic PC in the intact rat heart which cast doubt on the concept that the K_{ATP} channel is a universal mediator of ischemic PC in all animal species. However, recent data of Findlay[8] suggest that the pharmacokinetic properties of glibenclamide binding to its receptor in cardiac membranes may help explain this discrepancy between species. Findlay[8] found that glibenclamide had a slow onset of action and slow recovery in binding and unbinding to cardiac membranes and that this was concentration dependent. In the experiments performed by Liu and Downey,[7] glibenclamide was only given 5 minutes prior to the ischemic PC stimulus. If the slow kinetics of glibenclamide binding to cardiac cells in vitro has a counterpart in vivo, this time period may not have been sufficient to achieve the complete K_{ATP} channel blocking activity of glibenclamide prior to coronary artery occlusion in the rat.

In this regard, recent experiments in our laboratory addressed this possibility and the results are shown in Figure 10-1. In 4 groups of rats subjected to 30 minutes of left coronary artery occlusion and 2 hours of reperfusion, it was noted that 3 five-minute periods of PC ischemia interspersed with five-minute periods of reperfusion produced a marked reduction in infarct size from 53 + 3% to 8 + 1%, which further demonstrates the marked cardioprotective effect of PC in the intact rat heart. In agreement with Liu and Downey,[7] we found that a five-minute pretreatment with 0.3 mg/kg, iv of glibenclamide prior to PC did not block its cardioprotective effect (11 + 3% IS/AAR), however, when glibenclamide was administered 30 minutes prior to PC, this compound abolished the protective effect of ischemic PC to reduce infarct size (46 + 11%).

Thus, these results indicate that the K_{ATP} channel has an important role in mediating ischemic PC in the rat heart similar to that previously observed in other species and the data suggest that the K_{ATP} channel appears to be a universal mediator of ischemic PC in all species studied thus far.

Involvement of Endogenous Opioids in Ischemic PC

Recent evidence has revealed the involvement of the endogenous opioid system in protecting several organ systems from hypoxic or ischemic insults.[9,10] Mayfield and D'Alecy[9] showed that several intermittent brief periods of hypoxia induced an

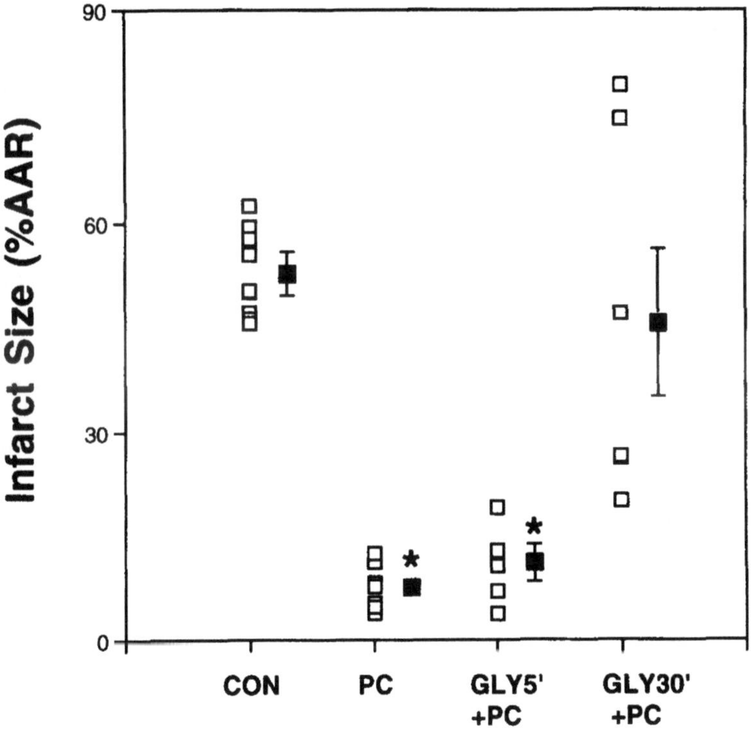

FIGURE 10-1. Infarct size (IS) in rat hearts subjected to vehicle treatment (controls, CON) and 3 five minute periods of ischemic preconditioning (PC) prior to a prolonged 30 minute period of coronary artery occlusion and 2 hours of reperfusion. In 2 additional groups, the K_{ATP} antagonist glibenclamide (GLY) was administered either 5 minutes prior to PC (GLY 5'+PC) or 30 minutes prior to PC (GLY 30' + PC). All open boxes represent values of IS expressed as a percent of the area at risk for each individual animal, whereas the closed boxes represent the mean + SEM for each group (N=6-8 rats/ group). *P<0.05 versus the CON group.

acute adaptive response to a subsequent more prolonged hypoxic challenge in mice and they presented evidence that an endogenous opioid pathway was responsible for this increased tolerance to hypoxia. Chien et al.[8] also demonstrated that opioids, most notably the synthetic enkephalin derivative [D-Ala2-D-Leu5] enkephalin, which activates δ-opioid receptors resulted in increased tissue preservation and survival time when administered to organs prior to transplantation. Based on these results, we proposed that endogenous opioids may also be involved in the ischemic PC response and tested this hypothesis in intact rats by using the nonselective opioid receptor antagonist naloxone.[11] It was found that naloxone administered at a dose of 3 mg/kg, iv 10 minutes prior to the 30 minute occlusion period had no effect on infarct size in nonpreconditioned rats (49 + 3%) as compared to controls (45 + 2%). However, when this same dose of naloxone was administered either 15 minutes prior to the first of 3 ischemic PC stimuli or following the last PC stimulus, it completely abolished the protective effect of ischemic PC which suggested a role for the endogenous opioid system in PC, at least in the rat. These results also suggest that opioid receptors are involved in both triggering and maintaining the PC response similar to that observed with the K_{ATP} channel in the dog.[5]

K_{ATP} Channels Mediate the Cardioprotective Effects of Opioid Receptor Activation in PC

Opioid receptors have been shown to be linked to various ion channels via G proteins. More specifically, the mu (μ) and delta (δ) opioid receptors have been shown to be linked via a Gi protein to several potassium channels[12] in atrial tissue which are regulated differently by both protein kinase A and protein kinase C. Recent evidence also indicates a possible interaction of μ and δ receptors to produce antinociception via the K_{ATP} channel.[13] These potential mechanisms and mediators which may be involved in theoretically transducing opioid receptor-induced cardioprotection are summarized in Figure 10-2.

Recent studies from our laboratory[14] have further addressed the role of some of these mechanisms in mediating opioid receptor-induced PC in the rat heart and these data are summarized in Figure 10-3. Interestingly, it was found that 3 five-minute infusions of the nonselective opioid agonist morphine at 100 μg/kg, iv interspersed with 3 five-minute drug-free periods prior to the prolonged 30 minute occlusion period in rats resulted in a reduction in infarct size similar to that of ischemic PC (12 + 5 versus 9 + 1%). This effect of morphine was completely blocked by glibenclamide pretreatment (Fig. 10-3). These data suggest that opioid receptors may be using the K_{ATP} channel as an important effector of the PC response in the rat myocardium. Obviously, more studies are necessary in the rat

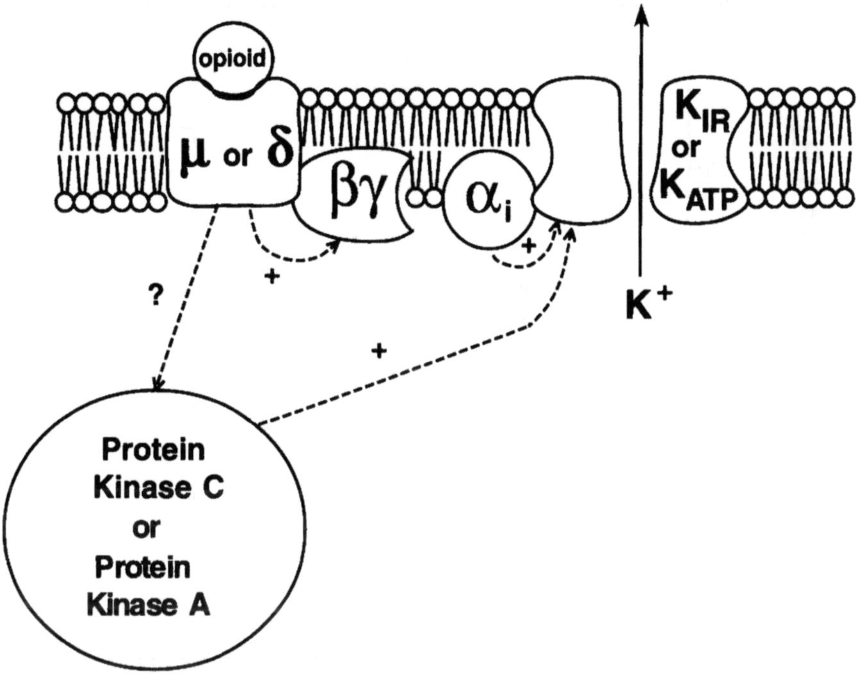

FIGURE 10-2. A schematic diagram representing possible signal transduction pathways by which stimulation of μ or δ opioid receptors may produce cardioprotection in the myocardium.

and other species using more specific receptor agonists and antagonists as well as bacterial toxins and certain molecular biological techniques to more clearly determine the signal transduction pathways involved in opioid receptor-mediated cardioprotection.

Conclusion

The ATP-gated potassium channel (K_{ATP}) has been clearly shown to be involved in both initiating and maintaining the cardioprotective effect of ischemic preconditioning (PC) in most animal species in which infarct size has been used as the endpoint of ischemic injury with the notable exception of the rat. However, recent evidence from our laboratory has demonstrated that the K_{ATP} channel antagonist glibenclamide blocks ischemic PC in the rat and that the inhibitory effect of glibenclamide is importantly dependent on the time interval between drug

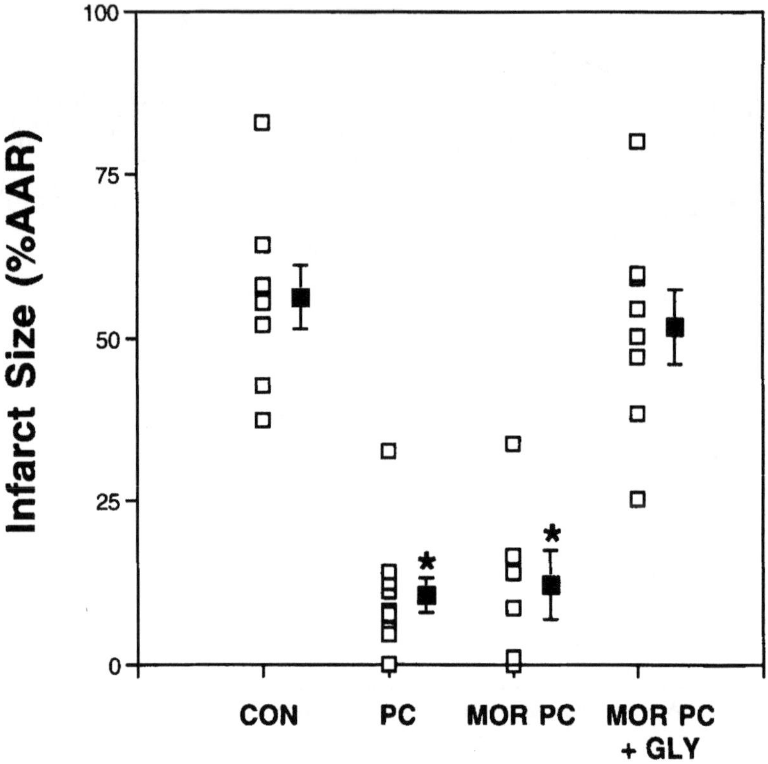

FIGURE 10-3. Infarct size (IS) in rat hearts subjected to vehicle treatment (CON), ischemic preconditioning (PC), morphine-induced preconditioning (3 x 100 μg/kg, 5 minute iv infusions, MOR PC) and glibenclamide (0.3 mg/kg, iv, GLY + MOR PC) given 30 minutes prior to MOR PC. Open squares indicate infarct sizes from individual hearts. Filled squares indicate the mean + SEM for each group (N=6-8 rats/group). *P<0.05 versus the CON group.

administration and the PC stimulus. Furthermore, we have identified a key role for the endogenous opioid system in mediating PC in this species and have evidence that K_{ATP} channels play an important role in opioid receptor-induced cardioprotection. These data suggest that the K_{ATP} channel may be a universal effector in the PC response and that currently available opioids such as morphine may be used clinically to elicit PC in man for therapeutic benefit.

Acknowledgments

The authors would like to thank Anna Hsu, Jeannine Moore and Carol Knapp for their excellent technical assistance and typing in the preparation of this chapter. The research results reported from the author's laboratory were supported by USPHS grant HL 08311 and an Advanced Predoctoral Fellowship from the Ph MRA Foundation.

References

1. Noma A. ATP-regulated K+ channels in cardiac muscle. Nature 1983;305: 147-148.
2. Nichols CG, Lederer WJ. Adenosine-triphosphate sensitive potassium channels in the cardiovascular system. Am J Physiol 1991;262:H1675-H1686.
3. Yao Z, Gross GJ. Effects of the K_{ATP} channel opener bimakalim on coronary blood flow, monophasic action potential duration and infarct size in dogs. Circulation 1994;89:1769-1775.
4. Grover GJ, D'Alonzo AJ, Parham CS et al. Cardioprotection with the K_{ATP} opener cromakalim is not correlated with ischemic myocardial action potential shortening. J Cardiovasc Pharmacol 1995;26:145-152.
5. Gross GJ, Auchampach JA. Blockade of ATP-sensitive potassium channels prevents myocardial preconditioning in dogs. Circ Res 1992;70:223-233.
6. Auchampach JA, Grover GJ, Gross GJ. Blockade of ischemic preconditioning in dogs by the novel ATP dependent potassium channel antagonist 5-hydroxydecanoate. Cardiovasc Res 1992;26:1054-1062.
7. Liu Y, Downey JM. Ischemic preconditioning protects against infarction in rat hearts. Am J Physiol1992;1 263:H1107-H-1112.
8. Findlay I. Inhibition of ATP-sensitive K+ channels in cardiac muscle by the sulfonyluyrea drug glibenclamide. J Pharmacol Exp Ther 1992;261: 540-545.
9. Mayfield KP, D'Alecy LG. Delta-1 opioid agonist acutely increases hypoxic tolerance. J Pharmacol Exp Ther 1994;268: 74-77.
10. Chien S, Oeltgen PR, Diana JN et al. Extension of tissue survival time in multiorgan block preparation with a delta opioid DADLE ([D-Ala2, D-Leu5]-enkephalin). J Thoracic Cardiovasc Surg 1994;107:964-967.
11. Schultz JJ, Rose E, Yao Z et al. Evidence for the involvement of opioid receptors in ischemic preconditioning in the rat heart. Am J Physiol 1995;268:H2157-H2161.
12. Chen Y, Yu L. Differential regulation by cAMP-dependent protein kinase and protein kinase C of the μ opioid receptor coupling to a G protein-activated K+ channel. J Biol Chem 1994;269:7839-7842.
13. Welch SP, Dunlow LD. Antinociceptive activity of intrathecally administered potassium channel openers and opioid agonists: a common mechanism of action? J Pharmacol Exp Ther 1993;267:390-399.
14. Schultz JJ, Hsu AK, Gross GJ. Morphine mimics the cardioprotective effect of ischemic preconditioning via a glibenclamide-sensitive mechanism in the rat heart. Circ Res 1996;78:1100-1104.

In: Mentzer, R.M., Jr., Kitakaze, M., Downey, J.M., Hori, M, eds. Adenosine, Cardioprotection and Clinical Application. Kluwer Academic Publishers, Norwell, MA, USA, 1997.

11. Bradykinin and Preconditioning Against Infarction

Tetsuji Miura
Jun Sakamoto
Takayuki Miki

Introduction

Bradykinin is a peptide consisting of nine amino acids, which is generated by the plasma kallikrein-kinin system as well as the glandular (tissue) kallikrein-kinin system and plasma aminopeptidase (Fig. 11-1). There are at least two classes of bradykinin receptors, i.e. B1 and B2 receptors, and bradykinin exerts its action on most of the cardiovascular system through B2 receptors. Although bradykinin production in ischemic myocardium was first reported almost 30 years ago, the significance of kinin in myocardial ischemic injury did not receive wide-spread attention for decades. Recently, a specific and potent B2 receptor antagonist Hoe 140 (icatibant) became available, and several important aspects of bradykinin in the pathophysiology of myocardial ischemia have been clarified in the past several years. Firstly, it has been suggested that activation of the B2 receptor before ischemia may protect the heart against ischemia/reperfusion injury, including arrhythmia, contractile dysfunction and necrosis. Secondly, bradykinin may play a role in an endogenous cardioprotective mechanism, ischemic preconditioning (i.e. cardioprotective effect of brief transient non-lethal ischemia). This article briefly reviews the involvement of bradykinin in the enhancement of myocardial tolerance against infarction by ischemic preconditioning.

Evidence for Involvement of Kallikrein-kinin System in Preconditioning

The first study suggesting the role of bradykinin in preconditioning was by Wall et al.[1] They found that infarct size limitation by preconditioning was blocked by

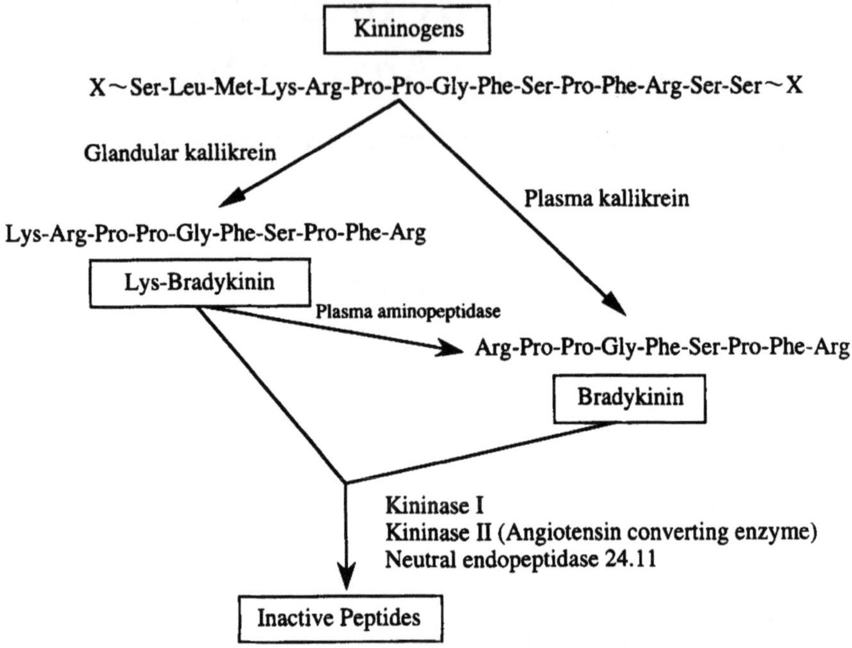

FIGURE 11-1. A simplified scheme of the kallikrein-kinin system

Hoe 140 administered before the preconditioning, and this observation was also confirmed in our laboratory (Fig. 11-2A). We also found that Hoe 140 does not modify preconditioning when administered after preconditioning, which suggests that the B2 receptor is important for triggering preconditioning, but its activation is not necessary during sustained ischemia for cardioprotection. Another line of evidence supporting the importance of bradykinin in preconditioning was obtained from experiments using aprotinin, an inhibitor of kallikrein. When rabbits were pretreated with aprotinin (2000 units/kg/min for 20 min plus 500 units/kg/min for 30 min), infarct size limitation by preconditioning was significantly attenuated as shown in Figure 11-2B. Aprotinin is a serine protease inhibitor, which is not very selective to kallikrein, and the inhibitory effect of aprotinin on preconditioning was not as potent as Hoe 140. Nevertheless, the attenuation of preconditioning by aprotinin supports the importance of bradykinin in the mechanism of preconditioning.

These results using Hoe 140 and aprotinin (Figs. 11-2A,B) suggest that the production of bradykinin and activation of B2 receptors play a crucial role in preconditioning. However, this does not necessarily mean that bradykinin is

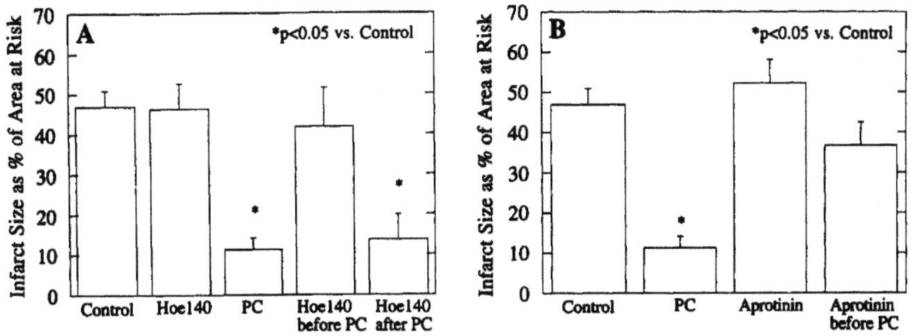

FIGURE 11-2: A) Effect of Hoe 140 (a B2 receptor antagonist) and aprotinin (a kallikrein inhibitor) on the infarct size limiting effect of preconditioning (PC) in the rabbit. Infarct was induced by 30 min coronary occlusion and 3 hr reperfusion. PC was performed with 5 min ischemia/5 min reperfusion. Hoe 140 (2μg/kg) was injected intravenously before or after preconditioning. B) Aprotinin was infused for 50 min (total dose = 55,000 units/kg) before the 30 min ischemia with or without PC. *$p<0.05$ vs Control. Bar represent 1 SE. See text for details.

produced in the myocardium during a brief period of preconditioning ischemia. To get an insight into this question, we took an indirect approach, since direct determination of bradykinin production in the myocardium undergoing preconditioning is technically impossible. If the level of bradykinin production during preconditioning is a critical determinant of preconditioning protection, kininase inhibitors should be able to lower the threshold of preconditioning ischemia for the preconditioning to be protective. To test this possibility, we assessed the effect of captopril, a kininase II inhibitor, on preconditioning with 2 min ischemia/5 min reperfusion.[2] Infarct size limitation by preconditioning with 2 min ischemia was very slight (approximately 20% reduction in infarct size). However, when the heart was pretreated with 1 mg/kg of captopril before 2 min-preconditioning, infarct size was limited by 50%, a level of protection which is equivalent to preconditioning with 5 min ischemia. This dose of captopril reduced systemic blood pressure by only 10 mmHg, which cannot explain its effect on preconditioning. Furthermore, the enhancement of 2 min-preconditioning by captopril was inhibitable by Hoe 140. Interestingly, the arterial bradykinin level was not changed by this dose of captopril with or without preconditioning, suggesting that production of bradykinin relevant to preconditioning occurs locally in the heart.

However, there are a number of questions regarding the contribution of the kallikrein-kinin system to preconditioning remain unanswered. Firstly, there is still no direct evidence of bradykinin production during preconditioning, although there have been a number of studies showing kinin release from the myocardium during a relatively long period of ischemia *in vitro* and *in vivo*. Secondly, it is not clear which of the two kallikrein systems (i.e. plasma or glandular) is mainly responsible for bradykinin production during preconditioning. The plasma kallikrein-kinin system in the vascular lumen in the ischemic myocardium might be able to produce sufficient bradykinin to trigger preconditioning. However, the contribution of a glandular, i.e. tissue kallikrein-kinin system in the cardiomyocytes and vasculature may also be important. Thirdly, the mechanism of the kallikrein system activation during myocardial ischemia is still unknown, although tissue acidosis might be a contributory factor.

Relationship Between Bradykinin and Adenosine in Preconditioning

In addition to bradykinin, at least four active substances (adenosine, free radicals, norepinephrine, and opioids) are currently proposed to be involved in preconditioning against infarction. Of these substances, adenosine has been most well characterized for its role in preconditioning.[3] Elevation of interstitial adenosine by preconditioning, inhibition of preconditioning by adenosine receptor blockers, and infarct limitation by adenosine receptor agonists have been confirmed in several animal models. All these findings support the importance of the adenosine receptor in triggering the preconditioning mechanism. Adenosine receptor activation may also play a crucial role during sustained ischemia for the preconditioning to be protective. This possibility was suggested by Thornton et al.[4] who found that inhibition of the adenosine receptor using PD115,199, *after* preconditioning significantly attenuated the infarct size limiting effect of preconditioning. We also confirmed their finding by using 8-sulphophenyl-theophylline as an adenosine receptor blocker (unpublished observation). These findings contrast the failure of Hoe140 to block preconditioning when it was given after preconditioning (Fig. 11-2A).

Findings that cardioprotection by preconditioning with 5 min ischemia is completely abolished by either adenosine or B2 receptor antagonists raise a following question: "Is there any dependence between adenosine-induced and B2 receptor-induced mechanisms in preconditioning?" Since the plasma kallikrein-kinin system has a considerable capacity for producing bradykinin, it appears unlikely that adenosine receptor activation is necessary for bradykinin production during ischemic preconditioning. Thus, we examined the possibility that B2 receptor activation may somehow augment adenosine production during preconditioning ischemia.[5] Using a microdialysis technique, we assessed the effect of Hoe 140, at a dose sufficient to abolish the infarct size-limiting effect of preconditioning, on the interstitial adenosine level in the heart *in vivo*. As shown

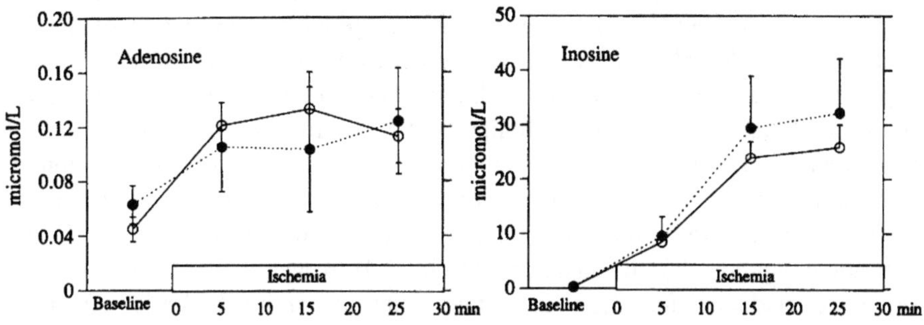

FIGURE 11-3. Profiles of adenosine and inosine in the dialysate before and during 30 min-coronary occlusion. Open circles are data from the controls (n = 9) and filled circles are those from the rabbits which received 2μg/kg of Hoe 140 before the onset of ischemia (n = 5). The time-course of the nucleoside levels was not significantly different between the two study groups (p = NS by two-way repeated measures analysis of variance). Bar represent 1 SE.

in Figure 11-3, ischemia-induced elevation of adenosine and inosine were not reduced by Hoe 140, which did not support our hypothesis. Rather these results suggest that activation of the adenosine and B2 receptors are probably independent during preconditioning.

Intracellular Mechanism of Preconditioning and the Role of the B2 Receptor

Although the intracellular mechanism of cardioprotection by preconditioning remains unclear, an attractive current hypothesis is activation of protein kinase C. This hypothesis was proposed by Downey and his colleagues from the findings that preconditioning against infarction was completely blocked by protein kinase inhibitors (staurosporine and polymyxin B), and conversely was mimicked by protein kinase C activators in a rabbit model of infarction. Recently, we obtained results suggesting that protein kinase C activation by preconditioning is through A1 receptor stimulation.[6] Administration of 1 mg/kg of R-phenylisopropyl-adenosine, an A1 receptor agonist, before ischemia limited infarct size by 50% in a rabbit model of infarction, and this cardioprotection was completely abolished by staurosporine and polymyxin B. These results support the existence of a link between the A1 receptor and protein kinase C in the mechanism of preconditioning.

The involvement of protein kinase C is also suggested in cardioprotection triggered by B2 receptor activation in preconditioning. Goto et al.[7] found that infarct size limitation by intracoronary injection of bradykinin before ischemia was completely blocked by protein kinase C inhibitors. In addition to protein kinase C activation, a number of cellular events are triggered by stimulation of the B2 receptor in endothelial cells and cardiomyocytes; activation of the inositol triphosphate pathway increases intracellular calcium release, which induces nitric oxide and activation of phospholipase A2, leading to the production of prostaglandins E2 and I2. However, both preconditioning and infarct limitation by bradykinin were not blocked by nitric oxide synthase inhibitors or by cyclooxygenase inhibitors, suggesting that nitric oxide and prostanoids do not contribute to preconditioning against infarction. However, it should be noted that there is evidence for their important roles in anti-arrhythmic effect of preconditioning.[8]

How does protein kinase C activation lead to enhancement of myocardial tolerance against ischemic necrosis? Intriguing metabolic features in the preconditioned myocardium are a reduction in ATP utilization rate and a slowed accumulation of protons, sodium and calcium during ischemia.[9,10] Reduced ATP utilization would preserve ATP and reduce the production of protons from degradation of ATP generated by anaerobic glycolysis. Suppression of proton accumulation during ischemia would attenuate sodium-proton exchange and consequently sodium-calcium exchange, leading to a delay in calcium overload in the ischemic myocytes. The effects of bradykinin on the energy metabolism in an ischemic myocardium appears similar to the effects of preconditioning. Linz et al.[11] and Zhu et al[12] found in isolated rat heart preparations that pre-ischemic administration of bradykinin suppresses the depletion of high energy phosphates and accumulation of lactate during ischemia. However, it remains unclear whether these apparently cardioprotective changes in metabolism is the cause or the result of cardioprotection and whether they are protein kinase C-mediated.

References

1. Wall TM, Sheehy R, Hartman JC. Role of bradykinin in myocardial preconditioning. J Pharmacol Exp Ther 1994;270:681-9.
2. Miki T, Miura T, Ogawa T et al. Captopril, a kininase II inhibitor, lowers the threshold of preconditioning through B2 receptor mediate mechanism. [Abstract] Circulation 1995;92 (suppl.I):I-455.
3. Downey JM, Miura T. "The role of adenosine in ischemic preconditioning." In Cardiac Adaptation and Failure, Hori M, Maruyama Y, Reneman RS, ed. Tokyo: Springer-Verlag, 1994.
4. Thornton JD, Thornton CS, Downey JM. Effect of adenosine receptor blockade: preventing protective preconditioning depends on time of initiation. Am J Physiol 1993;265:H504-8.
5. Miura T. Adenosine and bradykinin: Are they independent triggers of preconditioning? Basic Res Cardiol 1996;91:20-2.

6. Sakamoto J, Miura T, Goto M et al. Limitation of myocardial infarct size by adenosine A1-receptor activation is abolished by protein kinase C inhibitors in the rabbit. Cardiovasc Res 1995;29:682-8.
7. Goto M, Liu Y, Yang X-M et al. Role of bradykinin in protection of ischemic preconditioning in rabbit hearts. Circ Res 1995;77:611-21.
8. Parratt JR. Protection of the heart by ischemic preconditioning: mechanisms and possibilities for pharmacological exploitation. TiPS 1994;15:15-25.
9. Murry CE, Richard VJ, Reimer KA et al. Ischemic preconditioning slows energy metabolism and delays ultrastructural damage during a sustained ischemic episode. Circ Res 1990;66:913-31.
10. Steenbergen C, Perlman ME, London RE et al. Mechanism of preconditioning. Ionic alterations. Circ Res 1993;72:112-25.
11. Linz W, Wiemer G, Scholkens BA. Role of kinins in the pathophysiology of myocardial ischemia. In vitro and in vivo studies. Diabetes 1996;45 (Suppl.I):S51-8.
12. Zhu P, Zaugg CE, Simper D et al. Bradykinin improves postischaemic recovery in the rat heart: role of high energy phosphates, nitric oxide and prostacyclin. Cardiovasc Res 1995;29:658-63.

In: Mentzer, R.M., Jr., Kitakaze, M., Downey, J.M., Hori, M, eds. Adenosine, Cardioprotection and Clinical Application. Kluwer Academic Publishers, Norwell, MA, USA, 1997.

12. Preconditioning in Human Muscle and Myocytes

Cornelia S Carr
Derek M Yellon

Introduction

When the heart is subjected to brief periods of sublethal ischemia separated by reperfusion it becomes resistant to a more prolonged lethal ischemic insult, a phenomenon which has been shown to protect it against infarction, reperfusion arrhythmias, contractile dysfunction and contracture.[1-4] This endogenous protective mechanism has been termed ischemic preconditioning,[1] and appears to occur in all animal species studied,[2,5-7] including man.[8,9] The protection produced by ischemic preconditioning is very potent but is short lived and decreases with time, lasting for an hour in most species. However a delayed or second window of protection (SWOP) has also been observed as a consequence of ischemic preconditioning; this protection occurs many hours after the sublethal preconditioning ischemia.[10-14] The underlying mechanisms via which ischemic preconditioning protects the heart have been partly characterised in both animals and in the human, and appears to involve adenosine receptor activation, protein kinase C mediation and the possible opening of ATP-dependent-potassium (K_{ATP}) channels. If the exact mechanism of preconditioning in man could be determined, then it might be possible to develop preconditioning-like pharmacological therapies for patients at risk of certain cardiovascular disorders.

Although a limited number of human studies have been performed, it is not easy to adapt these in order to investigate the underlying mechanisms of ischemic preconditioning, therefore in vitro human muscle preparations have been developed which allow for the study of this phenomenon in greater detail. These have included isolated muscle and isolated cardiomyocyte preparations in which the investigation for the presence or absence of various ligand receptors and ion channels have been undertaken.

In addition, direct studies in patients undergoing coronary artery bypass surgery and percutaneous transluminal coronary angioplasty (PTCA) have been used to assess whether preconditioning could be of any advantage to patients. Finally, retrospective analysis of patients with pre-infarction angina has also been used to determine if prior ischemia has any beneficial effect on outcome.

In this chapter we shall briefly discuss each of these settings, with their limitations, and then concentrate on the use of the human muscle and myocyte preparations to ascertain the importance of using these models to assess preconditioning in man. Finally we conclude this chapter with the investigation of the underlying mechanisms associated with preconditioning in the human.

Human Models of Preconditioning: In Vivo Evidence

Angioplasty Model

Percutaneous transluminal coronary angioplasty provides an opportunity to study the human heart with respect to controlled regional ischemia and reperfusion. It has been shown that repeated balloon inflations cause less chest pain, less ST segment elevation and less lactate production than with the first balloon inflation.[15] However these studies must be interpreted with some caution, both because of the short periods of ischemia involved (less than 2 minutes) and the possible beneficial effects of increased collateral flow as a consequence of the first balloon inflation. Deutsch et al did show that cardiac vein flow was lower during the second balloon inflation suggesting that adaptation to ischemia was probably not due to an increase in coronary collateral blood flow.[15] These results have been confirmed by other groups. Tomai et al produced similar results but did not measure coronary collateral blood flow.[16] Although Cribier et al showed similar reductions in severity of angina and degree of ST segment elevation, they found that in 10 of the 17 patients the coronary collateral angiographic grade increased, so that acute recruitment of coronary collateral flow may have lead to the improvements observed.[17] There are however problems with the angioplasty model which need to be noted. The duration of the ischemia is often considered too small to precondition the myocardium. A further criticism is the selection of soft end points such as ECG changes and anginal pain. Pre-inflation ischemia should be avoided; this could occur as a consequence of an uninflated balloon lying across the lesion giving confounding results. Finally it is also important to allow for adequate reperfusion at the end of the first inflation in order to establish baseline haemodynamic and electrocardiographic conditions prior to the next inflation. Despite these points angioplasty does offer the possibility of controlled ischemia in the patient which mechanistically can be used to our advantage in the study of preconditioning in the clinical setting.

Prodromal Angina Model

Studies of pre-infarction angina 24-48 hours before an acute myocardial infarction have provided evidence for both a positive and negative effect on the outcome following myocardial infarction. Ottani et al[18] showed that infarct size as assessed by peak creatine kinase (CK) MB fraction was lower in patients with previous angina (within the preceding 24 hours) compared to those without. The number of hypokinetic segments was smaller in the angina group and angiography showed no evidence of collateral flow.[18] Data from the TIMI-4 study, showed that patients with angina preceding infarction by 48 hours or with a history of angina had a lower in-hospital death rate, decreased frequency of severe congestive heart failure and smaller infarct size using serial CK measurements. Again on angiography, no increased collateral blood flow was seen in these patients.[19] This data provides some supportive evidence for the possibility of preconditioning occurring in man. However it should be noted that patients with a history of angina preceding myocardial infarction are more likely to have multivessel coronary artery disease and some studies have shown worse long-term prognosis.[20]. Most of the studies showing a negative effect are from the period prior to the use of thrombolytic therapy, however as reperfusion is necessary for the preconditioning phenomenon to be triggered, these findings should be considered with caution. However there are indeed studies from the thrombolytic era which also fail to show benefit.[21]

'Warm-Up' Angina Model

A situation in which acute tolerance to angina can develop. An initial effort induces angina, followed by a subsequent, equivalent effort which produces no angina with increased exercise tolerance.[22] It has been suggested that this could be due to the recruitment of collaterals that have developed as the result of the coronary artery disease, although Okazaki found no change in cardiac vein blood flow on a second exercise test 15 minutes after the first; but interestingly they found increased adenosine release during the second test.[23] Wayne and colleagues also found that the second effort reproducibly exceeded the first effort provided that these two were separated by a rest of at least 2-5 minutes but not more than 30-60 minutes; these time intervals being consistent with the warm up phenomenon being a possible form of ischemic preconditioning.[24] Thus although it is possible that warm-up could represent preconditioning, it should be borne in mind that small collaterals which cannot be visualised by coronary angiography or that do not reflect a change in great cardiac vein flow might "open-up" between the 2 exercise periods and that this rather than true preconditioning might explain the benefit.

Cardiac Surgery Model

This setting allows for the direct examination of human myocardium taken at operation. The only in vivo prospective study using a model of global ischemia, thereby eliminating changes in collateral blood flow, was that of Yellon's group[25] who examined whether a preconditioning protocol prior to cross-clamp fibrillation during coronary artery bypass surgery protects the myocardium from prolonged ischemia. Twenty patients were randomized into two groups. Patients randomized to preconditioning received a preconditioning stimulus of two 3 minute periods of cross-clamping separated by 2 minutes of reperfusion prior to the long 10 minute ischemic insult with ventricular fibrillation. The control patients received 10 minutes of cross-clamping with fibrillation only. During the 10 minutes cross-clamping distal aortocoronary anastomoses were performed. Myocardial ATP was determined from biopsy specimens taken at the onset of cardiopulmonary bypass, at the end of preconditioning, and at the end of the 10 minute ischemic insult. Preconditioning resulted in a significant depletion of the myocardial ATP content. The 10 minutes ischemia resulted in a significant depletion of ATP in the controls. Preconditioning appeared to slow down the rate of myocardial ATP depletion in the preconditioned group to such an extent that at the end of the 10 minutes ischemic insult, preconditioned hearts had a significantly higher ATP content than the controls. This study showed that preconditioning ultimately led to the preservation of adenosine triphosphate (ATP) levels in preconditioned human hearts; this is in keeping with the metabolic changes seen in animal models.[26] Yellon's group has more recently investigated whether preconditioning alters the release of troponin T, a sensitive and specific marker of myocardial injury in patients undergoing coronary artery bypass surgery, and found that preconditioned patients released significantly less troponin T into the blood at 72 hours post surgery.[27] Although this cardiac surgery model can clearly be used to demonstrate the ability to precondition patients in this setting it is not easily adapted to investigate the underlying mechanisms of ischemic preconditioning in the human. Therefore various in vitro models have now been developed.

In Vitro Evidence

Human Atrial Trabeculae Model

An in vitro human model of preconditioning has been developed in our laboratory using isolated human right atrial trabeculae. This model allows the underlying mechanisms to be investigated with greater ease.[28,29]

Although the original definition of preconditioning related to infarct size,[1] many investigators use recovery of function as an index of myocardial injury. The main end-point in this human muscle model is the recovery of contractile function rather than limitation of infarction, but this model has shown consistent results, is reproducible between investigators and appears to follow the criteria used to examine preconditioning in animal models.[28] Although the evidence is incomplete, it appears likely that improved recovery of function following a prolonged ischemic insult is dependent on infarct size limitation, rather than an anti-stunning effect.[30] It seems likely therefore that the improved functional recovery seen in this isolated muscle model of preconditioning reflects improved myocyte viability.

This human muscle model uses a period of simulated ischemia with hypoxic, substrate-free superfusion and rapid pacing, rather than 'true' ischemia used in most models of ischemic preconditioning. There is evidence that in animal models of both regional and global hypoxia and in cell culture, that hypoxia is as effective as 'true' ischemia in inducing preconditioning.[31,32] There are important differences between such models and true ischemia, particularly in respect to the washout of ischemic catabolites and pH changes. It is assumed that in atrial tissue, recovery of global function is proportional to infarct volume. It has been shown that enhanced recovery of function due to preconditioning following prolonged ischemia is due to infarct size reduction rather than due to stunning.[33] The isolated human atrial preparation uses 90 minutes of ischemia as the prolonged ischemic insult which is more likely to lead to cell death than stunning, although this cannot be ruled out.

In this model preconditioned trabeculae had a significantly improved post-ischemic recovery of contractile function compared to the non-preconditioned trabeculae, and the results of these experiments are similar between investigators.[28,29,34]

The advantages of using an isolated human model are that the confounding factor of collateral flow is eliminated, in addition to there being no ethical considerations involved in the use of experimental drugs in vitro. Atrial tissue was chosen for these experiments because it is readily available (at cannulation of the right atrium during cardiopulmonary bypass procedures), provides a stable preparation and is of good quality (disease free). The main disadvantage of this model is the use of human atrial muscle and not ventricular muscle. Furthermore it is function as opposed to infarct size limitation that is being used as the end-point. However it has recently been shown that it is possible to precondition human ventricular tissue in a similar manner to that of the atrium.[35]

Cell Culture Evidence

Ikonomidis and colleagues have demonstrated that it is possible to directly precondition isolated human cardiomyocytes.[36] Human ventricular biopsy material was obtained from Tetralogy of Fallot patients undergoing corrective surgery, and then grown in culture. After stabilisation cells were exposed to simulated ischemia for 90 minutes followed by reoxygenation for 30 minutes. The preconditioning protocol involved 20 minutes of simulated ischemia followed by 20 minutes of reoxygenation. Cellular injury was assessed by the exclusion of uptake of the dye, trypan blue, and survival was assessed by culturing the cells for 24 hours post-intervention. Preconditioned cells had reduced cell injury to the subsequent longer 90 minutes of simulated ischemia: preconditioned cells had less uptake of trypan blue and increased survival. This group also examined the supernatant from the cells, and found that the preconditioned cells had a lower hydrogen ion, lactate and lactic dehydrogenase concentration.[36]

Curry et al[37] have shown that hypoxaemia from birth in immature rabbits increases the tolerance of isolated hearts to ischemia compared to age-matched normoxaemic rabbits. Rabbits raised from birth in hypoxic conditions, displayed a significantly enhanced recovery of left ventricular developed pressure (LVDP) during reperfusion compared to age-matched normoxaemic rabbits. Taking Curry's work into account, one must apply caution to the human cell studies, in that Ikonomidis and colleagues may have cultured cardiomyocytes that were destined to be more resistant to hypoxia and may not be representative of normal human myocardium as they were removed from patients with congenital cyanotic heart disease who had been exposed to chronic hypoxia for the whole of their lives.

Evidence for Specific Mechanisms Involved in Human Preconditioning

Adenosine is released from many cells under stress due to the breakdown of high energy phosphates, and it is thought that adenosine may act as a local regulator or trigger, modulating the function of the cell via a 'feedback' mechanism. The adenosine released from ischemic myocytes is thought to act on a subclass of adenosine receptors A_1 and/or A_3 that may mediate their protective effect via a G protein, leading to the activation of protein kinase C (PKC).[38] The activated PKC then phosphorylates a secondary effector protein so inducing protection, probably by slowing cell metabolism and reducing ATP consumption. It has been suggested that the ATP-dependent potassium (K_{ATP}) channel may be the final end-effector, since the opening of these channels causes an influx of potassium which shortens the cardiac action potential and limits ATP depletion and calcium influx.[29,39,40]

Activation of Adenosine Receptors

There is a substantial body of evidence suggesting that adenosine plays a part in the mechanism of ischemic preconditioning although it is not clear how it specifically acts and which receptor subtypes are directly linked in triggering its protective response.

In the angioplasty model Tomai and colleagues have shown that the selective A_1-adenosine receptor antagonist Bamiphylline was able to abolish the reduction in anginal pain and ST elevation seen with the second balloon inflation in those patients not receiving Bamiphylline.[41] This suggests that the adaptation to ischemia in man appears to involve adenosine A_1 receptors.

The adenosine agonist R-phenyl-isopropyl-adenosine (R-PIA) has been shown to protect human atrial trabeculae to a similar extent as preconditioning, whereas the non-selective adenosine antagonist 8-p-sulfophenyltheophylline (SPT) blocked the protective effect of preconditioning without adversely affecting controls.[28]

Using the isolated cardiomyocyte model it has been shown that the exogenous administration of adenosine can mimic the protection of preconditioning; administration of the supernatant from preconditioned cells can protect other cardiomyocytes that have not undergone a preconditioning protocol, and that this protection can be blocked by the administration of SPT the adenosine receptor antagonist.[42]

Taking all these data into consideration they appear to provide direct evidence for the involvement of the adenosine receptor in preconditioning the human myocardium.

ATP-dependent potassium (K_{ATP}) channels

The other major hypothesis for the mechanism of ischemic preconditioning involves the K_{ATP} channel. The evidence for the involvement of K_{ATP} channels comes from a number of studies specifically using drugs that block these channels: glibenclamide and 5-hydroxydecanoate (5-HD).

In vivo human evidence for the involvement of the K_{ATP} channel in preconditioning does exist: a clinical study showed that glibenclamide prevented the preconditioning effect normally seen during repeat balloon inflation in the angioplasty model.[8] Furthermore Taggart et al have shown, in patients undergoing PTCA, that on second balloon inflation there was reduced ST segment elevation, and an associated increased action potential duration shortening, consistent with activation of the K_{ATP} channels.[43]

Using in vitro human muscle preparations we have shown that cromakalim, a K_{ATP} channel opener conferred protection in a similar manner to that of preconditioning.[29] In addition using this in vitro human atrial model it has been shown that the protection against contractile dysfunction, post-simulated ischemia, can be induced by activation of PKC. Activation of PKC with the selective PKC activator 1,2-dioctanoyl-sn-glycerol (DOG) resulted in a similar degree of myocardial protection as seen with preconditioning and this effect could be prevented when the PKC inhibitor chelerythrine was used.[29] More importantly the protection conferred by preconditioning and by the activation of PKC could be prevented by blockade of the K_{ATP} channels with glibenclamide.[29] These findings suggest that the early preconditioning effect in human muscle may involve PKC and that the K_{ATP} channel may be the final effector mechanism.

A further study confirming that isolated human atrial trabeculae can be protected from an ischemic insult by a highly selective K_{ATP} channel opener BMS 180448 comes from our group.[34] This study demonstrated that this particular K_{ATP} channel opener elicited a similar degree of protection to that of 'ischemic preconditioning.' Importantly the use of this compound resulted in a non-significant decrease in the developed force prior to the 90 minutes simulated ischemic insult, unlike that of our previous study using cromakalim.[29] In that study the use of cromakalim lead to a significant reduction in the developed force which did not recover prior to the 90 minutes hypoxia, so potentially producing its protective effect via a 'cardioplegia-like' effect as opposed to that of a true preconditioning effect.[29]

Receptors / Ion Channels

Heidbuchel isolated cells from human right atrial appendages, and studied potassium channel activity using the patch-clamp technique, and was able to distinguish three different types of potassium channels; although disease state or medication of the patients was not mentioned.[44]

Bohm and colleagues have performed experiments on cell membrane preparations from human atrial and ventricular myocardium and on isolated electrically stimulated human right atrial or left ventricular papillary muscle strips.[45] The tissue they examined was obtained during mitral valve replacement or heart transplantation. The disease states and medication were both recorded, but as these varied it may have altered the results of these experiments. They showed that adenosine receptors are present in the human heart, that the receptor subtype was the A1 receptor, and that it was present in both the atrial and ventricular tissue.[45]

Adenosine receptors[45] as well as K_{ATP} channels[44] are present in both human atrium and ventricle, although it is not known how the density varies. It does seem likely that human atrial and ventricular tissue can respond in a similar manner to ischemic preconditioning. The studies to date do not demonstrate specifically what functional significance these receptors and channels play or whether they are involved in ischemic preconditioning in patients at risk of myocardial infarction.

Conclusion

There is now reasonable evidence for the existence of the phenomenon of ischemic preconditioning in the human. This evidence now includes a number of in vivo, as well as in vitro studies. It will however be necessary, in the future, to undertake controlled prospective studies in order to ascertain whether the phenomenon of preconditioning can be of direct benefit to those patients at risk of myocardial infarction.

References

1. Murry CE, Jennings RB, Reimer KA. Preconditioning with ischaemia: a delay of lethal cell injury in ischaemic myocardium. Circulation 1986;74(5):1124-1136.
2. Asimakis GK, Inners-McBride K, Medelin G et al. Ischaemic preconditioning attenuates acidosis and postischaemic dysfunction in isolated rat heart. Am J Physiol 1992;32(3):H887-H892.
3. Shiki K, Hearse DJ. Preconditioning of ischaemic myocardium: Reperfusion-induced arrhythmias. Am J Physiol 1987;253:H1470-H1476.
4. Cohen M, Liu G, Downey J. Preconditioning causes improved wall motion as well as smaller infarcts after transient coronary occlusion in rabbits. Circulation 1991;84:341-9.
5. Downey JM, Liu GS, Thornton JD. Adenosine and the anti-infarct effects of preconditioning. Cardiovas Res 1993;27:3-8.
6. Murry CE, Richard VJ, Reimer KA et al. Ischaemic preconditioning slows energy metabolism and delays ultrastructural damage during a sustain ischaemic episode. Circulation Res 1990;66:913-931.

7. Kida M, Yokota R, Tanaka M. Effect of ischaemic preconditioning on energy metabolism during short sustained ischaemia and reperfusion in pig hearts. J Moll Cell Cardiol 1992;24(Suppl II):II-S.5.
8. Tomai F, Crea F, Gaspardone A et al. Ischaemic preconditioning during coronary angioplasty is prevented by glibenclamide, a selective ATP-sensitive K^+ channel blocker. Circulation 1994;90(2):700-705.
9. Yellon DM, Alkhulaifi AM, Pugsley WB. Preconditioning the human myocardium. The Lancet 1993;342(July 31):276-277.
10. Sun JZ, Tank XL, Knowlton AA et al. Late preconditioning against myocardial stunning. An endogenous protective mechanism that confers resistance to postischaemic dysfunction 24 hour after brief ischaemia in conscious dogs. J Clin Invest 1995;95(1):388-403, 1995.
11. Vegh A, Papp JG, Parratt JR. Prevention by dexamethasone of the marked antiarrhythmic effects of preconditioning induced 20 hour after rapid cardiac pacing. Br J Pharmacol 1994;113:1081-1082.
12. Marber MS, Latchman DS, Walker JM et al. Cardiac stress protein elevation 24 hours following brief ischaemia or heat stress is associated with resistance to myocardial infarction. Circulation 1993;88(3):1264-1272.
13. Kuzuya T, Hoshida S, Yamashita N et al. Delayed effects of sublethal ischaemia on the acquisition of tolerance to ischaemia. Circ Res 1993;72(6):1293-9.
14. Yellon DM, Baxter GF. A "second window of protection" or delayed preconditioning phenomenon: future horizons for myocardial protection? J Mol Cell Cardiol 1995;27:1023-1034.
15. Deutsch E, Berger M, Kussmaul W et al. Adaptation to ischaemia during percutaneous transluminal coronary angioplasty: clinical, haemodynamic, and metabolic features. Circulation 1990;82:2044-2051.
16. Tomai F, Crea F, Gaspardone A et al. Mechanisms of cardiac pain during coronary angioplasty. Journal American College Cardiology 1993;22(7):1892-1896.
17. Cribier A, Lorsatz L, Koning R et al. Improved myocardial ischaemic response and enhanced collateral circulation with long repetitive coronary occlusion during angioplasty: a prospective study. J Am Coll Cardiol 1992;20(3):578-86.
18. Ottani F, Galvani M, Ferrini D et al. Prodromal angina limits infarct size: a role for ischaemic preconditioning. Circulation 1995;91:291-297.
19. Kloner R, Shook T, Przyklenk K et al. Previous angina alters in-hospital outcome in TIMI 4: c clinical correlate to preconditioning? Circulation 1995;91:37-47.
20. Cupples L, Gagnon D, Wong N et al. Pre-existing cardiovascular conditions and long-term prognosis after initial myocardial infarction: the Framingham Study. Am Heart J 1993;125:863-72.
21. Barbash G, White H, Modan M et al. Antecedent angina pectoris predicts worse outcome after myocardial infarction in patients receiving thrombolytic therapy: experience gleaned from the international tissue plasminogen activator/streptokinase mortality trial. J Am Coll Cardiol 1992;20(1):36-41.
22. Joy M, Cairns A, Springings D. Observations on the warm up phenomenon in angina pectoris. British Heart Journal 1987;58:116-21.
23. Okazaki Y, Kodama K, Sato H et al. Attenuation of increased regional myocardial oxygen consumption during exercise as a major cause of warm-up phenomenon. J Am Coll Cardiol 1993;21:1597-604.
24. Wayne E, Laplace L. Observations on angina of effort. Clin Sci 1:103-29, 1993.
25. Alkhulaifi A, Yellon D, Pugsley W. Preconditioning the human heart during aortocoronary bypass surgery. Eur J Cardio-thoracic Surg 1994;8:270-276.
26. Reimer KA, Murry CE, Yamasawa I et al. Four brief periods of ischaemia causes no cumulative ATP loss or necrosis. Am J Physiol 1986;251(Heart Circulation Physiology):H1306-1315.
27. Jenkins D, Pugsley W, Kemp M et al. Ischaemic preconditioning reduces troponin-T release in patients undergoing cardiac surgery. Heart 1996.

28. Walker D, Walker J, Pugsley W et al. Preconditioning in isolated superfused human muscle. J Mol Cell Cardiol 1995;27:1-9.
29. Speechly-Dick ME, Grover GJ, Yellon DM. Does ischaemic preconditioning in the human involve Protein Kinase C and the ATP-dependent K+ channel? Studies of contractile function following simulated ischaemia in an atrial in vitro model. Circ Res 1995;77(5):1030-1035.
30. Ovize M, Przyklenk K, Hale S et al. Preconditioning does not attenuate myocardial stunning. Circulation 1992;85:2247-2254.
31. Lasley R, Anderson G, Mentzer R. Ischaemic and hypoxic preconditioning enhance postischaemic recovery of function in the rat heart. Cardiovasc Res 1993;27:565-70.
32. Webster K, Discher D, Bishopric N. Cardioprotection in an in vitro model of hypoxic preconditioning. J Mol Cell Cardiol 1995;27:453-8.
33. Jenkins D, Pugsley W, Yellon D. Ischaemic preconditioning in a model of global ischaemia: infarct size limitation, but no reduction of stunning. J Mol Cell Cardiol 1995;27:1623-1632.
34. Carr C, Grover G, Yellon D. Comparison of ischaemic preconditioning and a highly selective ATP-dependent potassium channel opener in isolated human atrial muscle. Heart 1996; In press.
35. Wollmering M, Fullerton D, Walther J et al. Preconditioning protects function and viability in human ventricle. Circulation 1994;90(Abstract Suppl):I-477.
36. Ikonomidis J, Tumiati L, Weisel R et al. Preconditioning human ventricular cardiomyocytes with brief periods of simulated ischaemia. Cardiovascular Research 1994;28:1285-1291.
37. Curry B, Gross G, Baker J. Role of KATP channels in a rabbit model of chronic myocardial hypoxia. Circulation 1995;92(8(Supp I)):I-252(No1204).
38. Ytrehus K, Liu Y, Downey J. Preconditioning protects ischaemic rabbit myocardium by protein kinase C activation. Am J Physiol 1994;266:H1145-52.
39. Auchampach J, Grover G, Gross G. Blockage of ischaemic preconditioning in dogs by the novel ATP-dependent potassium channel antagonist sodium 5-hydroxydecanoate. Cardiovasc Res 1992;26:1054-62.
40. Gross GJ, Auchampach JA. Blockage of ATP-sensitive potassium channels prevents myocardial preconditioning in dogs. Circ Res 1992;70:223-233.
41. Tomai F, Crea F, Gaspardone A et al. Blockade of A1 adenosine receptors prevents myocardial preconditioning in man. European Heart J 1994;15(Suppl):553.
42. Ikonomidis J, Shirai T, Weisel R et al. Human cardiomyocyte preconditioning is adenosine A1 receptor dependent. Circulation 1994;90:I-477.
43. Taggart P, Sutton P, Oliver R et al. Ischaemic preconditioning may activate potassium ATP channels in humans? [abstract]. Circulation 1993;88(Suppl I(Pt 2)):I-569.
44. Heidbuchel H, Vereecke J, Carmeliet E. Three different potassium channels in human atrium: contribution to the basal potassium conductance. Circulation Research 1990;66(5):1277-1286.
45. Bohm M, Pieske B, Ungerer M et al. Characterization of A1 Adenosine receptors in atrial and ventricular myocardium from diseased human hearts. Circulation Research 1989;65(5):1201-1211.

In: Mentzer, R.M., Jr., Kitakaze, M., Downey, J.M., Hori, M, eds. Adenosine, Cardioprotection and Clinical Application. Kluwer Academic Publishers, Norwell, MA, USA, 1997.

13. Protein Kinase C and Adenosine Synergistically Activate ATP-Sensitive Potassium Currents: Implications for Ischemic Preconditioning

Yongge Liu
Wei Dong Gao
Brian O'Rourke
Eduardo Marban

Introduction

Several mechanisms have been proposed for the mechanism of ischemic preconditioning. Substantial evidence from studies involving rabbit hearts has shown that adenosine receptors, protein kinase C (PKC), and ATP-sensitive potassium (K_{ATP}) channels are involved.[1,2] Furthermore, it has been suggested that these three hypotheses may be interrelated, with the K_{ATP} channel as the final effector.[2] Opening of K_{ATP} channels shortens the action potential duration (APD). APD abbreviation reduces Ca^{2+} influx and contractility and thus conserves energy. If opening of K_{ATP} channels is the cause of the protection, the activity of K_{ATP} channels would need to be increased or primed by the initial preconditioning insult so that they would open more rapidly or to a greater extent during the subsequent ischemia. One explicit scheme[2] proposes that adenosine receptor activation stimulates PKC during preconditioning; PKC then phosphorylates K_{ATP} channels and the phosphorylation makes the channel open more readily during the second ischemia. The protective effect of adenosine has been linked to K_{ATP} channel opening: The protection induced by preconditioning, adenosine receptor agonists and PKC activators can be eliminated by K_{ATP} channel blockers.[2,3] Likewise, protection from preconditioning and adenosine receptor agonists can be blocked by PKC inhibitors.[3] The present chapter summarizes our results examining the effect of PKC and adenosine on K_{ATP} channels in heart cells. The reader is referred to the full-length paper[4] for details.

K_{ATP} current ($I_{K,ATP}$) modulation by PKC

The possible modification of the K_{ATP} channel by protein phosphorylation has been investigated most extensively in insulinoma cells. Dunne[5] showed that activation of PKC by PMA (phorbol 12-myristate 13-acetate) had a transient inhibitory effect on the K_{ATP} channel, while prolonged treatment with PMA (>5 min) increased the opening of K_{ATP} channels. In the same cell line, Ribalet et al.[6] reported that PKC activation can increase K_{ATP} channel activity directly or indirectly via a second messenger pathway. In myocytes, several studies have described the effect of PKC activation on K_{ATP} channels. Deutsch et al.[7] showed that phospholipase A_2, C, and D all modestly desensitize K_{ATP} channels to closure by ATP, although they did not investigate whether the desensitization is PKC-dependent. Using acetylcholine as an agonist, Wang et al.[8] demonstrated a PKC-related potentiation in glybenclamide-sensitive potassium conductance in cat atrial myocytes. Hu et al.[9] have shown that PKC activation abbreviates the time to $I_{K,ATP}$ activation when the intracellular ATP concentration is low (<0.5 mM) in rabbit and human ventricular myocytes. Light et al.[10] showed that a constitutively active PKC inhibits the opening of K_{ATP} channels in patches excised from rabbit ventricular myocytes at ATP concentration <0.1 mM, but at an ATP concentration of 1 mM, PKC increases the open probability.[10] To further investigate the possible modulation of $I_{K,ATP}$ by PKC, we used pinacidil, a direct channel opener, and metabolic inhibition to elicit $I_{K,ATP}$.

PKC activation increases pinacidil induced $I_{K,ATP}$

$I_{K,ATP}$ can be induced by K_{ATP} channel openers such as pinacidil. As shown in Figure 13-1A, pinacidil induced a small $I_{K,ATP}$ measured by whole-cell configuration of patch clamps with 1 mM MgATP in the recording pipette. The pinacidil-induced current during a second application of the drug was not significantly different from the first one. Figure 13-1B illustrates the very different response of a cell that was treated with PMA, a phorbol ester which directly activates PKC, for 10 min prior to the second exposure to pinacidil. PMA treatment alone did not significantly change the membrane currents, but the subsequent response to pinacidil (Fig. 13-1B, "repeat pinacidil") in the absence of PMA was markedly increased. This large outward current reversed at the K^+ equilibrium potential and was partially blocked by glybenclamide. Figure 13-1C

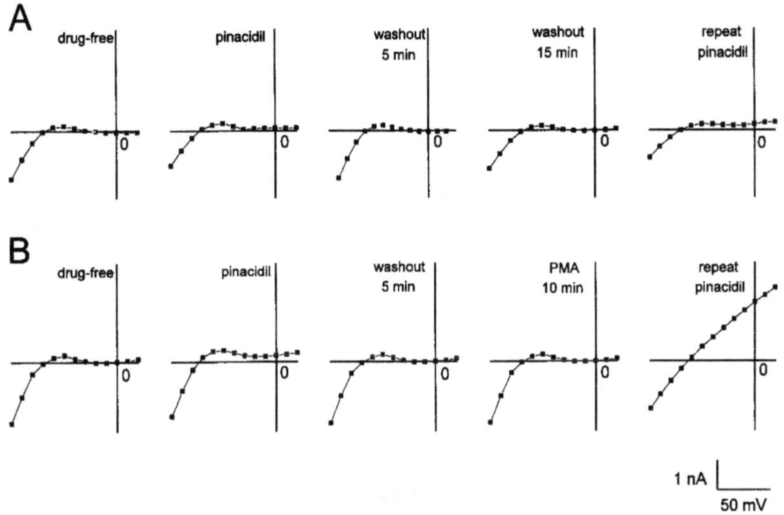

FIGURES 13-1 A, B. Current and voltage relations for two representative cells (one from the control group (A) and one from the PMA group (B)). Currents were elicited by 400 msec steps from the holding potential (-80 mV) to test potentials from 20 mV to -100 mV (10 mV increments), measured 200 msec after the onset of the step, and shown as black squares. In the control cell, 100 mM pinacidil induced a small outward current ($I_{K,ATP}$). This current was complete reversible after washout of pinacidil. A second exposure to the same concentration of pinacidil (repeat pinacidil) activated a similar $I_{K,ATP}$ as that seen in the first pinacidil (A). In contrast, if the cell was treated with 100 nM PMA prior to the second pinacidil exposure, the drug activated a much greater $I_{K,ATP}$ (repeat pinacidil) than that induced by the first pinacidil) (B).

summarizes the currents measured at 0 mV at each stage of the experiment in the control group and the PMA group. The critical comparison is between the first and second pinacidil exposure in the control versus the PMA-treated cells. The first pinacidil-activated currents at 0 mV were 0.48 ± 0.25 nA for the control group and 0.55 ± 0.32 nA for the PMA group. The second exposure to pinacidil activated a comparably sized current in the control group. However, if the cells were treated with PMA, the current increased greatly during the second pinacidil exposure to 3.25 ± 0.47 nA ($p < 0.01$ vs. first pinacidil). These data indicate that PKC activation increases currents induced by a K_{ATP} channel opener. Because pinacidil appears to act directly on the channel, rather than via second messengers or intermediary pathways, the elevated drug responsiveness does not necessarily imply that PKC activation will suffice to potentiate $I_{K,ATP}$ during metabolic stress (e.g., ischemia). For this reason, we next determined the effects of PMA treatment on $I_{K,ATP}$ during metabolic inhibition.

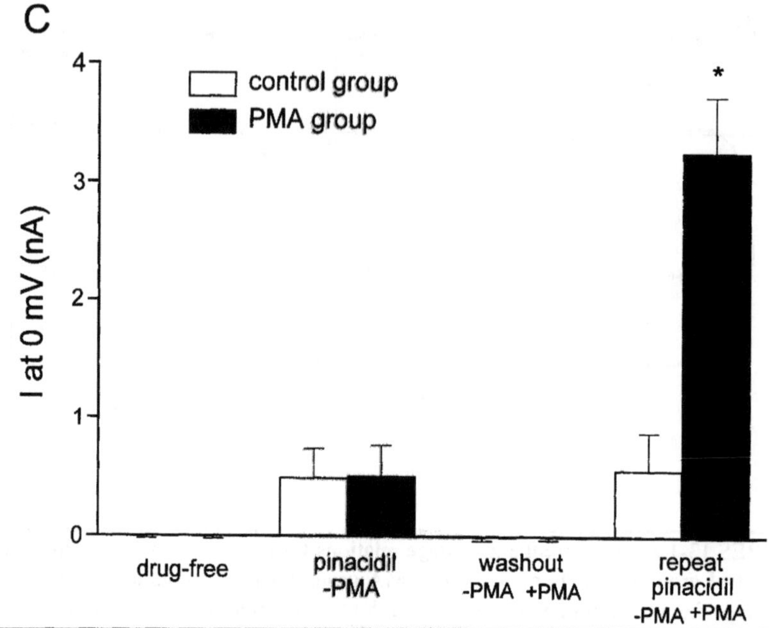

FIGURE 13-1C. Pooled data from membrane currents measured at 0 mV for both control and PMA groups, using the protocols illustrated in Figs. 13-1A and B. * = $p < 0.01$ vs the current activated by the first pinacidil.

PKC activation shortens the time to turn on $I_{K,ATP}$ during metabolic inhibition

Figure 13-2A shows the time course of membrane currents (measured at -100 mV and 0 mV) during metabolic inhibition from a representative cell. When exposed to 2 mM sodium cyanide (CN) and zero glucose (MI group), the currents measured at -100 mV did not change over time. Nevertheless, currents at 0 mV ($I_{K,ATP}$) started to increase after a delay of approximately 15 min. Prior activation of PKC did not alter this response: when cells were treated with 100 nM PMA before metabolic inhibition (PMA+MI), the current changes were similar to those in the MI group (Fig. 13-2B).

Adenosine accumulates in tissues and in the interstitial space during ischemia, and adenosine receptor activation has been shown to act as both initiator and mediator of ischemic preconditioning. In our protocol, cells were continuously superperfused, making it impossible for adenosine to accumulate around the cell as it would during ischemia. To mimic ischemia more faithfully, 10 mM adenosine was added during metabolic inhibition. Cells exposed to 2 mM CN, 0 glucose and

10 μM adenosine (MI+Ado) developed a gradually increasing current at 0 mV similar to the responses in the MI and PMA+MI groups (Fig. 13-2C). However, if PMA-treated cells were subjected to metabolic inhibition including adenosine (PMA+MI+Ado), the time required to increase the current at 0 mV was markedly abbreviated (Fig. 13-2D).

Figure 13-2E summarizes the pooled data for the times required for $I_{K,ATP}$ activation. This latency was 15.1±2.4 min in the MI group, and was not significantly altered in the PMA+MI (11.9±2.0 min) or the MI+Ado groups (12.3±1.5 min). However, the latency to develop $I_{K,ATP}$ in the PMA+MI+Ado group decreased to only 5.5±1.6 min ($p<0.05$ vs the other three groups). Inactive PMA analog 4α-phorbol did not significantly affect the time course of $I_{K,ATP}$ development during metabolic inhibition in the presence of 10 mM adenosine (13.9±2.5 min) (4α-phorbol+MI+Ado). This would exclude the possibility of phorbol ester effects unrelated to PKC. The non-selective adenosine receptor

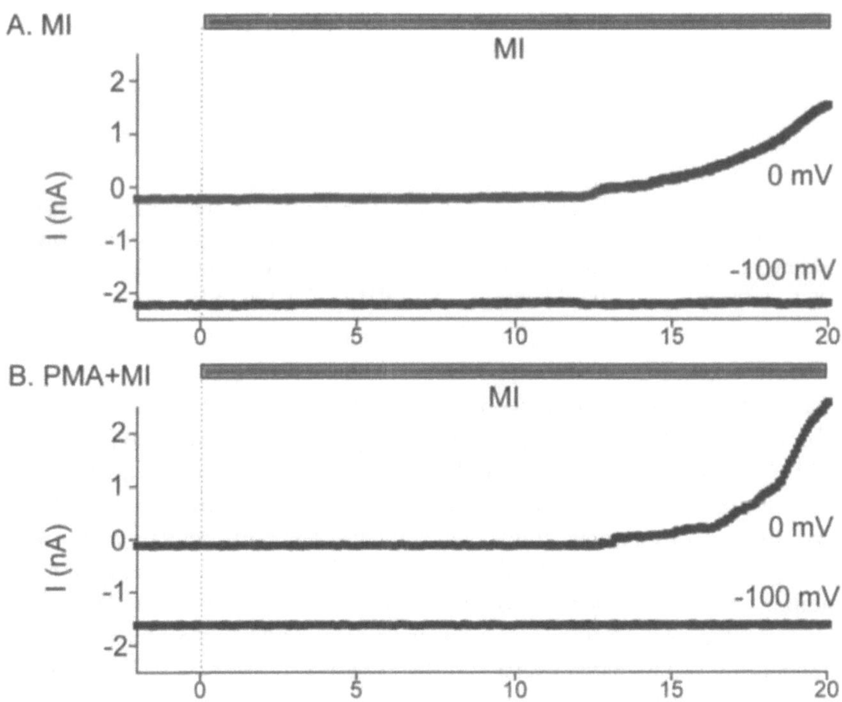

FIGURES 13-2 A, B. Time courses of membrane current development during metabolic inhibition from four representative cells (one from each of the four groups). Currents were measured at -100 mV and 0 mV. Gray bars indicate the period of metabolic inhibition. A: results from a MI cell. B: results from a PMA+MI cell.

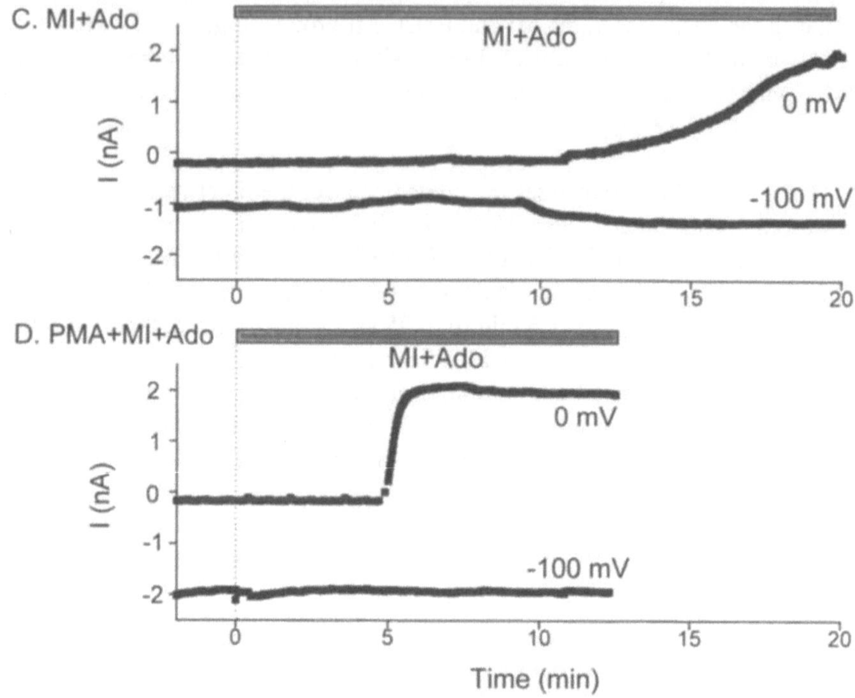

FIGURES 13-2C, D. Time courses of membrane current development during metabolic inhibition from four representative cells (one from each of the four groups). Currents were measured at -100 mV and 0 mV. Gray bars indicate the period of metabolic inhibition. C: results from a MI+Ado cell. D: results from a PMA+MI+Ado cell.

antagonist 8-(p-sulfophenyl)-theophylline (SPT, 100 mM), completely blocked the abbreviation of the time to $I_{K,ATP}$ activation by PMA and adenosine (14±3.5 min; PMA+MI+Ado+SPT), suggesting that the effect from adenosine is mediated by adenosine receptors. The current activated by metabolic inhibition was not blocked very effectively by glybenclamide, which is consistent with previous work showing that $I_{K,ATP}$ loses its glybenclamide sensitivity during metabolic inhibition.[11] As another check on the identity of the channels activated by PMA+MI+Ado, we compared the properties of single channels induced by this protocol to those of channels evoked by patch excision or by exposure to pinacidil. They all showed properties characteristic of K_{ATP} channels.

Our results indicate that PMA pretreatment shortens the time required to develop $I_{K,ATP}$, but only if adenosine is included during metabolic inhibition. This

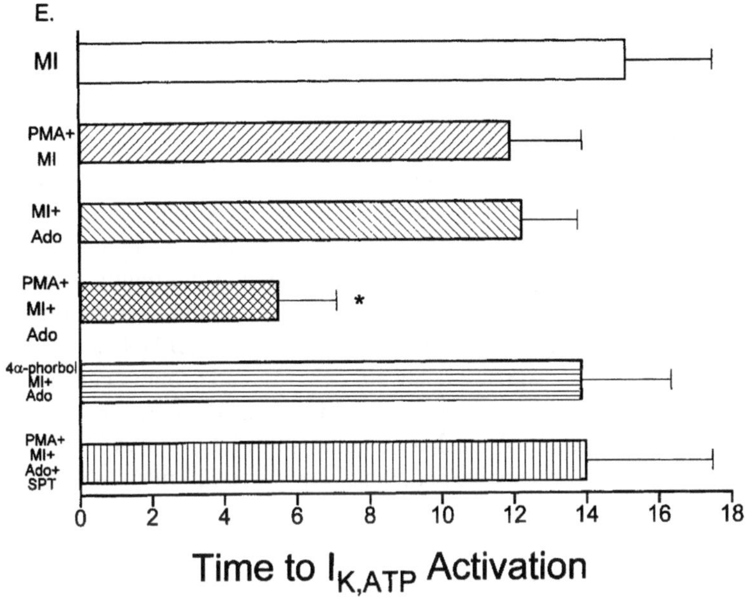

FIGURE 2 E: Pooled data for the time required to activate $I_{K,ATP}$ (determined by the time required to induce a clearly measurable outward current (>0.1 nA at 0 mV)) during metabolic inhibition. Cells in the 4α-phorbol+MI+Ado group were treated the same way as PMA+M+Ado except PMA was replaced by 100 nM 4α-phorbol. The PMA+MI+Ado+STP group was similar to the PMA+MI+Ado group, except that 100 mM of SPT was added into the superperfusate during metabolic inhibition.. * = $p < 0.05$ vs each of the other five groups.

finding has important implications for the role played by adenosine in ischemic preconditioning. A prevailing concept holds that adenosine receptor activation plays a dual role: it initiates as well as mediates the protection.[1] This conclusion was drawn from experimental evidence that adenosine receptor antagonists could abolish the protection from ischemic preconditioning when given during the preconditioning phase as well as during the subsequent prolonged ischemia. The protection provided by direct PKC activators such as PMA could also be abolished by blocking adenosine receptors during ischemia. Thus, adenosine receptors have to be activated during both the preconditioning and the prolonged ischemia to provide protection. In our experimental setting, cells were continually superperfused. Therefore, adenosine was not able to accumulate and activate its receptors. When we added 10 μM adenosine during metabolic inhibition, PMA pretreatment greatly abbreviated the time to activation of $I_{K,ATP}$. A concentration of 10 μM was chosen because it mimics the adenosine levels reached in the myocardium during ischemia.

PKC activation accelerates APD shortenings during metabolic inhibition

Action potentials shorten during ischemia or metabolic inhibition, and myocytes become electrically inexcitable when the duration of ischemia or metabolic inhibition is prolonged. In isolated cells, one of the major reasons that APD shortens is because of the increase in $I_{K,ATP}$. Nichols et al.[12] suggested that even very small increases in $I_{K,ATP}$ would result in significant shortening of APD. We investigated whether PMA treatment and/or adenosine could alter the time course of APD shortening during metabolic inhibition. Because APD depends critically on the balance between inward and outward currents, and calcium currents tend to run down in the whole-cell configuration, we accelerated the metabolic inhibition by adding the glycolytic inhibitor 2-deoxyglucose (2-DG). Therefore, metabolic inhibition in the action potential experiments consisted of 10 mM 2-DG, 2 mM CN and zero glucose.

Figure 13-3 summarizes the APD_{50} (APD at 50% repolarization) and APD_{90} (APD at 90% repolarization) data. PMA pretreatment alone did not alter APD_{50} and APD_{90}, nor did it affect the time course of APD shortening during metabolic inhibition. When 10 μM adenosine was added during metabolic inhibition, it did not significantly affect the time course of APD shortening. Nevertheless, cells pre-exposed to PMA exhibited significantly accelerated APD shortening (PMA+MI+Ado group). Five of 6 cells in the PMA+MI+Ado group became inexcitable after 7 min metabolic inhibition, while none of the cells from the other three groups were inexcitable at this time (they eventually failed to fire action potentials in about 10 min). We measured $I_{K,ATP}$ by switching from current clamp to voltage clamp mode in the cells that had turned inexcitable, and confirmed that $I_{K,ATP}$ had developed in every cell.

Time to develop rigor during metabolic inhibition

The activation of $I_{K,ATP}$ is energy-dependent. The modulation of $I_{K,ATP}$ and the acceleration of APD shortening could simply reflect a change of cellular energy metabolism induced by PMA pretreatment and/or adenosine. In particular, these interventions may decrease energy stores before metabolic inhibition or increase the rate of energy utilization during metabolic inhibition. We used the transition to rigor as a bioassay of cellular energy stores. The transition to rigor has been shown to correlate with the depletion of intracellular energy, particularly with the cessation of anaerobic ATP production. PMA pretreatment and/or including

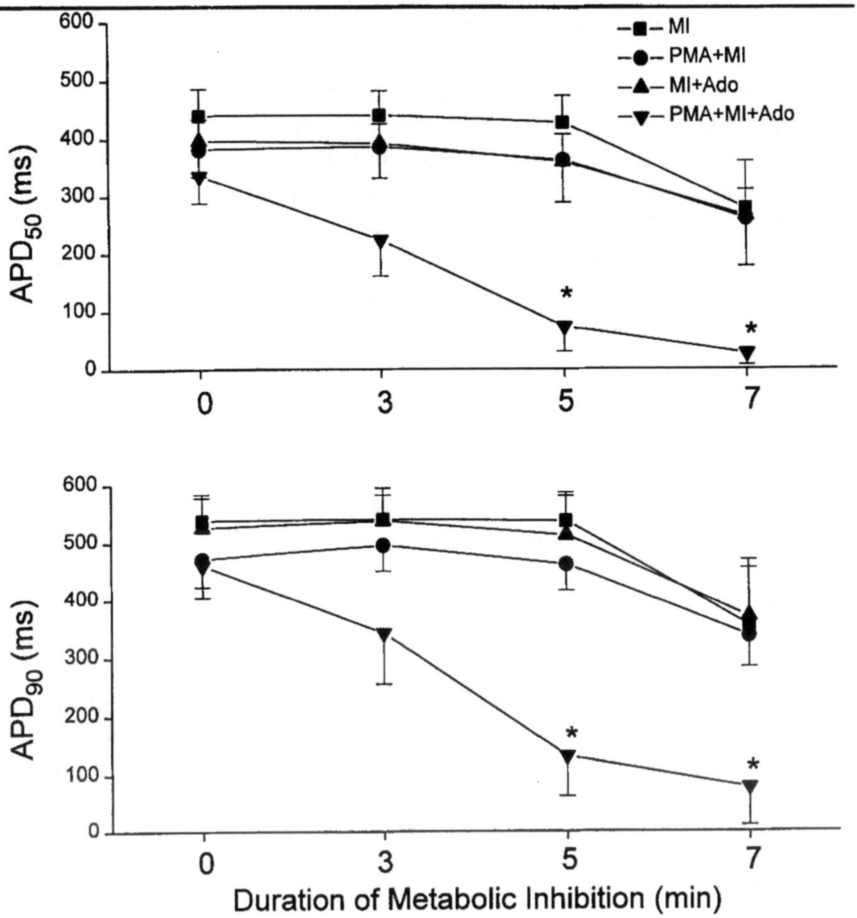

FIGURE 13-3. Summarized data for APD_{50} and APD_{90} during metabolic inhibition. Note that APD_{50} and APD_{90} in the PMA+MI+Ado group were significantly shorter after 5 min metabolic inhibition than in the other three groups. Action potentials were stimulated every 5 second in current-clamp mode, and were initiated by short (25-ms) depolarizing current pulses (25 pA). Group names as in Fig. 13-2 legend. * = $p < 0.05$ vs each of the other three groups.

adenosine during metabolic inhibition did not alter the time to induce rigor, suggesting that they do not affect the net rate of energy depletion.

Can the effect of PMA be reproduced by adenosine?

An important part of the PKC theory is that adenosine receptor activation during preconditioning stimulates PKC. Adenosine receptors are capable of activating PKC isoform δ in rat myocytes.[13] In preliminary results, we found that 10 μM adenosine was unable to potentiate the pinacidil-induced $I_{K,ATP}$ by using the same protocol as in the PMA group (PMA was substituted by adenosine). This could be due to the intracellular dialysis (including Ca^{2+} buffering) which is a consequence of our whole-cell recordings. Perforated patch recordings will be useful in examining this possibility.

Conclusion

Our results demonstrate that PMA increases $I_{K,ATP}$ induced by direct opener pinacidil, and by metabolic inhibition in the presence of adenosine. This provides an explicit basis for the current paradigm of ischemic preconditioning. Although the protective effect of opening K_{ATP} channels during ischemia has been proposed to relate to APD shortening, it is not clear whether such an effect would suffice to mediate the protection. Further investigation is required to test this idea rigorously. Recently, K_{ATP} channels have been cloned, which will greatly enhance our understanding of this channel. The availability of this cloned channel opens new prospects for investigating the protective effect of K_{ATP} channels at the molecular level.

Acknowledgments

This work was supported by a grant (RO1 HL 44065) from the National Institutes of Health.

References

1. Downey JM, Cohen MV, Ytrehus K et al. Cellular mechanisms in ischemic preconditioning: the role of adenosine and protein kinase C, in Das DK (ed): Cellular, Biochemical, and Molecular Aspects of Reperfusion Injury. New York Academy of Sciences 1994;82-98.
2. Gross GJ, Yao Z, Auchampach JA. Role of ATP-sensitive potassium channels in ischemic preconditioning, in Przyklenk K, Kloner (ed). Ischemic Preconditioning: the Concepts of Endogenous Cardioprotection, Develop Cardiovasc Med. Vol 148. Boston:Kluwer Academic Publishers, 1994:125-135.
3. Speechly-Dick ME, Grover GJ, Yellon DM. Does ischemic preconditioning in the human involve protein kinase C and the ATP-dependent K^+ channel? - Studies of contractile function after simulated ischemia in an atrial in vitro model. Circ Res 1995;77:1030-1035.

4. Liu Y, Gao WD, O'Rourke B et al. Synergistic modulation of ATP-sensitive K^+ currents by protein kinase C and adenosine: implications for ischemic preconditioning. Circ Res 1996;78:443-454.
5. Dunne MJ. Phorbol myristate acetate and ATP-sensitive potassium channels in insulin-secreting cells. Am J Physiol 1994;267:C501-C506.
6. Ribalet B, Eddlestone GT. Characterization of the G protein coupling of a somatostatin receptor to the K^+ ATP channel in insulin-secreting mammalian HIT and RIN cell lines. J Physiol 1995;485:73-86.
7. Deutsch N, Weiss JN. ATP-sensitive K^+ channel modification by metabolic inhibition in isolated guinea-pig ventricular myocytes. J Physiol 1993;465:163-179.
8. Wang YG, Lipsius SL. Acetylcholine activates a glibenclamide-sensitive K^+ current in cat atrial myocytes. Am J Physiol 1995;268:H1322-H1334.
9. Hu K, Duan D, Nattel S. Protein kinase C activates ATP-sensitive K^+ current in human and rabbit ventricular myocytes. Circ Res 1996;78:492-498.
10. Light PE, Sabir AA, Allen BG, et al. Protein kinase C-induced changes in the stoichiometry of ATP binding activated cardiac ATP-sensitive K+ channels: A possible mechanistic link to ischemic preconditioning. Circ Res 1996; 79:399-406.
11. Findlay I. Sulphonylurea drugs no longer inhibit ATP-sensitive K^+ channels during metabolic stress in cardiac muscle. J Pharmacol Exp Ther 1993;266:456-467.
12. Nichols CG, Ripoll C, Lederer WJ. ATP sensitive potassium channel modulation of the guinea pig ventricular action potential and contraction. Circ Res 1991;68:280-287.
13. Henry P, Puceat M, Demolombe S et al. Adenosine A_1 stimulation activates δ-protein kinase C in rat ventricular myocytes. Circ Res 1996;78:161-165.

In: Mentzer, R.M., Jr., Kitakaze, M., Downey, J.M., Hori, M, eds. Adenosine, Cardioprotection and Clinical Application. Kluwer Academic Publishers, Norwell, MA, USA, 1997.

IV. CLINICAL APPLICATION OF NEW STRATEGIES TO PROTECT THE ISCHEMIC HEART

14. Adenosine and Myocardial Protection in Humans

Robert M. Mentzer, Jr.
Robert D. Lasley

The purine nucleoside adenosine appears to exert similar cardiovascular effects in humans as it does in most laboratory animal species. These include coronary and systemic vasodilation,[1,2] renal vasoconstriction,[3,4] slowing of atrial-ventricular (AV) conduction,[5,6] inhibition of norepinephrine release from sympathetic nerves,[7] and inhibition of platelet aggregation.[8,9] These properties provide the basis for the current use of adenosine in the clinical arena to diagnose and treat supraventricular arrhythmias and enhance radionuclide perfusion imaging scans. Intravenous adenosine has also been used in humans after cardiac surgery to control postoperative systemic and pulmonary hypertension.[10,11] Recent reports also indicate that systemic adenosine infusion reduces pain and the requirements for various anesthetics.[12] These findings indicate that adenosine can be administered safely to patients.

Despite numerous studies in many animal species that demonstrate adenosine has cardioprotective properties, there is little information available describing adenosine's use to treat reversible postischemic myocardial dysfunction or limit myocardial infarct size clinically. This is due in part to the lack of specific information that adenosine is cardioprotective in humans. However, there are several reports of the beneficial effect of adenosine in human tissue in in vitro "simulated ischemia" models.[13,14] There are also reports that human myocardium contains adenosine receptors and their associated signal transduction mechanisms that are found in numerous animal models.[6,15] These observations suggest that adenosine may exert a cardioprotective effect in humans.

One of the potential reasons for the paucity of data on adenosine cardioprotection in humans may be concern over the safety and tolerance of high doses of adenosine which, based on animal studies, appear to be necessary to exert a cardioprotective effect. There are several studies in humans that peripheral adenosine infusions at doses $\leq$ approximately 70 μg/kg/min are well tolerated, but higher doses may produce undesirable side-effects.[1,2,10] However, since adenosine is rapidly metabolized by red blood cells and endothelial cells, this dose may not be sufficient to reach the cardiac myocytes. Utterback et al[16] measured plasma adenosine levels during peripheral and central infusions of adenosine in humans undergoing elective coronary artery bypass surgery. They reported that approximately 75% of peripherally administered adenosine (infusions of 75-150 μg/kg/min) was extracted during passage through the pulmonary vascular bed. However Utterback et al[16] also reported that central administration of adenosine (right ventricle) at a dose of 45 μg/kg/min was associated with a significant increase in left atrial plasma adenosine levels without any systemic hemodynamic effects. These findings suggest that if adenosine is infused centrally or when patients are on cardiopulmonary bypass, it may be possible to safely administer doses high enough to exert a cardioprotective effect.

Adenosine Cardioprotection Studies in Humans

There are in fact 3 recent clinical studies indicating that adenosine may be administered safely, and possibly efficaciously, as an adjunct to cardioplegia in humans during coronary artery bypass surgery.[17-19] In 1995, Lee et al[17] tested whether an adenosine infusion in patients prior to undergoing coronary artery bypass grafting would improve postbypass myocardial hemodynamics. Seven patients were pretreated with adenosine and 7 served as controls. Adenosine was infused incrementally prior to the initiation of cardiopulmonary bypass at a rate of 50 μg/kg/min every minute until a dose of 350 μg/kg/min was reached. The total duration of the adenosine infusion lasted for ten minutes or until the patient developed systemic arterial pressures less than 70 mmHg at which time the infusion was discontinued. Five minutes after the completion of adenosine or the saline control infusion, patients were placed on cardiopulmonary bypass and then underwent the standard bypass operation using cold blood cardioplegia to facilitate arrest. Patients that received adenosine exhibited immediate post-bypass and 40 hour postoperative improvements in cardiac index (CI) and left ventricular stroke work index (LVSWI) and lower creatine phosphokinase (CPK) release during the first 24 hour postoperative period. The investigators concluded that adenosine treatment prior to the initiation of bypass was associated with improved postoperative myocardial function.

Fremes et al[18] reported the results of an open-label, non-randomized Phase I adenosine dose-ranging study in patients scheduled for elective coronary artery bypass surgery. Antegrade warm blood potassium cardioplegia was administered in the routine fashion with adenosine added to the initial 1000 ml dose and final 500 ml dose. Adenosine concentrations of 0, 15, 20, and 25 μM were tested.

Although the authors reported that hypotension during cardioplegic induction was more prevalent with the higher doses, they concluded that adenosine can be safely administered as a supplement to cardioplegic formulations when used in the range of 15 to 25 μM.

We have recently tested the efficacy of adenosine as an additive to cold blood cardioplegia in a single center, open label, randomized study in sixty-one patients.[19] The study was performed in patients with ejection fractions greater than 0.30 and who were undergoing elective coronary artery bypass surgery. Patients were randomized to standard cold blood cardioplegia without adenosine or to one of five adenosine doses, i.e., 100 μM, 500 μM, 1 mM, 2 mM, and 2 mM cardioplegia plus an intravenous pretreatment infusion of 140 μg/kg/min. In the preischemic adenosine treatment group the aortic cross-clamp was applied after continuously infusing the agent for ten minutes into the venous reservoir. Subsequent cardioplegic infusions and their durations were left to the surgeon's discretion, however there were no differences in cardiopulmonary bypass time or aortic cross-clamp time among the groups. Multiple measurements of ventricular performance and rhythm were obtained preoperatively, prebypass, and then at 1, 2, 4, 8, 16, and 24 hours after cessation of cardiopulmonary bypass. In addition to standard hemodynamic measurements and derived values such as cardiac index (CI), systemic vascular resistance (SVR), and LVSWI, non-invasive evaluations of cardiac function included transesophageal echocardiography (TEE) and transthoracic echocardiography (TTE). Regional wall motion was scored using the American Society of Echocardiography 16-Segment Model and a wall-motion score index was calculated by dividing the sum of segmental point scores by the number of segments analyzed. The use of inotropic agents (dopamine, dobutamine, norepinephrine, epinephrine, and amrinone) and vasoactive drugs (nitroglycerin, nitroprusside, phenylephrine, ephedrine) were also recorded for 24 hours after cessation of cardiopulmonary bypass. The institutional preference was to use dopamine to treat patients with a cardiac index less than 2.0 L/min. Vasodilators and vasoconstrictors were administered to treat ischemia or hypertension, respectively. Each patient's average drug dose over 24 hours was estimated as the area under the dose response curve (AUC).

Although there are several reports of plasma adenosine measurements in humans as a marker of myocardial ischemia,[20-22] the human adenosine cardioprotection studies by Lee et al[17] and Fremes et al[18] did not measure adenosine levels. Therefore we measured plasma levels of adenosine and its degradation products, inosine and hypoxanthine, during bypass and immediately post-bypass. During bypass, blood samples were drawn for the measurement of nucleoside levels before and after the first, second and last dose of cardioplegia. Plasma adenosine and total purine (Σ adenosine + inosine + hypoxanthine) concentrations are illustrated in Figures 1A and 1B.

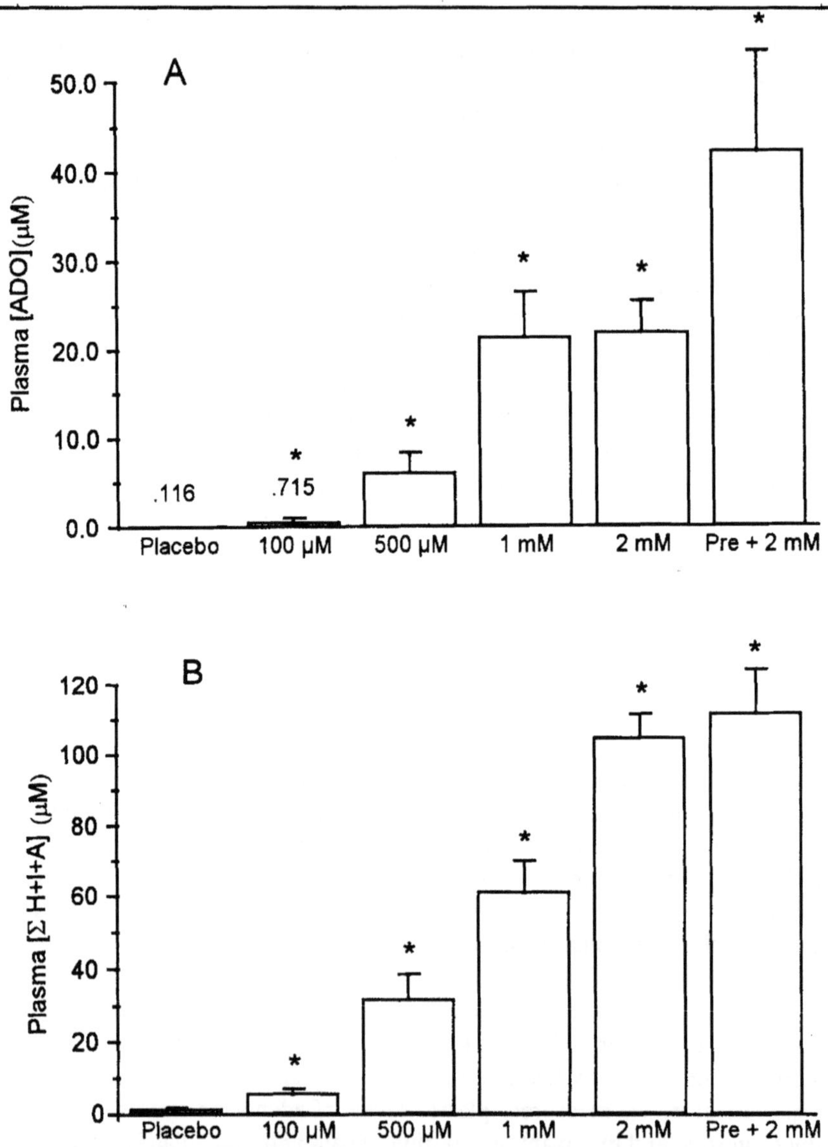

FIGURE 14-1. Effects of increasing doses of adenosine (ADO) in cold blood cardioplegia on venous plasma adenosine (Panel A) and total purines (Σ H+I+A) (Panel B). H, hypoxanthine; I, inosine; A, adenosine; Pre, preteatment with i.v. adenosine prior to aortic cross-clamping. N > 9 per group; * $p < 0.05$ vs placebo group.

Plasma adenosine levels increased with each concentration of adenosine additive, from a baseline (pre-cardioplegia) value of 0.12 ± 0.04 μM in the placebo group to 0.72 ± 0.32 μM with 100 μM adenosine and to 42.3 ± 11.2 μM in the pretreatment + 2 mM adenosine. Total plasma purine concentrations increased from a baseline value of 1.72 ± 0.19 μM to 5.92 ± 1.13 μM with 100 μM adenosine and to 111.9 ± 12.5 μM in the pretreatment + 2 mM adenosine.

The addition of adenosine to blood cardioplegia had no effect on cardiopulmonary bypass time, aortic cross-clamp time, or post-bypass systemic hemodynamic parameters. Similarly, there were no significant changes in regional wall motion detected by TEE. In terms of inotropic and vasoactive drug use adenosine treatment had no effect on dobutamine, amrinone, epinephrine, nitroprusside, phenylephrine or ephedrine use. However, among the 61 patients, only eight received dobutamine, seven received amrinone, four received epinephrine, and six patients were administered ephedrine. In contrast, adenosine treatment resulted in a significant reduction in the use of dopamine and nitroglycerin within the first 24 hours of surgery. In contrast 67% (41/61) and 88% (54/61) of the patients received dopamine and nitroglycerin within the first 24 hours of surgery. In these patients, increasing doses of adenosine were associated with a 65% (P = 0.003) and 67% (P = 0.001) probability of receiving less dopamine and nitroglycerin, respectively. Also, the number of patients who received dopamine and nitroglycerin in the postoperative period decreased as the adenosine concentration increased. For example, in the placebo treated patients, 12 of 13 patients administered dopamine whereas in the high dose adenosine treatment group (Pre +2 mM) only 2 of 9 patients received dopamine. The 24 hour average doses for dopamine and nitroglycerin in the placebo group was 28 fold and 2.6 fold greater than the respective high dose adenosine treatment cohorts.

With respect to the TTE results, the regional wall motion analyses revealed improvement in the inferior, posterior, and anterolateral regions with the 1 mM (p = 0.063), 2 mM (p = 0.002), and pre + 2 mM adenosine (p = 0.032). When the data were analyzed in the context of global function seven days postoperatively and the treatment groups collated into three cohorts, i.e., low dose, intermediate dose, and high dose adenosine, the low dose adenosine group was associated with a lower postoperative ejection fraction compared to the preoperative value, i.e. 61% versus 54%, respectively. The results of this Phase I Adenosine Myocardial Protection Trial suggest that adenosine as an additive to cold blood cardioplegia is safe and effective and supports the hypothesis that the nucleoside is a cardioprotective agent in humans. The limitations of this trial include that the number of patients in each cohort was relatively small and the indications for the administration of inotropic agents and vasodilators were not well-defined. Certainly, additional clinical trials are needed to determine the optimal dose, timing and efficacy of adenosine in protecting the human heart during cardiac surgery and heart preservation for transplantation.

Adenosine and Ischemic Preconditioning in Humans

The use of adenosine as cardioprotective agent in humans has also received much recent interest due to its potential role in mediating ischemic preconditioning. There are several reports that ischemic preconditioning may occur in clinical settings,[23-32] some of which also implicate the involvement of adenosine.[25-29] One of the earliest such reports was that by Deutsch et al.[23] These investigators reported that electrocardiographic changes and lactate release after the first balloon occlusion were reduced after subsequent balloon inflations during coronary angioplasty. Inoue et al[24] reported that in patients undergoing percutaneous transluminal coronary angioplasty (PTCA), the ST-segment changes and anginal chest pains were less after the third balloon occlusion. Subsequent studies in humans undergoing PTCA indicate that adenosine may play a role in this aspect of ischemic preconditioning. This hypothesis is supported by findings observed with exogenous adenosine,[25] dipyridamole,[26,27] and the adenosine receptor antagonists aminophylline[28] and bamiphylline.[29] Whether these forms of preconditioning are mediated by the same mechanism as preconditioning against more severe forms of ischemia remains to be determined however.

There are at least three reports of the effects of ischemic preconditioning in humans during cardiac surgery.[33-35] Alkhulafi et al[33] reported that human hearts preconditioned with two three-minute periods of aortic cross-clamping separated by two minutes of reperfusion, prior to ten minutes of ischemia and normothermic ventricular fibrillation exhibited a reduced rate of myocardial ATP depletion when compared to non-preconditioned hearts. However, in a subsequent study by the same group[34] when the patients were cooled to 32°C this preconditioning protocol did not alter ATP catabolism. Perrault et al[35] reported that three-minutes of aortic cross-clamping and two minutes reperfusion prior to warm cardioplegia arrest (31-32°C) in patients undergoing coronary artery bypass surgery did not enhance myocardial protection. However, these authors' conclusions were also based purely on their metabolic findings, and in two recent experimental studies ischemic preconditioning's beneficial postischemic effects could be dissociated from its metabolic effects.[36,37] In terms of ischemic preconditioning's potential clinical use during cardiac surgery, it must also be pointed out that there are several reports in experimental animal models that ischemic preconditioning does not attenuate reversible postischemic ventricular dysfunction.[38-40] In fact in the only species in which ischemic preconditioning consistently improves reperfusion function, i.e. the rat, this effect may be due to reduction of irreversible injury. In addition there are conflicting reports on the protective effect of ischemic preconditioning in rat myocardium when applied in conjunction with cardioplegia.[41-43]

Conclusion

In conclusion, the substantial experimental data and the corroborating clinical findings obtained to date, support the hypothesis that adenosine and ischemic preconditioning may be cardioprotective in the clinical arena. However, several aspects of these treatment regimens must be addressed in both experimental and clinical studies. In experimental studies the exact mechanisms of action must be determined, and the protective effects of adenosine and preconditioning must be assessed in animal models that more closely mimic clinical conditions. With respect to clinical studies the optimal dose, timing, and route of administration of adenosine remain unknown. The question of whether combining adenosine with an adenosine metabolism inhibitor (draflazine) or enhancer (acadesine or PD 81,723) should be addressed. The development of very specific adenosine A_1 receptor analogs may also hold therapeutic promise. The ultimate potential benefit of ischemic preconditioning may be in mimicking its protective effect with a pharmacological agent. In terms of their use during cardiac surgery the beneficial effects of these treatments on post-bypass cardiac function, inotrope use, and duration of hospital stay must be demonstrated. Both treatments may also prolong heart preservation times for transplantation and be of benefit in the setting of minimally invasive direct coronary artery bypass (MIDCAB) surgery.

References

1. Wilson RF, Wyche K, Christensen BV et al. Effects of adenosine on human coronary arterial circulation. Circulation 1990;82:1595-606.
2. Edlund A, Sollevi A, Linde B. Haemodynamic and metabolic effects of infused adenosine in man. Clin Science 1990;79:131-8.
3. Edlund A, Sollevi A. Renal effects of i.v. adenosine infusion in humans. Clin Physiol 1993;13:361-71.
4. Marraccini P, Fedele S, Marzilli M et al. Adenosine-induced renal vasoconstriction in man. Cardiovasc Res 1996;32:949-953.
5. Conti JB, Belardinelli L, Utterback DB et al. Endogenous adenosine is an antiarrhythmic agent. Circulation 1995;91:1761-7.
6. Bertolet BD, Belardinelli L, Franco EA et al. Selective attenuation by N-0861 (N-6-endonorboran-2-YL-9-methyladenine) of cardiac A(1) adenosine receptor-mediated effects in humans. Circulation 1996;93:1871-1876.
7. Rongen GA, Lenders JWM, Lambrou J et al. Presynaptic inhibition of norepinephrine release from sympathetic nerve endings by endogenous adenosine. Hypertension 1996;27:933-938.
8. Soderback U, Sollevi A, Wallen NH et al. Anti-aggregatory effects of physiological concentrations of adenosine in human whole blood as assessed by filtragometry. Clin Sci 1991;81:691-4.

9. Mentzer RM, Rahko PS, Canver CC et al. Adenosine reduces postbypass transfusion requirements in humans after heart surgery. Ann Surgery 1996;224:523-529.
10. Owall A, Ehrenberg J, Brodin LA et al. Effects of low-dose adenosine on myocardial performance after coronary artery bypass surgery. Acta Anaesthesiol Scand 1993;37:140-148.
11. Fullerton DA, Jones SD, Grover FL et al. Adenosine effectively controls pulmonary hypertension after cardiac operations. Ann Thorac Surg 1966;61:1118-1123.
12. Segerdahl M, Ekblom A, Sandelin K et al. Peroperative adenosine infusion reduces the requirements for isoflurane and postoperative analgesics. Anesth Analg 1995;80:1145-9.
13. Speechly-Dick ME, Grover GJ, Yellon DM. Does ischemic preconditioning in the human involve protein kinase C and the ATP-dependent K+ channel? Studies of contractile function after simulated ischemia in an atrial in vitro model. Circ Res 1995;77:1030-5.
14. Walker DM, Walker JM, Pugsley WB et al. Preconditioning in isolated superfused human muscle. J Mol Cell Cardiol 1995;27:1349-57.
15. Bohm M, Pieske B, Ungerer M et al. Characterization of A1 adenosine receptors in atrial and ventricular myocardium from diseased human hearts. Circ Res 1989;65:1201-11.
16. Utterback DB, Staples ED, White SE et al. Basis for the selective reduction of pulmonary vascular resistance in humans during infusion of adenosine. J Appl Physiol 1994;76:724-30.
17. Lee HT, Lafaro RJ, Reed GE. Pretreatment of human myocardium with adenosine during open heart surgery. J Cardiac Surg 1995;10:665-676.
18. Fremes SE, Levy SL, Christakis GT et al. Phase 1 human trial of adenosine-potassium cardioplegia. Circulation 1996;94(Suppl II):370-375.
19. Mentzer RM, Rahko PS, Molina-Viamonte V et al. Safety, tolerance, and efficacy of adenosine as an additive to blood cardioplegia in humans during coronary artery bypass surgery. Int J Cardiol (In Press), 1997.
20. Feldman MD, Ayers CR, Lehman MR et al. Improved detection of ischemia-induced increases in coronary sinus adenosine in patients with coronary artery disease. Clin Chem 1992;38:256-62.
21. Nissinen J, Raatikainen MJ, Karlqvist K et al. Efflux of adenosine and its catabolites during cold blood cardioplegia. Ann Thorac Surg 1993;55:1546-52.
22. Vlessis AA, Ott G, Cobanoglu A. Purine efflux from transplanted human cardiac allografts. Correlation with graft function. J Thorac Cardiovasc Surg 1994;107:482-6.
23. Deutsch E, Berger M, Kussmaul WG et al. Adaptation to ischemia during percutaneous transluminal coronary angioplasty: clinical, hemodynamic, and metabolic features. Circulation 1990;82:2044-2051.
24. Inoue T, Fujito T, Hoshi K et al. A mechanism of preconditioning during percutaneous transluminal coronary angioplasty. Cardiology 1996;87:216-223.
25. Kerensky RA, Kutcher MA, Braden GA et al. The effects of intracoronary adenosine on preconditioning during coronary angioplasty. Clin Cardiol 1995;18:91-96.
26. Pasini FL, Guideri F, Ferber D et al. Pharmacological preconditioning of ischemic heart disease by low-dose dipyridamole. Int J Cardiol 1996;56:17-27.
27. Strauer BE, Heidland UE, Heintzen MP et al. Pharmacologic myocardial protection during percutaneous transluminal coronary angioplasty by intracoronary application of dipyridamole - impact on hemodynamic function and left ventricular performance. J Am Coll Cardiol 1996;28:1119-1126.
28. Claeys MJ, Vrints CJ, Bosmans JM et al. Aminophylline inhibits adaptation to ischaemia during angioplasty - role of adenosine in ischaemic preconditioning. Eur Heart J 1996;17:539-544.
29. Tomai F, Crea F, Gaspardone A et al. Effects of A(1) adenosine receptor blockade by bamiphylline on ischaemic preconditioning during coronary angioplasty Eur Heart J 1996;17:846-853.
30. Ottani F, Galvani M, Ferriai D et al. Prodromal angina limits infarct size: A role for ischemic preconditioning. Circulation 1995;91:291-297.
31. Ottani F, Galvani M, Ferrini D et al. Prodromal angina limits infarct size. A role for ischemic preconditioning. Circulation 1995;91:291-7.

32. Kloner RA, Shook T, Przyklenk K et al. Previous angina alters in-hospital outcome in TIMI 4: A clinical correlate to preconditioning? Circulation 1995;91:37-45.
33. Alkhulafi AM, Yellon DM, Pugsley WB. Preconditioning the human heart during aortocoronary bypass surgery. Eur J Cardiothorac Surg 1994;8:270-275.
34. Di Salvo C, Hemming A, Jenkins D et al. Can the human myocardium be preconditioned with ischaemia under hypothermic conditions? Proc Eur Assoc Cardiothorac Surg Paris September 25-7,1995:324.
35. Perrault LP, Menasche P, Bel A et al. Ischemic preconditioning in cardiac surgery - a word of caution. J Thorac Cardiovasc Surg 1996;112:1378-1386.
36. Goto M, Cohen MV, Van Wylen DGL et al. Attenuated purine production during subsequent ischemia in preconditioned rabbit myocardium is unrelated to the mechanism of protection. J Mol Cell Cardiol 1996;28:447-454.
37. Cave AC, Garlick PB. Ischemic preconditioning and intracellular pH - a P-31 NMR study in the isolated rat heart. Am J Physiol 1997;41:H544-H552.
38. Ovize M, Przyklenk K, Hale SL et al. Preconditioning does not attenuate myocardial stunning. Circulation 1992;85:2247-54.
39. Miyamae M, Fujiwara H, Kida M et al. Preconditioning improves energy metabolism during reperfusion but does not attenuate myocardial stunning in porcine hearts. Circulation 1993;88:223-34.
40. Jenkins DP, Pugsley WB, Yellon DM. Ischaemic preconditioning in a model of global ischaemia: infarct size limitation, but no reduction of stunning. J Mol Cell Cardiol 1995;27:1623-32.
41. Cave AC, Hearse DJ. Ischaemic preconditioning and contractile function: studies with normothermic and hypothermic global ischaemia. J Mol Cell Cardiol 1992;24:1113-1123.
42. Kolocassides KG, Galinanes M, Hearse DJ. Ischemic preconditioning, cardioplegia or both? Differing approaches to myocardial and vascular protection. J Mol Cell Cardiol 1996;28:623-634.
43. Valen G, Takeshima S, Vaage J. Preconditioning improves cardiac function after global ischemia, but not after cold cardioplegia. Ann Thorac Surg 1996;62:1397-1403.

In: Mentzer, R.M., Jr., Kitakaze, M., Downey, J.M., Hori, M, eds. Adenosine, Cardioprotection and Clinical Application. Kluwer Academic Publishers, Norwell, MA, USA, 1997.

15. Clinical Applications of Ischemic Preconditioning

Yochai Birnbaum
Robert A. Kloner

Introduction

The term "Ischemic preconditioning" is used to describe the phenomenon of protection of the myocardium from ischemic-reperfusion injury by preceding short sublethal ischemic episodes. Ischemic preconditioning is one of the most powerful means known to protect the myocardium during subsequent ischemic-reperfusion insult. However, its mechanisms are still unknown. Understanding its mechanisms and development of "preconditioning-mimetic" drugs may allow myocardial protection in various clinical situations in which the heart is exposed to ischemia. In the following chapter we shall discuss human myocardial preconditioning by brief ischemic episodes in four major clinical situations:

1. Cardiopulmonary bypass: ischemic preconditioning as an alternative method to cardioplegia for the preservation of the myocardium.

2. Percutaneous transluminal coronary angioplasty: changes in severity of pain and electrocardiographic manifestations of ischemia during repeated balloon occlusion.

3. Acute myocardial infarction: the effects of previous angina on infarct size, left ventricular function, ventricular arrhythmias, and prognosis.

4. Adaptation to angina: augmentation of maximal effort during repeated exertion.

The protection afforded by ischemic preconditioning in the experimental setting is dependent on three important variables:[1,2] 1) The duration and numbers of the preconditioning ischemic episodes. The minimal duration of ischemia for achieving protection is species dependent (2 to 10 min). There is evidence that numerous repeated ischemic episodes may induce tolerance or a refractory period and even augment myocardial necrosis. 2) A period of reperfusion between the initial preconditioning and sustained ischemia is mandatory to confer protection. When this period is too short, no protection is induced. However, the protective effect is short lived and is lost after 60 to 120 minutes. A second window of protection was described 24 hours after the first preconditioning stimulus. However, it is still unclear for how long it lasts. 3) The duration of the sustained occlusion. If the ischemia is extended beyond three hours in the dog model, the effect of preconditioning is lost. In humans all of these time frames are unknown. Thus, we do not know the minimal and maximal time limits of the preconditioning stimulus, the time limits of the protection conferred, and whether there are tolerance, refractory period, and a second window of protection. Moreover, most of the clinical situations in which ischemic preconditioning is suspected to occur differ from the experimental models used to investigate ischemic preconditioning. In the experimental models a controlled occlusion of a normal coronary artery supplying a normal myocardium is commonly applied. However, in the clinical acute ischemic syndromes (acute myocardial infarction and unstable angina) the coronary artery is occluded by a thrombus. In many cases there are repeated spontaneous episodes of recanalization and reocclusion of variable duration, with episodes of ischemic pain interposing with silent ischemia. Hence, the exact timing of the preconditioning episodes are difficult to assess. It is still unknown whether silent ischemia can precondition the heart, whether continuation of silent ischemia after resolution of pain is sufficient for the mandatory "intervening reperfusion period", or whether prolonged periods of silent ischemia may exceed the upper limit of ischemic preconditioning and may induce tolerance. It might be that the composition of the intracoronary thrombus is different in patients with and without antecedent angina before infarction and thus the thrombus may react differently to thrombolytic therapy.[3] Other situations, such as controlled balloon occlusion during elective percutaneous transluminal coronary angioplasty, differ from the experimental models because there is a preexisting coronary stenosis and the myocardium is exposed to previous ischemic episodes of variable length and severity, which may confer protection or induce tolerance. In addition, the metabolic effects of ischemic preconditioning should be distinguished from the protection afforded by recruitment of collaterals.[4] Gradual progression of coronary narrowing and repeated short ischemic episodes may augment recruitment of collaterals. Some studies, but not all have found that patients with preinfarction angina tend to have a higher degree of collateral circulation. Well developed collateral circulation attenuates the ischemic insult upon coronary occlusion.

Cardiopulmonary bypass

Ischemic preconditioning, by either brief aortic cross clamping or by preconditioning-mimicking agents, may become an alternative technique for preservation of the myocardium during cardiac surgery and cardiac transplantation. Yellon et al[5] studied human myocardial biopsies obtained from the left ventricle during coronary artery bypass surgery. Seven patients were preconditioned by two ischemic periods of three minutes each, separated by two minutes of reperfusion, and seven patients served as controls. All patients were subjected to ten minutes of cross clamping of the aorta with electrical ventricular fibrillation (the period of test ischemia). Myocardial biopsies were taken before, after the two preconditioning episodes, and after the 10 minutes of ischemia, and analyzed for ATP content. At the start of cardiopulmonary bypass ATP concentrations were similar in both groups. Ischemic preconditioning resulted in a decrease in tissue ATP content compared with controls. However, ATP content after 10 minutes of ischemia was higher in the preconditioned group compared with controls. Thus, this study showed that ischemic preconditioning slows the rate of ATP depletion during ischemia.

Ischemic preconditioning has been used for many years in cardiac bypass surgery.[6] In this technique, several brief (3-10 minutes) periods of aortic cross-clamping with the heart fibrillating separated by reperfusion periods are induced to allow connection of the distal aorto-coronary anastomosis. However, except for a few centers this technique has not gained much popularity, particularly in cases with extensive aorto-coronary bypass procedures. Preconditioning mimetic agents such as adenosine are now being tested in cardiopulmonary bypass patients.

Percutaneous transluminal coronary angioplasty

In elective angioplasty, the onset and duration of ischemia is well controlled. Thus, angioplasty seems to be a good model to study the effects of ischemic preconditioning on the magnitude of pain, severity of electrocardiographic changes, lactate production, and changes in hemodynamics and global and regional wall motion scores. However, as mentioned above, patients undergoing elective angioplasty suffer from active ischemia (painful or silent) that may modulate the initial ischemic response. Hence, patients may be either in a period of tolerance, or protected by the first or second window due to recent ischemia by the time of the first balloon inflation. Moreover, some of the patients have already developed collateral circulation that might attenuate the ischemic response. In addition, the severity of pain is influenced not only by the severity of ischemia but by stretching the vessel wall by balloon inflation. Changing the inflation pressure may result in alteration of the severity of pain.[4] Nevertheless several studies have shown decrease in the intensity of chest pain and the magnitude of ST segment deviation following repeated balloon occlusion, especially if >90 seconds of balloon inflations were employed.[4,7,8]

Tomai et al assessed the magnitude of ST segment deviation during the first balloon occlusion in patients with stable (n=33) or unstable (n=29) angina pectoris.[9] All patients had no previous myocardial infarction and had 1-vessel disease. Mean ST segment shift was smaller in patients with unstable than stable angina, despite a similar prevalence of collateral vessels. The adaptation to repeated ischemia may be ascribed in some but not all patients to recruitment of collaterals. Hence, a metabolic adaptation, or preconditioning by ischemia may be the underlying mechanism.[4] It has been demonstrated that glibenclamide (an ATP-sensitive K^+ channel blocker that prevents preconditioning in animal models) and selective A_1-adenosine receptor inhibition by either bamiphylline or aminophylline, prevented the reduction of the magnitude of ST segment shift during the second, compared with the first balloon occlusion.[7]

Acute myocardial infarction

Numerous studies have assessed the effects of antecedent angina on myocardial infarct size, global left ventricular function, and prognosis. However, the time definitions of preinfarction angina in the different studies ranged from a few hours to several months.[3] As mentioned above, all the time frames of ischemic preconditioning of the human heart are unknown. Hence, it is difficult to verify whether a preconditioning effect was actually assessed in some of the studies. The effects of silent ischemia have not been investigated. Moreover, not all studies excluded patients without timely proven reperfusion. In addition, only the minority of the studies evaluated the collateral circulation before reperfusion occurred. Thus, in most studies, the effect of recruitment of collaterals on outcome was not taken into consideration.[8] None of the previous studies has evaluated patients on medications that might interfere with preconditioning (such as glibenclamide and theophyllines) separately.

Most of the studies, evaluating the effect of antecedent angina on outcome of acute myocardial infarction, have found that patients with a history of long standing angina are older, have more risk factors, have more extensive coronary artery disease, and higher residual coronary artery stenosis after thrombolytic therapy than patients without a history of angina. In addition, the incidence of post-infarction angina and recurrent infarction is higher in patients with a history of prior angina. All of these factors may adversely affect long term outcome. And indeed, several studies of patients with acute myocardial infarction who did not undergo reperfusion therapy demonstrated adverse and more complicated in-hospital and long term outcome in patients with antecedent angina.

Iwasaka et al assessed left ventricular function in patients with first acute Q wave anterior myocardial infarction due to proximal occlusion of the left anterior descending coronary artery. All patients were admitted within 3 hours from onset of infarction and underwent successful percutaneous transluminal coronary angioplasty.[10] Twenty eight patients had, and 25 patients did not have unstable angina prior to infarction, respectively. Baseline clinical characteristics and the percentage of patients with demonstrable collaterals were similar in both groups. The number of LV cords with akinesis or dyskinesis, 4 to 5 weeks after infarction, was greater in patients without antecedent angina, while left ventricular ejection fraction was lower.

Anzai et al reported that in patients with first Q wave myocardial infarction, the subgroup without preinfarction angina had higher peak creatine kinase, higher in-hospital incidence of ventricular tachyarrhythmias, pump failure and cardiac mortality.[11] Among patients with anterior myocardial infarction, angina was associated with a lower incidence of cardiac rupture and less incidence of heart failure within one year after infarction. The prevalence of multivessel coronary artery disease and the extent of coronary collaterals filling at emergency coronary angiography were comparable among patients with or without angina. Patients with anterior myocardial infarction and angina had higher left ventricular ejection fraction, lower left ventricular end diastolic volume, and lower prevalence of left ventricular aneurysm.

Kloner et al, in a retrospective analysis of the TIMI-4 trial patients, have found that the subgroup with previous angina had lower in-hospital mortality (3% vs. 8%, p=0.03), lower incidence of severe congestive heart failure or shock (1% vs. 7%, p=0.004), and lower creatine kinase release over 24 hours (119 vs. 154 CK integrated units, p=0.01) than the subgroup without angina.[12] More patients with prior angina had previous myocardial infarction and multivessel coronary artery disease. However, there was no difference in the collateral score, as assessed 90 minutes after initiation of thrombolytic therapy, between the groups. The subgroup of patients experiencing anginal pain within 48 hours before infarction, compared to the patients who did not had a trend towards less in-hospital mortality (3% vs. 6%, p=0.09), a lower incidence of severe congestive heart failure or shock (1% vs. 6%, p=0.008), and smaller creatine kinase release over 24 hours (115 vs. 151 CK integrated units, p=0.03). In contrast to the better clinical outcome, opacified collateral vessels at the 90 minute coronary angiography were found less frequently in patients with than those without angina within 48 hours of infarction (9% versus 23%, respectively).

Nakagawa et al evaluated 84 patients with first anterior wall acute myocardial infarction who achieved reperfusion by either thrombolytic therapy or angioplasty within 6 hours from onset of symptoms.[13] Thirty seven patients had no antecedent angina, while 22 and 25 patients had angina that started less than 7 days, and > 7 days before infarction, respectively. Episodes of chest pain within the 24 hours before infarction were more frequent in patients with new onset angina (82%) than in those with long standing angina (28%). All patients underwent left ventriculography on the day of admission and 28 days later. Collateral score was higher in the long standing angina group than in the groups with new onset or no angina. While left ventricular ejection fraction was comparable among the groups on the first day, at 28 days after infarction left ventricular function improved by 6±10% in patients with long standing angina and by 7±10% in patients with new onset angina. No improvement in ejection fraction (0±8%) was observed in patients without angina. Late regional wall motion in the infarcted zone was improved more in patients with new onset and long standing angina than in patients without angina. When only patients without visible collaterals were assessed, only the 19 patients with new onset angina, but not the 31 patients without angina and the 10 patients with long standing angina, had significant improvement in regional wall motion in the infarcted zone. Thus, increased collateral circulation may explain protection in patients with long standing angina, but not in patients with new onset angina.

The study by Haider et al is probably the study that most resembles the experimental models of the "first window of protection".[14] A group of 57 patients with evolving acute myocardial infarction underwent holter ST segment monitoring before thrombolytic therapy was initiated. Spontaneous two or more episodes of transient decline in ST elevation to within 0.05 mV of baseline, lasting over 1 minute myocardial reperfusion (an electrocardiographic marker of intermittent reperfusion) occurred in 28 patients. There was no difference in mean time from onset of pain to initiation of therapy. However, time to 50% resolution of the ST segment elevation (an estimation of the time to reperfusion) was longer in patients without intermittent ST segment reduction. Patients with spontaneous intermittent ST segment decline had lower CK-MB and higher left ventricular ejection fraction. Coronary patency, assessed by coronary angiography at 90 minutes after initiation of therapy, was similar. Thus, it might be that the early intermittent spontaneous reperfusion preconditioned the heart and reduced infarct size. Alternatively, perhaps these patients reperfused earlier, as judged by the time to 50% ST segment resolution, and thus were subjected to shorter ischemic periods. The study by Andreotti et al[3] supports the latter assumption. They found that in patients with acute myocardial infarction preceded by unstable angina, thrombolytic therapy resulted in more rapid reperfusion and smaller infarct size, as estimated by creatine kinase release. Although baseline hemostatic factors before thrombolytic therapy were similar in both groups, the percentage of patients treated with aspirin in each group was not reported.[3] It is plausible that more patients with preceding angina received aspirin. Aspirin may enhance spontaneous reperfusion and decrease infarct size.[8] However, it might be that the composition of the occlusive thrombus is different in patients with than without antecedent angina, and that the thrombus of patients with angina is more amenable to thrombolysis.[8]

In summary, most studies showed beneficial effects of prior angina. It seems that short term angina (<7 days) is probably associated with protection by either ischemic preconditioning or enhanced propensity to thrombolysis, while longer duration of angina (>7 days) may be associated also with recruitment of collateral vessels. Benefits of short term angina may include both classic preconditioning, if ischemia occurs just prior to infarction, as well as "the second window of protection"- type preconditioning. However, long term prognosis is hampered by the higher prevalence of risk factors and a tendency to reinfarction in patients with prior angina.

Adaptation to angina

"Walk through" angina and "warm-up" angina are two phenomena that may represent a form of myocardial preconditioning by ischemia.[4] "Walk through" angina refers to the paradoxical disappearance of anginal pain despite continuation of exertion. However, there is no intervening rest, thus the mandatory reperfusion period probably does not occur. The second term, "warm-up" angina, describes the phenomenon of augmentation of maximal effort following rest after initial effort was terminated due to ischemia.[4]

Jaffe and Quinn subjected 34 patients to an initial exercise test, followed by 30 min of walking, 20 minutes of rest and a second exercise test.[4] During the peak exercise of the second test patients reached a higher rate-pressure product. Yet, the magnitude of ST segment deviation was smaller on the second than on the first exercise test. Williams et al evaluated eleven patients with effort induced angina and isolated >70% narrowing of the left anterior descending coronary artery. Patients were subjected to two identical bouts of rapid cardiac pacing separated by a 5-15 minute rest period. During the second stress there was less anginal pain and ST segment depression, and lactate extraction was improved.[4] Peak coronary blood flow during the first and second pacing periods were comparable. However, regional myocardial oxygen consumption was lower during the second stress.

Thus, relative reduction in myocardial oxygen consumption, a form of metabolic adaptation to ischemia, and not an augmentation of coronary blood flow, is responsible for the improved tolerance to pacing-induced ischemia. The findings of Okazaki et al are similar. They evaluated 13 patients with exertional angina and >90% stenosis of the proximal left anterior descending coronary artery, without >50% stenosis of other coronary arteries. Patients underwent two consecutive supine exercise tests separated by 15 minutes of rest in the catheterization laboratory. Exercise time was longer and the magnitude of ST segment deviation at the time of angina onset was smaller during the second exercise test. Hemodynamic variables and great cardiac vein flow were comparable during the first and second exercise. However, at 3 minutes of exercise regional myocardial oxygen consumption was smaller, and adenosine release was higher in the second test. Thus, the "warm-up" phenomenon is not related to an increase in collateral flow but rather to a reduction in myocardial oxygen consumption, perhaps mediated by adenosine A_1 receptors. Maybaum et al studied the effect of three exercise tests separated by 30 minute intervals, and reported that patients could exercise longer until 1 mm ST depression was reached during the second and third exercise tests than at the first one.[15] Furthermore, exercise duration was longer and the rate-pressure product at 1 mm ST depression was greater during the second and third than the first tests.

In conclusion, brief ischemic periods protect the human heart in various clinical situations by at least three independent mechanisms: recruitment of collateral flow, ischemic preconditioning, and perhaps increased propensity to reperfusion.[8] A limiting factor to utilization of ischemic preconditioning in the clinical practice is that ischemia is mandatory to exert protection. Thus, the clinical applicability of ischemic preconditioning by brief ischemic episodes may be limited to several situations such as training patients with effort induced angina to better perform exercise by a short "warm-up" pre-effort; facilitation of long balloon inflation during complicated cases of percutaneous transluminal coronary angioplasty; and as a technique to preserve myocardial function during cardiac surgery. However, development of "preconditioning-mimetic" agents may enable us to confer long term protection for susceptible patients, and maybe even to limit injury after sustained ischemia already started (for example- on admission of patients with acute myocardial infarction). These future agents may be used to increase tolerance to effort induced angina, limitation of infarct size in susceptible patients, better preservation of myocardial function during iatrogenic ischemia (cardiac surgery and angioplasty), and may even decrease the incidence of sudden death and ischemic and reperfusion ventricular tachyarrhythmias. Another aspect that should be extensively evaluated is whether chronic use of therapeutic agents with presumed preconditioning-blocking effects, such as glibenclamide and theophyllines, may adversely affect prognosis in patients with coronary artery disease.

References

1. Przyklenk K, Kloner RA. Preconditioning: a balanced perspective. Br Heart J 1995;74:575-577.
2. Lawson CS, Downey JM. Preconditioning: State of the art myocardial protection. Cardiovasc Res 1993;27:542-550.
3. Andreotti F, Pasceri V, Hackett DR et al. Pereinfarction angina as a predictor of more rapid coronary thrombolysis in patients with acute myocardial infarction. N Engl J Med 1996;334:7-12.
4. Kloner RA, Yellon D. Does ischemic preconditioning occur in patients? J Am Coll Cardiol 1994; 24:1133-1142.
5. Yellon DM, Alkhulaif AM, Pugsley WB. Preconditioning the human myocardium. Lancet 1993;342:276-277.
6. Abd-Elfattah AS, Wechsler AS. Myocardial preconditioning: a model or a phenomenon? J Card Surg 1995;10:381-388.
7. Tomai F, Crea F, Gaspardone A et al. Ischemic preconditioning during coronary angioplasty is prevented by glibenclamide, a selective ATP-sensitive K^+ channel blocker. Circulation 1994;90:700-705.
8. Braunwald E. Acute myocardial infarction- the value of being prepared. N Engl J Med 1996;334:51-52.
9. Tomai F, Crea F, Gaspardone A, et al. Determinants of myocardial ischemia during percutaneous transluminal coronary angioplasty in patients with significant narrowing of a single coronary artery and stable or unstable angina pectoris. Am J Cardiol 1994;74:1089-1094.
10. Iwasaka T, Nakamura S, Karakawa M et al. Cardioprotective effect of unstable angina prior to acute anterior myocardial infarction. Chest 1994;105:57-61.
11. Anzai T, Yoshikawa T, Asakura Y et al. Preinfarction angina as a major predictor of left ventricular function and long-term prognosis after a first Q wave myocardial infarction. J Am Coll Cardiol 1995;26:319-327.
12. Kloner RA, Shook T, Przyklenk K et al. Previous angina alters in-hospital outcome in TIMI 4. A clinical correlate to preconditioning? Circulation 1995;91:37-47.
13. Nakagawa Y, Ito H, Kitakaze M et al. Effect of angina pectoris on myocardial protection in patients with reperfused anterior wall myocardial infarction: retrospective clinical evidence of "preconditioning". J Am Coll Cardiol 1995;25:1076-1083.
14. Haider AW, Andreotti F, Hackett DR et al. Early spontaneous intermittent myocardial reperfusion during acute myocardial infarction is associated with augmented thrombogenic activity and less myocardial damage. J Am Coll Cardiol 1995;26:662-667.
15. Maybaum S, Ilan M, Mogilevsky J et al. Repeated exercise induced ischemia causes myocardial preconditioning (abstract). J Am Coll Cardiol 1995;25:22A.

In: Mentzer, R.M., Jr., Kitakaze, M., Downey, J.M., Hori, M, eds. Adenosine, Cardioprotection and Clinical Application. Kluwer Academic Publishers, Norwell, MA, USA, 1997.

16. Clinical Pharmacology of Preconditioning and Adenosinergic Drugs

Herman Van Belle

Introduction

On an array of cells and organs adenosine may exert a multitude of effects, all apparently serving one purpose: restore and maintain the balance between energy supply and demand (for recent reviews, Refs. 1,2). Its rapid formation in response to ischemia constitutes a natural defense system which appears to be extremely efficient, hence very attractive, for three reasons:

1. Adenosine's formation is the simple consequence of a disequilibrium between dephosphorylation of ATP (≈ energy demand) and rephosphorylation (mitochondrial oxidative metabolism ≈ energy supply). AMP, adenosine's immediate precursor, is a most sensitive sensor of energy shortage.
2. Adenosine's formation is local and temporarily. It is limited to the ischemic area within most vital organs and only when oxygen supply is insufficient to cope with the demand. Nature has even taken precautions to prevent spreading of this potent messenger to normoxic regions or organs by providing rapid catabolism in the endothelial cells lining the microvessels, and in erythrocytes.
3. Adenosine's production initiates a cascade of effects. Its most prominent activity, microvascular vasodilatation, will be a first-aid measure to restore the balance. If not sufficient, more adenosine will accumulate and more receptors within reach may be triggered: demand will be moderated and there will be a delay in the start of a vicious circle of events leading to major organ damage.

It should be emphasized that endogenous adenosine does not prevent ischemia (it is the product of ischemia) but may limit the deleterious consequences of ischemia and reperfusion.

With the ever increasing knowledge of the pharmacology of adenosine there is the continuing interest to explore - and exploit - the adenosinergic system for therapy. The strategies that can be used will be briefly discussed in this paper (for many details, see Refs. 1, 2).

Preconditioning

From many experimental studies it is known that a short period (or a few periods) of ischemia and reperfusion prior to a sustained ischemia results in impressive protection.

Less ST-segment shift, chest pain and lactate production on a second than on a first balloon inflation during angioplasty provides clinical evidence for preconditioning in humans. Significant reduction in hospital death (from 8% to 3%; $p=0.03$) and severe heart failure or shock (from 7% to 1%; $p<0.01$) in acute myocardial infarction patients with ($n=218$), respectively without previous angina ($n=198$), has been regarded as clinical correlate to preconditioning.[3]

Besides the fact that this induction of ischemia is of course the most direct way to raise tissue adenosine levels, there are other good reasons nowadays to believe that adenosine plays a major role in the protection seen with preconditioning.[4]

Because nobody knows exactly when infarction will strike, preconditioning can hardly become daily practice and, most probably, it will remain restricted to the surgical room with PTCA as the most obvious opportunity.

Enhancement of receptor binding

PD81723, 2-amino-3-benzylthiophene, has been reported to be a prototype drug enhancing the binding of adenosine to its receptor(s). In the meantime it has been found that the enhancement is confined to the A_1-receptor, limiting the expression of the entire spectrum of adenosine's beneficial effects (see Ref. 5 for details). The appeal of this approach is that the effect, if any, is dependent on the presence of endogenous adenosine, making potential therapy site- and event-specific. However, until now this strategy has not yielded a clinically relevant therapeutic.

Exogenous Adenosine or Adenosine Agonists?

Exogenous adenosine

At first glance, mimicry of the natural system by systemic administration of adenosine is appealing but there are some problems. First, the half-life of adenosine in human circulation is a few seconds. Hence, to achieve a relatively sustained effect, huge quantities have to be infused and, even more of a problem, that should be done exactly in time. Second, indiscriminate triggering of adenosine receptors all over the body will create unwanted, and even harmful, effects.

Nevertheless, there may be room for this approach in the surgical setting and a trial is ongoing indeed on the use of intracoronary adenosine during coronary artery bypass surgery. Preliminary data, also with intracoronary adenosine, but before primary angioplasty in patients with acute myocardial infarction, illustrate feasibility and tolerability of the approach with, associated, a lower incidence of angiographically assessed no-reflow in the dilated infarct-related artery (Picano's team, Pisa; abstr. 920-30; JACC 1996). Equally during PTCA, Bolli's group (Kentucky, US; Abstr. 901-89; JACC 1996) was able to show preconditioning in patients by infusion of adenosine 10 min. prior to balloon inflation (significantly less ST-segment shifts and chest pain scores).

Adenosine agonists

Chemical modification of the adenosine molecule has yielded products much less prone to catabolism and, more interestingly, products with widely different pharmacological effects. The availability of such "agonists" marked a big step forwards in the pharmacology/receptorology of adenosine with, in turn, stimulated new syntheses.

The return, thus far, for the pharmaceutical industry, which sponsored this evolution to a great extent and with interest, of course, beyond the pharmacology, is scanty. As therapeutics only a few are in preclinical stage and development has been discontinued for many.

Confounding factors that could explain why the exceptional progress in the preclinical area, both chemical and biological, has not been paralleled in the clinic are: first, receptor subtype specificity is often obscured by overlap in pharmacological activity; second, confusion often exists (especially in animal models) between direct effects at the cellular level and those which are secondary to cardiovascular changes; and, third, agonist activity at receptors frequently changes when administration is chronic. Needless, of course, to emphasize again that administration exactly in time, remains a major problem.

Acadesine, AICA-riboside

The introduction of AICA-riboside as a drug beneficial in coronary artery bypass surgery has created a lot of fuss. The original idea behind its use was that, as a natural precursor in the biosynthesis of purines (not of adenosine!), it would help the heart to recover the purines lost during ischemia and reperfusion. It was soon realized, however, that it did not work that way *in vivo*. However, in the meantime a study in dogs revealed some transient accumulation of adenosine early during ischemia with infusion of AICA-riboside. The lower incidence in these animals of arrhythmias and of leukocyte sequestration during reperfusion was ascribed to this adenosine. The evidence appeared sufficient to start an ambitious study in humans in the setting of bypass surgery, a trial which in the meantime has been terminated because of lack of significant benefit.

More recent biochemical studies in different species have failed to reveal any effect from this compound on myocardial adenosine.

Interference with adenosine catabolism

Inhibition of adenosine deaminase

Adenosine deaminase, present intracellularly in endothelial cells and, abundantly, in human erythrocytes, is the first enzymatic step in the breakdown of adenosine.

In experimental conditions EHNA and deoxycoformycin, known as tight-binding, almost irreversible inhibitors of adenosine deaminase, have been reported to prevent indeed the rapid deamination of adenosine to pharmacologically inactive inosine, but success, as to major benefit, has been equivocal. Furthermore, whenever there should be excessive production of adenosine, the peripheral concentrations of adenosine may rise and could create the problems discussed above with exogenous adenosine. In addition, long-term prophylactic use of these drugs can hardly be envisaged because of their marked toxicity.

Nucleoside transport inhibition

Before discussing nucleoside transport inhibitors, the role of the transporter in the fate of adenosine should be addressed. This protein is, within the myocardium (and probably in most other organs), almost exclusively located on the membrane of endothelial cells. These cells line the microvessels and constitute a strong physical and chemical barrier against passage of many products, including the nucleosides. The transporter facilitates the diffusion of the nucleosides according to the existing gradient. When during ischemia, adenosine accumulates in the interstitial space, the transporter will enhance its influx into the endothelial cells because of the gradient created by adenosine deaminase activity intracellularly. In other words, the transporter at the endothelial cell surface is the truly first step in adenosine's catabolism. During reperfusion, the gradient created by the tremendous expansion of the luminal compartment will favor facilitation by the transporter of the efflux, thus bypassing the barrier function and accelerating the washout.

Several biochemical studies in different species have documented a marked prolongation of adenosine's presence in myocardial tissue in both isolated hearts and *in vivo* when the nucleoside transporter is inhibited.

Nucleoside transport inhibition is an extremely rare property within organic molecules, at least when considering products active at micromolar or submicromolar concentrations.

Known already for decades is dipyridamole, mainly used as an antiplatelet agent, an activity related more to nucleoside transport inhibition than to inhibition of platelet phosphodiesterase as claimed. Dilazep is more potent and much more specific as a transport inhibitor than dipyridamole but its clinical development lagged far behind, most probably because of poor oral bioavailability (if any) and its very short half-life in systemic circulation. The lidoflazine-family of compounds was added to the list several years later, the most recent analogue being draflazine, which has been shown to be a very potent and stereospecific inhibitor of the transporter with no other known activity thus far and with very interesting pharmacokinetics in humans.[1]

Despite its long-standing clinical use, the output of studies revealing marked cardioprotection in humans by dipyridamole is very limited. Reasons for relative failure may be poor - and irreproducible - oral bioavailability, a relatively short duration of action and the neglect, in designing clinical trials, to focus on events with ischemia (= endogenous adenosine) as underlying pathology.

In a randomized double-blind study on patients undergoing thrombolysis (rtPA) within 6 hours of an acute myocardial infarction, treatment with dipyridamole (400 mg/day i.v. followed by 300 mg/day orally) was found to improve the recovery of left-ventricular function after 1 month as illustrated in Table 16-1 (adapted from Ref. 6).

More recently,[7] pharmacological protection by dipyridamole has been reported during PTCA. Intracoronary application (0.5 mg/kg in the artery to be dilated; 5 min. before angioplasty; n=10) resulted in a significant preservation of systolic and diastolic left ventricular performance during PTCA, when compared to placebos (n=10). Most prominent was an unaffected global ejection fraction (deterioration of 29% in placebos), an increment of diastolic stiffening of 13% versus 57%, and a significant prolongation of achievable balloon-inflation time by 48%. In a third group of 10 patients dipyridamole pretreatment per se (no PTCA) induced significant amelioration of angiographically assessed left ventricular systolic performance. It was concluded from this study that intracoronary application of dipyridamole might result in the induction of myocardial preconditioning.

A recent preliminary report on the results of the 2nd European Stroke Prevention Study[8] revealed potential for therapy with nucleoside transport inhibitors as prophylactics in patients with history of stroke or transient ischemic attack (TIA). As illustrated in Table 16-2, combining dipyridamole (DIP) with aspirin shows a marked additive effect on stroke prevention. In this respect it may be worthwhile to look for brain protection by transport inhibitors in the setting of coronary bypass grafting where cerebral complications may be quite common and intracoronary adenosine will hardly be effective because of its pharmacokinetics.

Table 16-1. LV-function recovery 1 month after MI

	tPA + PLAC n=39	**+DIP n=44**
LVEF	42%	47%*
EDV	71 ml/m2	60 ml/m2
LVEDP	26mm Hg	22mm Hg*

*p<0.05 versus PLAC

Adapted from Rousseau MF, Van Eyll C, Hayashida W et al. Circulation 1995;88: Abstr. 0841.

At the time draflazine was cleared for clinical studies it was decided to jump on the AICA-riboside train which was hoped to reach soon its goal: prevention of death and/or perioperative infarction during surgery in patients at high cardiac risk.

In a first study the outcome was assessed of patients undergoing coronary artery bypass grafting when given placebo (n=17) or 2.5 mg (n=17) or 5 mg (n=18) of draflazine (bolus injection over 5 min. just before cardiopulmonary bypass). Preliminary data, illustrated in Figure 1, show a better left ventricular function post-surgery in patients receiving the drug. Left ventricular tissue levels of adenosine were also increased, dose-dependently, just before removal of the clamp.

A more extended Phase II-trial including some 200 patients in the same setting and in three different centers is being analyzed these days. The number of events (hard endpoints being perioperative infarction or death) is definitely too small to achieve sufficient power for a final conclusion. In this respect it should also be stressed that at least half of these events are due to mechanical/surgical problems for which a pharmacological cure can not be expected. Apart from a significant improvement of the cardiac index (much alike the one mentioned above) in the 3 centers, another interesting finding came out of one center which contributed 100 patients and where the release of CK_{MB} was measured at 4 hour intervals for 2 days following surgery. As illustrated in Figure 2, the second peak of enzyme release, frequently seen in placebo-treated patients (n=47), was much less prominent in patients receiving draflazine (n=48). Because absolute values of enzymatic activities released are meaningless in the setting of surgery, the

Table 16-2. European Stroke Prevention Study -2(ESPS-2)

6602 patients - history of stroke or TIA

	Incidence Stroke	Death
aspirin (50 mg/d)	↓18%	↓13%
DIP (400mg/d)	↓16%	↓15%
asp. + DIP (50mg/400mg)	↓37%	↓24%
PLACEBO		

Treatment for 2 years

Adapted from Ferguson JJ. Circulation 1996;93:399.

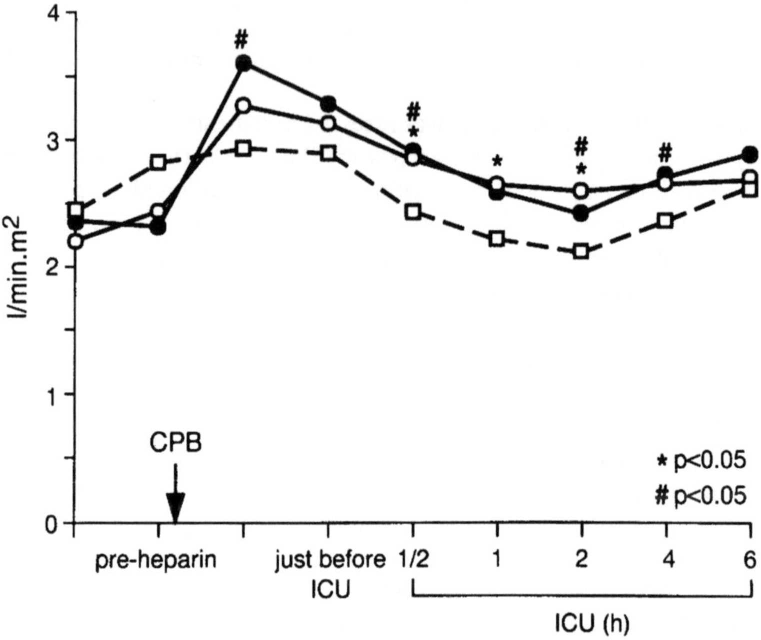

FIGURE 16-1. Cardiac index following coronary artery bypass grafting in patients receiving placebo (n=17) (□), and 2.5 mg (n=17) (○) or 5 mg (n=18) (●) respectively of draflazine as a bolus injection at the time indicated
Taken from a study by P.J.A. van der Starre et al., Zwolle, The Netherlands.

percentage of patients is shown who exhibit values equal to or above the values at 12 hours (when the activities due to surgical damage start to decline). The exact meaning of these data remains to be elucidated.

A six way cross-over trial, double blind and placebo controlled, has been conducted in 6 healthy volunteers using doubling doses of draflazine (i.v.) from 0.25 mg to 4 mg and assessing left-ventricular performance by measuring systolic time intervals. The ratio between the pre-ejection period and the left ventricular ejection time decreased significantly and dose-dependently (from 0.345 to 0.305, 0.285 and 0.26, at 1,2 and 4 mg respectively; peak effects at around 20 min.) suggestive, according to the investigators, of an overall improvement of left ventricular function (J. De Cree, personal communication). The degree of ex vivo nucleoside transport inhibition in these patients completely paralleled the functional response. These results in healthy volunteers resemble to some extent the outcome of the study with dipyridamole mentioned above. Interestingly, if oral treatment with draflazine would achieve a more sustained effect, as it does for nucleoside

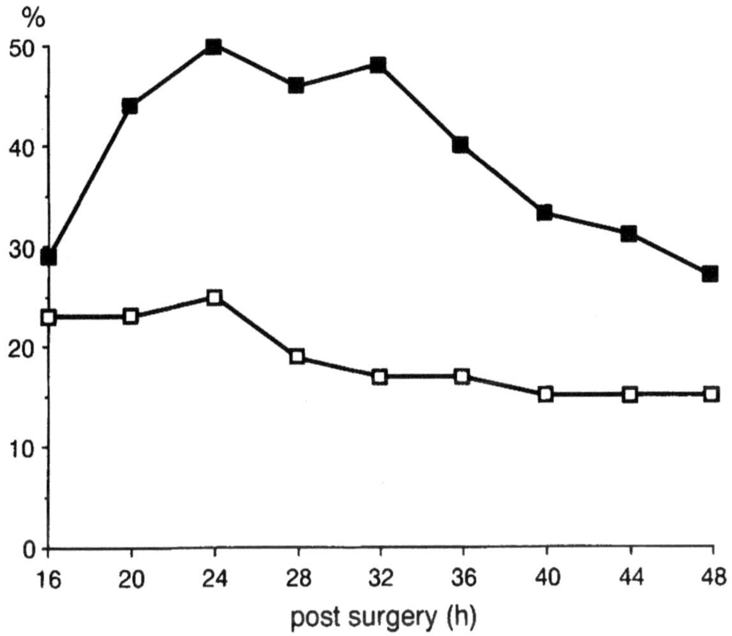

FIGURE 16-2. Percentage of patients undergoing coronary artery bypass surgery showing CK_{MB} values (units of activity) equal to or higher than the values at 12 hours post surgery.
■ Placebo's (n=47).
□ Treated with draflazine, 2.5 mg bolus just before bypass followed by infusion of 1 mg/h. for 2 hours.
Taken from a study by W. Flameng et al., Leuven, Belgium.

transport inhibition, the drug may well become an attractive, prophylactic therapy for patients with progressive congestive heart failure.

Conclusions

As therapy, preconditioning and local administration of adenosine may have limited application in the surgical setting. Adenosine agonists may find their way provided they can be pointed at specific target cells or organs which, as yet, has not been achieved. Remain the nucleoside transport inhibitors which strengthen the natural system, retaining the latter's major advantages being a whole spectrum of beneficial activities expressed exactly when and where needed.

References

1. Van Belle H. Specific metabolically active anti-ischemic agents: adenosine and nucleoside transport inhibitors. In Singh BN, Dzau VJ, Vanhoutte PM et al, eds. Cardiovascular Pharmacology and Therapeutics; Churchill Livingstone,1993:217-235.
2. Van Belle H: Adenosine promotors: An overview of existing strategies. Curr Opin Invest Drugs 1993;2 :1191-1199.
3. Kloner RA, Shook T, Przyklenk K et al. Previous angina alters in-hospital outcome in TIMI-4. A clinical correlate to preconditioning ? Circulation 1995;91:37-47.
4. Miura T, Iimura O. Infarct size limitation by preconditioning: its phenomenological features and the key role of adenosine. Cardiovasc Res 1993;27:36-42.
5. Kollias-Baker C, Ruble J, Dennis D et al. Allosteric enhancer PD81723 acts by novel mechanism to potentiate cardiac actions of adenosine. Circ.Res. 1994;75:961-971.
6. Rousseau MF, Van Eyll C, Hayashida W et al. Intravenous dipyridamole infusion during thrombolysis improves the recovery of left ventricular function. Circulation 1995;88: Abstr. 0841.
7. Strauer BE, Heidland HE, Heintzen MP et al. Pharmakologische Myokardprotektion während perkutaner transluminaler Koronarangioplastie (PTCA) durch Dipyridamole intrakoronär: Hämodynamische, Kontraktile und Ventrikeldynamische Konsequenzen. Z.Kardiol. 1995;84: 898-910.
8. Ferguson JJ. Research News: Second European Stroke Prevention Study. Circulation 1996;93: 399.

In: Mentzer, R.M., Jr., Kitakaze, M., Downey, J.M., Hori, M, eds. Adenosine, Cardioprotection and Clinical Application. Kluwer Academic Publishers, Norwell, MA, USA, 1997.

17. Clinical Application of Ischemic Preconditioning by ATP-Sensitive Potassium Channel Openers

Naoshi Arakawa
Motoyuki Nakamura
Ken-ichi Fukami
Katsuhiko Hiramori

Introduction

Prognosis after myocardial infarction is dependent on infarct size, which reflects left ventricular dysfunction. It is therefore important to explore a strategy for reducing infarct size in patients with acute myocardial infarction. It has been reported that infarct size derived from regional wall motion of the left ventricle or calculated from total release of cardiac enzymes and the rate of incidence of cardiogenic shock after acute myocardial infarction was significantly decreased in patients with a history of angina pectoris compared to those without pre-infarction angina.[1]

This reduction of cardiac damage and infarct size after prolonged myocardial ischemia appears to be caused by the preceding transient myocardial ischemia.

Ischemic preconditioning and the K^+_{ATP} channel

Murry and co-workers[2] first observed a reduction in myocardial infarct size in dogs when transient myocardial ischemia had been preceded by prolonged myocardial ischemia and reperfusion but not when this brief ischemic episode was absent. They termed this phenomenon "ischemic preconditioning." Many studies have subsequently been performed to clarify the mechanisms responsible for this phenomenon. It has been reported that a receptor agonist of adenosine, a precursor of adenosine triphosphate (ATP), induces ischemic preconditioning, and that ATP-sensitive potassium (K^+_{ATP}) channel blocker inhibits the effect, whereas K^+_{ATP} channel opener enhances it. As a result, adenosine receptor activation with subsequent K^+_{ATP} channel activation has been suggested as an important mechanism underlying ischemic preconditioning which protects the myocardium from ischemia and damage.

The existence of K^+_{ATP} channels in cardiomyocytes was identified by Noma. [3] A decrease in the intracellular concentration of ATP during myocardial ischemia leads to opening of the K^+_{ATP} channel. The intracellular mechanism(s) underlying ischemic preconditioning remain unclear, however, so the following mechanism is presumed. Transient myocardial ischemia induces opening of the K^+_{ATP} channel. This activation in turn results in a reduction in calcium overload during ischemia with a decrease in membrane action potential. The reduction of cytosolic free calcium levels leads to inhibition of contractile activity and preservation of ATP, which would be expected to delay myocardial cell death and thus to reduce myocardial infarct size.

K^+_{ATP} channel openers and blockers

Intracoronary infusion of the K^+_{ATP} channel blocker glibenclamide has been shown to decrease coronary blood flow and myocardial oxygen consumption in a dose dependent manner in dogs.[4] Glibenclamide has also been shown to decrease resting coronary blood flow and to attenuate coronary reactive hyperemia blood flow induced by 20-second coronary occlusion.[4] These findings indicate that the K^+_{ATP} channel modulates coronary vasomotor tone and contributes to coronary vasodilation during myocardial ischemia.

Gross and Auchampach[5] demonstrated that a brief coronary occlusion and subsequent short-term reperfusion in dogs markedly reduced the size of infarct caused by prolonged (1 hour) ischemic insult followed by 5-hour reperfusion compared to infarct size in dogs where ischemic preconditioning was absent. In this investigation, administration of glibenclamide before or immediately after preconditioning completely abolished the protective effect.

A different type of K^+_{ATP} channel blocker, sodium 5-hydroxydecanoate, has also been demonstrated as inhibiting the preconditioning-related cardioprotective effects in dogs. In contrast, pretreatment with the K^+_{ATP} channel opener aprikalim caused a significant reduction in infarct size. It has also been reported that bimakalim, another type of K^+_{ATP} channel opener, mimics the effects of ischemic preconditioning and potentiates the effects of reduction in infarct size.[6] An important inference may be drawn from these findings; that the mechanism of myocardial preconditioning in the canine heart is mediated by activation of K^{+}_{ATP} channels. However, another report was unable to prove the contribution of K^{+}_{ATP} channels to myocardial preconditioning in rats.[7] Although the reason for this inconsistency is not known, the discrepancy may be due to differences between the species concerned or to differing experimental conditions.

The effect of ischemic preconditioning varies when the duration of pre-ischemia is brief. It was reported that a 3-minute period of coronary artery occlusion with a subsequent 10-minute reperfusion before a more prolonged (60 minute) occlusion followed by a 4-hour reperfusion was insufficient to produce ischemic preconditioning in dogs. However, a 10-minute occlusion with a 10-minute reperfusion period markedly reduced myocardial infarct size (by one quarter) after sustained coronary arterial occlusion and reperfusion injury compared to a single 60-minute ischemic insult.[8] It is interesting to note that even where the pre-ischemia duration was short, intracoronary infusion of the K^{+}_{ATP} channel opener bimakalim and a 3-minute preconditioning period reduced myocardial infarct size to a marked extent that was comparable to that resulting from a 10-minute period of ischemic preconditioning.[8] These results suggest that K^{+}_{ATP} channel activation with a K^{+}_{ATP} channel opener may produce and enhance ischemic preconditioning effects.

The prospects for clinical application of K^{+}_{ATP} channel openers

It has been suggested that ischemic preconditioning may occur in humans as it does in animal models. It is known that during percutaneous transluminal coronary angioplasty (PTCA), myocardial ischemia during the second balloon inflation is less severe than during the first inflation, an effect that may be related to the phenomenon of ischemic preconditioning. However, it is unclear whether the mechanism underlying the cardioprotective effect of ischemic preconditioning in humans is identical to that in other species. The influence of the K^{+}_{ATP} channel blocker glibenclamide on ischemic preconditioning during PTCA has been studied recently by Tomai et al.[9] They have demonstrated that, in glibenclamide-treated patients, the mean ST-segment shift on 12-lead ECG during the second balloon inflation was similar to that observed during the first inflation, while the severity of cardiac pain was greater than during the first inflation. In contrast, placebo-treated patients demonstrated a lower mean ST-segment shift and less severe cardiac pain during the second inflation than during the first inflation. This indicates that ischemic preconditioning caused by brief repeated coronary occlusion is abolished by pretreatment with glibenclamide. These findings suggest that K^{+}_{ATP} channels may be significantly implicated in ischemic preconditioning in humans.

Nicorandil is a new hybrid drug which has two pharmacological properties; it is a nitrate and K^+_{ATP} channel opener,[10] and it partially dilates coronary resistant vessels by virtue of its effect on K^+_{ATP} channels. We have studied the ischemic myocardial protective effect of intracoronary infusion of nicorandil during PTCA. The subjects in this study were 23 patients (male/female ratio 16:7, mean age 65 years) undergoing PTCA for a lesion of the left anterior descending artery. After a successful first dilatation (<50% degree of stenosis), the patients were randomly assigned to either nicorandil or a placebo group in a double blind fashion (Table 1). Chest pain score, ST-segment shift on surface 12-leads and intracoronary ECG, and left ventricular anterior wall motion score by echocardiogram were determined during the second inflation as a control. Intracoronary administration of nicorandil (1 mg) or vehicle (physiological saline) for 20 seconds was then carried out, and the ischemic parameters during the third inflation were compared with those during the control inflation. Intra-balloon pressure and balloon inflation time were the same for both inflations.

The rates of reduction for chest pain, maximum ST-segment shift on 12-lead and intracoronary ECG, and wall motion score were higher in the nicorandil group than in the placebo group (Table 17-2). Moreover, the augmentation of heart rate and rate-pressure product during balloon inflation was significantly less in the

Table 17-1. Clinical Characteristics of Two Patient Groups

	nicorandil group (n=13)	placebo group (n=10)	difference
Age (years)	65 ± 3	65 ± 2	ns
Male/female	10 / 3	7 / 3	ns
Duration of AP (months)	36 ± 14	27 ± 10	ns
Previous MI (%)	54	20	ns
Number of stenotic vessels			
1 vessel	31	60	ns
2 vessels	38	20	ns
3 vessels	31	20	ns
Intraballoon pressure (atm)	7.0 ± 0.3	7.0 ± 0.3	ns
Inflation time (sec)	115 ± 5	111 ± 6	ns
Severity of stenosis			
before PTCA	82 ± 3	79 ± 2	ns
after PTCA	19 ± 3	26 ± 4	ns

Mean ± SE
AP = angina pectoris; MI = myocardial infarction; PTCA = percutaneous transluminal coronary angioplasty

Table 17-2. Reduction Rates for ST-segment, Chest Pain, and Wall Motion Score in Two Patient Groups

	nicorandil group	placebo group
Reduction of max ST-seg on S-ECG	23%	15%
Reduction of Σ ST-seg on S-ECG	26%	18%
Reduction of ST-seg on IC-ECG	23%	17%
Reduction of chest pain score	25%	-6%
Reduction of wall motion score	6%	-10%

S-ECG = surface 12-lead ECG; IC-ECG = intracoronary ECG

nicorandil group than in the placebo group (Table 17-3). Heart rate and systemic arterial blood pressure did not change significantly as a result of intracoronary infusion of nicorandil, nor were there any ventricular arrhythmias or other adverse effects during the infusion.

These results indicate that myocardial ischemia during balloon inflation tended to be reduced by intracoronary infusion of nicorandil. This suggests that this K^+_{ATP} channel opener may have a cardioprotective effect by enhancing ischemic preconditioning, a contention supported by its suppressive effect on heart rate increase and rate-pressure product during PTCA. These beneficial effects of nicorandil may be clinically useful due to their potential for improving the safety of PTCA, especially in cases of balloon inflation of lengthy duration.

It may be also predicted that the enhancement of ischemic preconditioning by K^+_{ATP} channel openers might limit the detrimental effects of myocardial ischemia or infarction in clinical settings such as unstable angina pectoris and cardiac surgery which induce prolonged myocardial ischemic insult.

Table 17-3. Changes in Heart Rate and Rate-Pressure Product During Balloon Inflation in Two Patient Groups

	nicorandil group		placebo group	
	2nd Infl	3rd Infl	2nd Infl	3rd Infl
Heart rate change (bpm)	4.3 ± 1.5	-1.5 ± 1.2*	2.8 ± 3.6	2.3 ± 4.8
RPP changes (mmHg/min x 100)	5.3 ± 0.4	-2.6 ± 3.4*	5.6 ± 7.6	1.8 ± 8.0

Mean ± SE, * $p < 0.05$ versus 2nd inflation
RPP = rate-pressure product
Infl = inflation

References

1. Kloner RA, Shook T, Przyklenk K et al. for the TIMI 4 investigators. Previous angina alters in-hospital outcome in TIMI 4: a clinical correlate to preconditioning? Circulation 1995;91:37-47.
2. Murry CE, Jennings RB, Reimer KA. Preconditionig with ischemia: a delay of lethal cell injury in ischemic myocardium. Circulation 1986;74:1124-1136.
3. Noma A. ATP-regulated K^+ channels in cardiac muscle. Nature 1963;305:147-148.
4. Duncker DJ, Van Zon NS, Altman JD et al. Role of K^+_{ATP} channels in coronary vasodilation during exercise. Circulation 1993;88:1245-1253.
5. Gross GJ, Auchampach JA. Blockade of ATP-sensitive potassium channels prevents myocardial preconditioning in dogs. Circ Res 1992;70:223-233.
6. Mizumura T, Nithipatikom K, Gross GJ. Bimakalim, an ATP-sensitive potassium channel opener, mimics the effects of ischemic preconditioning to reduce infarct size, adenosine release, and neutrophil function in dogs. Circulation 1995;92:1236-1245.
7. Liu Y, Downey JM. Ischemic preconditioning protects against infarction in rat heart. Am J Physiol 1992;263:H1107-H1112.
8. Yao Z, Gross GJ. Activation of ATP-sensitive potassium channels lowers threshold for ischemic preconditioning in dogs. Am J Physiol 1994;36:H1888-1894.
9. Tomai F, Crea F, Gaspardone A et al. Ischemic preconditioning during coronary angioplasty is prevented by glibenclamide, a selective ATP-sensitive K^+ channel blocker. Circulation 1994;90:700-705.
10. Taira N. Nicorandil as a hybrid between nitrates and potassium channel activators. Am J Cardiol 1989;63:18J-24J.

In: Mentzer, R.M., Jr., Kitakaze, M., Downey, J.M., Hori, M, eds. Adenosine, Cardioprotection and Clinical Application. Kluwer Academic Publishers, Norwell, MA, USA, 1997.

18. Potassium Channel Openers and Cardiac Surgery

Louis P. Perrault
Philippe Menasché

Introduction

Cardiac operations offer the unique possibility of precisely planning the time at which the aortic crossclamp will be applied, thereby initiating the period of global ischemia. This provides the opportunity of using the timely implementation of preconditioning strategies as a novel approach to intraoperative myocardial protection based on the therapeutic exploitation of the heart's natural defense mechanisms against ischemic injury. Efficacy, safety and practicality issues have lead to shift attention from ischemic to pharmacologic preconditioning regimens, the underlying rationale being to take advantage of the cardioprotective mediators of ischemic preconditioning whilst eliminating the detrimental effects inherent to any ischemic insult. Among these mediators, potassium channel openers (PCO) are receiving a growing deal of attention because of the recognition (reviewed in another chapter of this book) that they might act as the effectors of the intracellular signaling pathway leading to ischemic preconditioning. Since one of the drugs is currently available this reinforces the interest of establishing their potential role in the armamentarium of our myocardial preservation techniques. This role might indeed be important as, depending on the timing and modalities of their administration, PCO may play a multiplicity of roles and can be considered as preconditioning agents (if given before standard potassium arrest), hyperpolarizing cardioplegic agents (if given instead of potassium cardioplegia) or simple potentiators of arrest (if given as additives to potassium cardioplegia). In this review, these three potential applications will be successively discussed.

Potassium Channel Openers as Preconditioning Agents

The interest of PCO as agents of inducing preconditioning stems from the awareness that the use of ischemic preconditioning in surgical practice is fraught with serious limitations. These limitations will first be reviewed from both experimental and clinical standpoints.

Experimental Limitations of Ischemic Preconditioning

Two major conclusions emerge from the bulk of experimental data on preconditioning: First, this adaptive phenomenon reduces infarct size after regional ischemia in animal preparations across a wide variety of species but its effect on arrhythmias and on preservation of function after global ischemia is less consistent. Second, regardless of the various components of the intracellular signaling pathway elicited by the preconditioning stimulus, it seems that a major mechanism by which this pathway leads to cardioprotective effects is a slowing of the rate of depletion of adenosine triphosphate (ATP) during the protracted period of ischemia. Paradoxically, these two events may account for the observation that preconditioning, at least of the ischemic type, is not as readily suited for use in clinical cardiac surgery as one would expect.

Namely, in most cases, postbypass pump failure is due to reversible contractile dysfunction (stunning), not to a discrete myocardial infarct.[1] The question then arises: can preconditioning alleviate stunning independently of the reduction of infarct size? Only a few studies that have *concomitantly* assessed function and infarct size can shed some light on this problem.[2] Indeed, their findings conclusively demonstrate that preconditioning improves postischemic function only by reducing infarct size, not by reducing stunning of reversibly injured myocardium. Importantly, this conclusion applies both to regionally ischemic preparations which have been preconditioned by a transient coronary artery occlusion and to models of global ischemia where preconditioning has been induced by a transient period of aortic crossclamping.[3] These data are further supported by a recent study from our laboratory in which isolated buffer-perfused rabbit hearts were subjected to 60 minutes of normothermic potassium arrest. This ischemic insult caused only minimal necrosis (< 10% of the left ventricle), as assessed by triphenyl tetrazolium chloride staining. Preconditioning, achieved with 5 minutes of total (zero-flow) ischemia followed by 5 minutes of reperfusion before arrest, failed to improve recovery of function or coronary flow over that seen in nonpreconditioned hearts (unpublished data). It is most likely that infarct size was too small in these controls to be further reduced by any intervention. Conversely, Hendrikx and coworkers[4] have reported that a similar protocol of preconditioning improved functional recovery of rabbit hearts subjected to 45 minutes of *unprotected* global ischemia. Unfortunately, in this study, infarct size was not measured. Consequently, we have duplicated these experiments and found that the type of injury used by Hendrikx and his co-authors caused a massive infarction of the left ventricle, thereby offering some room for preconditioning to reduce the extent of necrosis and confirming that the beneficial effects of this phenomenon on function were achieved through its infarct size-limiting capacity.

Furthermore, if the cardioprotection due to preconditioning is ultimately due to a slowing of the rate of ATP depletion during ischemia, then, it can be reasonably predicted that this energy-sparing effect may become redundant to that of cardioplegia. This hypothesis is indeed confirmed by the observations, made in isolated rat hearts subjected to 35 minutes of global ischemia, that both ischemic preconditioning and cardioplegia *independently* improve the recovery of function over that seen in control unprotected hearts, but without additive effects.[5] Likewise, preconditioning combined with magnesium-based cardioplegia fails to ameliorate the recovery of hearts compared with cardioplegia alone.[6] Indeed, there are only two situations in which preconditioning has been shown to add protection beyond that yet provided by hypothermia and cardioplegia: Long ischemic times[7] and inhomogeneous delivery of cardioplegia due to proximal coronary artery occlusion.[8] It is likely that in these two settings, the beneficial effects of preconditioning are due to a reduction of the amount of necrosis that may have resulted from suboptimal cardioplegic protection.

Clinical Limitations of Ischemic Preconditioning

If we except intermittent aortic crossclamping whose long standing good clinical results may have resulted from some unintentional form of preconditioning,[9] the deliberate clinical use of ischemic preconditioning has been pioneered by Alkhulaifi and coworkers[10,11] in patients undergoing coronary artery bypass operations. These authors have shown that patients subjected to two cycles of preconditioning (each consisting of 3 minutes of aortic crossclamping followed by 2 minutes of reperfusion) had higher myocardial levels of ATP at the end of a subsequent 10-minute episode of global ischemia than their nonpreconditioned counterparts. These data, however, are far from being convincing for at least two reasons: first, ATP measurements were not correlated with function or clinical outcome. Second, during the period of sustained global ischemia (which was used for the construction of the distal anastomosis), hearts fibrillated at normothermia, which is a suboptimal method of myocardial "protection" that it is not unexpected that it let some room for preconditioning to provide some improvement. In support of this hypothesis is the finding, by the same group but in another study published in an abstract form,[12] that simply lowering the temperature during fibrillation was sufficient for eliminating between-group differences in ATP levels. Our experience with ischemic preconditioning before normothermic cardioplegic arrest has been equally disappointing.[13] Not only did a brief prearrest episode of aortic crossclamping fail to improve clinical outcome, but preconditioned patients tended to demonstrate a greater release of CK-MB and lactate in the coronary sinus at the end of cardioplegia, thereby suggesting that the detrimental effects of the preconditioning ischemia largely offset its putative cardioprotective action.

Ischemic preconditioning has also been shown to provide protection against an ischemic insult occurring 24 hours after the initial challenge. Whereas immediate protection is due to activation of membrane receptors, this delayed ("second window") protection is thought to involve the overexpression of stress, or heat shock, proteins (HSP).[14,15] A tight relationship has been established between the myocardial content of HSP and postischemic mechanical recovery, i.e., the higher the content, the better the function,[16] hence the concept that any intervention that would elevate myocardial tissue levels of HSP should be cardioprotective. Furthermore, the time course of expression of these proteins has been reported to be shorter than what initially thought and, indeed, consistent with a surgically relevant time frame. Thus, in the study of Liu and associates[17] using a pig model of 3-hour hypothermic cardioplegic arrest, a brief period of prebypass hyperthermia was shown to increase myocardial levels of HSP 70 as early as 2 hours after the onset of reperfusion. Consequently, in our aforementioned clinical study,[13] right atrial biopsies have been performed and processed by Northern blotting for the expression of the ribonucleic acid messenger (mRNA) coding for HSP 70. At the end of the crossclamping period, HSP 70 mRNA levels in preconditioned patients were not different from those measured at baseline (before bypass), nor were they different from those measured in control patients at the same time point. One could argue that this last biopsy was taken immediately before removal of the aortic crossclamp and that this timing may have led to miss a delayed increase in HSP occurring during reperfusion. This is unlikely as in the study of McGrath and coworkers[18] where HSP 72 levels were measured at different time points in patients undergoing cardiac operations, postbypass values were unchanged from those measured both before bypass and at the end of the crossclamping period.

One possible explanation why ischemic preconditioning may be ineffective in standard clinical practice is that cardiopulmonary bypass, by itself, could act as a preconditioning stimulus, possibly through the release of membrane-activating mediators like adenosine or catecholamines. This hypothesis is based on the observation that the reduction in infarct size achieved by short bursts of preconditioning ischemia can be duplicated by a period of cardiopulmonary bypass, whereas this cardioprotective effect of bypass is abolished by antagonists of adenosine A_1 and α-1 adrenoreceptors.[19-21] If this hypothesis is correct, it would imply that "control" patients are indeed already preconditioned to the point that any further intraoperative preconditioning intervention is likely to be redundant and ineffective. The only clinical situation in which ischemic preconditioning remains logical would be « off-pump » minimally invasive coronary artery bypass surgery as the occlusion of the target vessel during construction of the distal anastomosis most closely mimics the experimental scenario that has turned out to result in reduction of regionally-induced ischemic damage.[22]

From the above considerations, it appears that the clinical use of ischemic preconditioning is fraught with both conceptual and practical difficulties. These problems should not imply that the mechanisms underlying myocardial endogenous protection should not be exploited therapeutically. It simply emphasizes the importance of identifying these mechanisms in an attempt to pharmacologically duplicate the protective action of ischemically induced preconditioning. If adenosine is now recognized as a major trigger of the intracellular signaling pathway that links the preconditioning stimulus to its cardioprotective effects,[23] ATP-sensitive potassium channels have been increasingly reported as end effectors of this pathway in a wide variety of species, including guinea pig,[24] rat,[25,26] rabbit,[27] dog,[23,28,29] pig[30] and human,[31-33] although other mechanisms might also be involved.

Potassium Channel Opener-Based Pharmacologic Preconditioning

Over these past years, the role of ATP-sensitive potassium channels as mediators of the cardioprotective effects of preconditioning has been largely based on the observations that these effects could be duplicated by PCO whereas they were abolished by potassium channel blockers.[34] Recently, more direct evidence has been brought for the involvement of potassium channels as it has been shown[35] that protein kinase C, which can be activated by the stimulation of various membrane receptors known to be involved in ischemic preconditioning, in particular $\alpha\text{-}_1$ adrenoreceptors and adenosine receptors, activated the ATP-sensitive potassium current (I_{KATP}) in rabbit and human ventricular myocytes by reducing channel sensitivity to intracellular ATP. It is noteworthy that a direct link between activation of adenosine receptors and opening of ATP-sensitive potassium channels has not been established in rat hearts.[36] These hearts, however, can be successfully preconditioned by PCO, which raises the possibility that, in this species, the pathway leading to activation of protein kinase C and, subsequently, of potassium channels would be preferentially initiated by stimulation of $\alpha\text{-}_1$ adrenoreceptors.[19,20] Such an hypothesis would be consistent with the role attributed to these receptors in the mediation of the cardioprotective effects of ischemic preconditioning in the rat heart.[19,20]

The initial observations, made in regionally ischemic preparations,[37] that pharmacologic preconditioning with PCO could mimic ischemic preconditioning have now been extended to the more surgically relevant setting of global ischemia and cardioplegia. Thus, using an isolated rat heart model of 45-minute normothermic potassium arrest, we[38] have shown that the protective effects of ischemic preconditioning (achieved by 5 minutes of zero-flow ischemia followed by 5 minutes of reperfusion before arrest) on postcardioplegia systolic and diastolic function could be duplicated by preconditioning with nicorandil, given (at the dose of 10 FM/L) over 5 minutes (followed by 5 additional minutes of drug-free buffer perfusion before arrest). Also, both forms of preconditioning similarly lengthened the time to peak contracture during arrest as well as the magnitude of this peak. The potassium channel blocker glibenclamide completely abolished the cardioprotective effects of nicorandil preconditioning, thereby confirming that the drug acted through modulation of potassium channel activation, whereas it only partially blunted those of ischemic preconditioning, which suggests that, at least in rat heart, other end effectors may be involved. Subsequently, we[39] have duplicated these results under more clinically relevant conditions of hypothermic cardioplegic arrest. Other studies[40,41-43] have further confirmed the ability of PCO given before potassium arrest to enhance functional recovery during reperfusion (although, in these studies, the drug was infused until the onset of cardioplegia, which defines pretreatment rather than true preconditioning as the latter involves a period of intervening reperfusion between the initial preconditioning challenge and the subsequent period of prolonged ischemia).

The mechanism by which myocardial cells keep the "memory" of their transient exposure to PCO before arrest remains unclear. One possibility is that the persisting effect of the drug is to lower the threshold beyond which potassium channels open so that they might be more readily activated during the subsequent period of global ischemia.[43] Such a mechanism could provide significant protection as the opening of less than 1% of all available channels would result in a 50% reduction of action potential duration.[44] However, the relationship between such a shortening and the cardioprotective action of potassium channel opening has been recently questioned.[36,45,46] Additional studies are therefore required to further clarify the mechanism of PCO-based preconditioning and also to define the optimal timing of administration and dosage regimen of these drugs. Notwithstanding, our observations[38] and those of Grover et al[7] have confirmed the cardioprotective effects of nicorandil and cromakalim preconditioning seem to be independent of the temperature of the subsequent cardioplegia and are of clinical relevance as they should allow to widen the surgical applications of this therapeutic approach. Currently, however, those applications would probably be hampered (in particular, in the context of surgery without cardiopulmonary bypass) by the fact that the anti-ischemic effects of PCO are obtained at much higher doses than those required for relaxation of smooth muscle, so that it is a concern that important hemodynamic changes due to vasodilation occur before the cardioprotective effects become apparent.[47]

Potassium Channel Openers as Alternatives to Potassium-Based Cardioplegia

There is a strong rationale for using PCO as cardioplegic agents that would substitute for potassium. First, the pharmacologic opening of potassium channels shifts membrane voltage towards more negative values, at or near the equilibrium potential for potassium. This causes the resting membrane potential to hyperpolarize by just a few millivolts because it is already close to this equilibrium potential. At these potentials, transmembrane ion concentration gradients are largely abolished and few voltage-dependent ion channels are open. This, in turn, reduces energy expenditure associated with ion pump activity. Thus, in rat hearts, nonischemic tetrodoxin-induced membrane polarized arrest yields a significantly lower myocardial oxygen consumption than that associated with nonischemic depolarized arrest,[48] a finding that correlated with a reduced diastolic pressure during arrest. This sparing of energy is thought to result primarily from a limitation of calcium overload which occurs during potassium-induced membrane depolarization in exchange for intracellular sodium. However, other cardioprotective functions of the potassium channel cannot be excluded and, in particular, the role of the mitochondrial channel for this ion[49] in the regulation of calcium fluxes remains to be defined. In addition, PCO have potent vasodilatory effects which raises the possibility that hyperpolarized arrest may cause better distribution of cardioplegia during arrest and higher coronary blood flow during reperfusion. The latter hypothesis is supported by the finding that ATP-sensitive potassium channels seem to mediate coronary hyperhemia following cardioplegic arrest.[50] In addition, a recent study has shown that PCO may prevent calcium loading of cardiomyocytes after reperfusion which could offer interesting advantages in clinical surgery.[51] Of note, the purported superiority of PCO-based arrest over potassium-based arrest is unlikely to be due to the sole shortening of the action potential as the latter has been shown, in blood-perfused papillary muscle preparations, to be the consequence of increased extracellular potassium concentration, as would occur following exposure to an hyperkalemic solution, rather than the opening of ATP-sensitive potassium channels.[52]

These theoretical considerations are actually supported by the experimental studies of two independent investigators. Thus, using the parabiotic blood-perfused rabbit heart, Maskal,[45] Lawton[53] and their coworkers have shown that aprikalim (100 μM/L) and pinacidil (50 μM/L) cardioplegia, respectively, afforded a better recovery of systolic function (and coronary flow in the case of pinacidil) than standard hyperkalemic (20 mM/L) cardioplegia after 30 minutes of normothermic global ischemia and 30[45] or 60[53] minutes of reperfusion. Of note, in these *blood*-perfused isolated heart models, none of the two PCO significantly improved postischemic diastolic function compared with potassium-arrested controls. This observation contrasts with the previous finding made in a *crystalloid*-perfused preparation[54] that aprikalim-induced hyperpolarized arrest was associated with a lengthening of the time to contracture and a significant reduction in postischemic diastolic pressure compared with potassium-induced depolarized arrest. Such a discrepancy only reemphasizes how much experimental results can be confounded by the type of experimental preparation used.

However, the use of PCO in this setting has two potential drawbacks: First, a prolongation of the time to electrical arrest; this concern may, in fact, be of minor importance because electrical activity only accounts for 1% of total myocardial oxygen consumption. This component of energy expenditure could therefore be easily compensated for by the energy-sparing effect inherent to hyperpolarized arrest; second, an increased incidence of reperfusion arrhythmias. This finding is not surprising in view of the effect of PCO on the shortening of action potential duration and the subsequent decrease in the refractory period.[55] It is noteworthy that, in the study of Lawton and coworkers,[56] 50% of the pinacidil-treated hearts underwent ventricular fibrillation during the early phase of reperfusion (with no subsequent recurrence over the 60-minute observation period) whereas the aprikalim study[53] failed to show a significant difference in the occurrence of ventricular fibrillation at reperfusion between hearts arrested with the PCO and those arrested with potassium. Although, intraoperatively, these reperfusion arrhythmias could be easily treated by cardioversion, they still represent a potential limitation to a safe clinical use. Likewise, it remains to be determined whether the "cardioplegic" doses of PCO that would be required to induce and maintain cardiac arrest are compatible with clinically relevant drug regimens. In summary, the concept of hyperpolarized arrest seems sound and attractive but the appropriate compounds for clearly establishing its clinical feasibility have yet to become available.

Potassium Channel Openers as Additives to Potassium Cardioplegia

This combination may, at first glance, appear surprising in view of the seemingly opposite effects of PCO and potassium on membrane voltage. Indeed, the rationale, if any, for the inclusion of PCO in cardioplegic solutions is not yet clear and the currently available experimental data are far from being convincing. Thus, in the previously mentioned study of Sugimoto and associates,[43] guinea pig papillary muscle that were superfused with nicorandil-enriched cold cardioplegic solution had a significantly better recovery of developed tension than those exposed to drug-free cardioplegia (119% ± 19% of baseline vs 54% ± 6%, $p < 0.01$). However, this result is flawed by several confounding variables: First, the dose of nicorandil was very high (1 mM/L), far greater than the clinically acceptable range; second, the drug was given both before and during arrest and, as the results are not different from those of another group in which it was only given as a pretreatment, it is impossible to determine to what extent the addition of nicorandil to cardioplegia contributed to the successful recovery of isometric contractility; third, the model itself is convenient for screening myocardial preservative strategies but its clinical relevance is debatable. These negative concerns are indeed supported by the negative results of three subsequent studies. Thus, Galinanes and coworkers[57] failed to document any benefit of adding levakalim to St Thomas' cardioplegic solution infused into rat hearts exposed to 35 minutes of normothermic global ischemia. In other experiments performed by another group[58] in the same model and with the same solution, addition of cromakalim was also unable to favorably affect recovery of contractile function or enzyme leakage. Similarly negative conclusions were reached by Irie and coworkers[59] in a dog model of hypothermic cardioplegic arrest during which a nicorandil-enriched cardioplegic solution was delivered in a multidose fashion.

Slightly more encouraging results seem to emerge, however, from three other studies. Thus, Pignac and associates[40] have reported that addition of aprikalim to St Thomas' solution resulted in a better function after 90 minutes of hypothermic cardioplegic arrest in isolated rabbit hearts. However, a careful analysis of their data shows that this conclusion is based on relatively weak end-points. Namely, the improvement attributed to the drug is derived from the observation that, within this group, there is no significant difference in left ventricular systolic pressure between reperfusion and baseline values whereas this index significantly decreased in control hearts. However, if one looks at absolute values, there is no significant difference between the two groups during reperfusion, nor is there any effect of drug supplementation on postischemic diastolic pressures. Hosoda and coworkers[60] have reported a significantly better recovery of aortic flow (but not of aortic pressure or coronary flow) in isolated rat hearts receiving an hyperkalemic solution supplemented with pinacidil (at three different doses) and delivered intermittently throughout an 80-minute arrest period at 25°C. Of note, hearts exposed to the 10 μM/L dose of pinacidil had, after 30 minutes of reperfusion, a myocardial calcium content which was not different from the preischemic value, in contrast to the 5 μM/L and 50 μM/L groups in which the calcium concentration had significantly increased over baseline. In a different setting, Qiu and associates[61] have tried to mimic the scenario of continuous warm cardioplegia by perfusing isolated rat hearts at low flow (0.7 ml/min) and for 100 minutes with a cardioplegic solution at 37EC containing, or not, nicorandil (10 FM/L). The results show a slightly (but significantly) better recovery of left ventricular developed pressure in the drug-treated group than in the controls, without any additional between-group difference in the other end points (diastolic pressure, coronary flow, myocardial ATP levels and creatine kinase leakage during reflow).

Put together, these data lead one to be cautious about the purported advantages of supplementing cardioplegic solutions with PCO. First, Qiu and coworkers[61] make the argument that nicorandil added to cardioplegia reduced the resumption of electrical activity during arrest and could thereby potentiate the cardioplegic effects of the St. Thomas' solution. We believe that this observation is of limited clinical relevance. During continuous warm blood cardioplegic perfusion, recurrences of electromechanical activity are uncommon, except for patients with marked left ventricular hypertrophy, and, in any case, they are easily controlled, whether they feature rhythmic contractions that respond to increased delivery of potassium or disorganized "creeping" waves that are effectively ablated by procaine.[62] Indeed, current cardioplegic solutions do not require additional arresting agents to induce cardiac quiescence[57] and one would expect this to be even more true under hypothermic conditions (the shortening of the time to arrest reported by Sugimoto[43] is more likely due to the high dose of nicorandil and the type of experimental preparation). Second, there is no conclusive evidence that addition of PCO in cardioplegic solutions can improve postreperfusion coronary flow as in the pinacidil[60] and nicorandil[61] studies, the improvement in postischemic aortic flow and developed pressure yielded by the drug-treated hearts, respectively, was not paralleled by an increase in coronary flow. This is consistent with the idea that vasodilation is not a major component of the cardioprotective action of PCO.[46] A third reason for the use of PCO in this setting could be more convincing: These drugs, in particular bimakalim[63] and nicorandil[60,61,64-66] have been shown to reduce neutrophil infiltration into myocardium submitted to ischemia-reperfusion, whether given before and throughout a period of sustained regional ischemia or just before reperfusion and over the ensuing hours. This effect (that might not be a direct consequence of potassium channel opening, but rather of increased coronary blood flow and subsequently increased shear rate) could be relevant to postcardioplegia reperfusion during which a substantial component of myocardial tissue damage is attributed to neutrophil adhesion and emigration of bypass-activated neutrophils.[67] The inhibitory action of PCO on neutrophil function might contribute to their ability to attenuate stunning,[68] an effect that has been attributed to the drug-induced persistence of potassium channel opening during early reperfusion.[45] A last, conceptually attractive, argument for the supplementation of cardioplegic solutions with PCO is that membrane hyperpolarization could prevent opening of voltage-dependent calcium channels on exposure to depolarizing stimuli. The hypothesis is based on the opposite finding, made in rat mesenteric resistance vessels, that prior depolarization by norepinephrine does not preclude membrane hyperpolarization and vessel tone relaxation upon subsequent exposure to pinacidil.[69] This possibility, however, has yet to be confirmed in a more surgically relevant model of potassium arrest.

Additional studies, in particular in large animal blood-perfused models, are thus warranted to clarify these issues and, to be clinically relevant, their design will have to take into account several potentially confounding factors, either PCO-related (type of drug, dosage regimen) or cardioplegia-related (temperature, duration of infusion). The latter variable may be important because of the time required for these drugs to reach their active sites, which increases the likelihood for them to be effective when added to[60,61] perfused cardioplegic solutions continuously or intermittently as opposed to single-dose cardioplegia deliveries. The type of arrest (ischemic versus aerobic) should also be considered as the finding that PCO are more effective in opening potassium channels when intracellular ATP levels decline[68] rather favors their use in the former setting.

Conclusion

In conclusion, it is sound to predict that PCO may find a place among future myocardial preservation strategies. This place still needs to be defined since, experimentally, the use of these drugs for achieving pharmacologic preconditioning and/or hyperpolarized arrest is yet to be associated with a substantial improvement compared with conventional cardioplegic approaches. Whether these effects will translate into better clinical outcomes will require additional studies that would be greatly facilitated by a more thorough understanding of the involvement of ATP-sensitive potassium channels in myocardial ischemia-reperfusion injury and from the development of more cardioselective drugs.

Acknowledgments

We would like to thank Roselyne Prioux for aid in the preparation of the manuscript.
Dr. Perrault is supported by the Clinician-Scientist program of the Medical Research Council of Canada.

References

1. Kloner RA, Przyklenk K, Kay GL. Clinical evidence for stunned myocardium after coronary artery bypass surgery. J Card Surg 1994;9[Suppl]:397-402.

2. Bolling SF, Olszanski DA, Childs KF, et al. Stunning, preconditioning , and functional recovery after global myocardial ischemia. Ann Thorac Surg 1994;58:822-7.
3. Ovize M, Kloner RA, Przyklenk K. Preconditioning and myocardial contractile function. In: Przyklenk K, Kloner RA, Yellon DM. eds. Ischemic preconditioning: the concept of endogenous cardioprotection. Boston:Kluwer Academic Publishers, 1994: 41-60.
4. Hendricx M, Toshima Y, Mubagwa K, et al. Improved functional recovery after ischemic preconditioning in the globally ischemic rabbit heart is not mediated by adenosine A_1 receptor activation. Bas Res Cardiol 1993;88:576-593.
5. Kolocassides KG, Galinanes M, Hearse DJ. Ischemic preconditioning, cardioplegia or both? J Mol Cell Cardiol 1994;26:1411-1414.
6. Steenbergen C, Perlman ME, London RE, et al. Mechanism of preconditioning; ionic alterations. Circ Res 1993;72:112-125.
7. Cave AC, Hearse DJ. Ischaemic preconditioning and contractile function: studies with normothermic and hypothermic global ischaemia. J Mol Cell Cardiol 1992;24:1113-1123.
8. Galiñanes M, Argano V, Hearse DJ. Can ischemic preconditioning ensure optimal myocardial protection when delivery of cardioplegia is impaired? Circulation 1995;92(suppII): II-389-II394.
9. Abd-Elfattah AS, Ding M, Wechsler AS. Intermittent aortic cross-clamping prevents cumulative adenosine triphosphate depletion, ventricular fibrillation, and dysfunction (stunning):is it preconditioning? J Thorac Cardiovasc Surg 1995;110:328-329.
10. Alkhulaifi AM, Yellon DM, Pugsley WB, et al. Preconditioning the human heart during aorto-coronary bypass surgery. Eur J Cardiothorac Surg 1994;8:270-276.
11. Yellon DM, Alkhulaifi AM, Pugsley WB. Preconditioning the human myocardium. The Lancet 1993;342:276-277.
12. Di Salvo C, Hemming A, Jenkins D, et al. Can the human myocardium be preconditioned with ischaemia under hypothermic conditions? Proceedings of the 9th annual meeting of the European Association for Cardiothoracic Surgery, Paris 25-27 September 1995 page 324 (abstract).
13. Perrault LP, Menasché P, Bel A, et al. Ischemic preconditioning in cardiac surgery: a word of caution. J Thorac Cardiovasc Surg 1996; (in press).
14. Marber MS, Latchman DS, Walker JM. Cardiac stress protein elevation 24 hours after brief ischemia or heat stress is associated with resistance to myocardial infarction. Circulation 1993;88:1264-1272.
15. Sun JZ, Tang XL, Knowlton AA, et al. Late preconditioning against myocardial stunning. An endogenous protective mechanism that confers resistance to postischemic dysfunction 24h after brief ischemia in conscious pigs. J Clin Invest 1995;95:388-403.
16. Robinson BL, Morita T, Toft DO, et al. Accelerated recovery of postischemic stunned myocardium after induced expression of myocardial heat-shock protein (HSP 70). J Thorac Cardiovasc Surg 1995;109:753-764.
17. Liu X, Engelman RM, Moraru II, et al. Heat shock. A new approach for myocardial preservation in cardiac surgery. Circulation 1992;86(suppl II):II-358-II-363.
18. McGrath LB, Locke M, Cane M, et al. Heat shock protein (HSP 72) expression in patients undergoing cardiac operations. J Thorac Cardiovasc Surg 1995;109:370-376.
19. Burns PG, Krukenkamp IB, Caldarone CA, et al. Does cardiopulmonary bypass alone elicit myoprotective preconditioning? Circulation 1995;92(supplII):II447-II451.
20. Winter CB, Mitchell MB, Locke-Winter CR, et al. Adenosine-induced cardiac preconditioning is dependent upon α1-adrenoreceptor activation. Circulation 1992;86(suppl I):I-25, (abstract).
21. Tsuchida A, Miura T, Miki T, et al. Role of adenosine receptor activation in myocardial infarct size limitation by ischemic preconditioning. Cardiovasc Res 1992; 26:456-461.
22. Subramanian VA, Sani G, Benetti FJ. Minimally invasive coronary bypass surgery: a multicenter report of preliminary clinical experience. Circulation 1995; 92(suppl I): I-645.

23. Yao Z, Gross GJ. A comparison of adenosine-induced cardioprotection and ischemic preconditioning in dogs. Efficacy, time course and role of Katp channels. Circulation 1994;89:1229-1236.
24. Hecquet C, Mestre M, Cavero I. Synergistic cardioprotective effect of a subtreshold concentration of aprikalim and a subtreshold ischemic preconditioning stress. Circulation 1994;90(suppl I):I-48.
25. Grover GJ, Dzwonczyk S, Sleph PG. Reduction of ischemic damage in isolated rat hearts by the potassium channel opener RP 52891. Eur J Pharmacol 1990;191:11-18.
26. Grover GJ, Sleph PG. Protective effect of Katp openers in ischemic rat heart treated with a potassium cardioplegic solution. J Cardiovasc Pharmacol 1995;26:698-706.
27. Cohen NM, Wise RM, Wechsler AS, et al. Elective cardiac arrest with a hyperpolarizing adenosine triphosphate-sensitive potassium channel opener; a novel form of myocardial protection. J Thorac Cardiovasc Surg 1993;106:317-328.
28. Gross GJ, Auchampach JA. Blockade of ATP-sensitive potassium channels prevents myocardial preconditioning in dogs. Circ Res 1992;70:223-233.
29. Yao Z, Gross GJ. Role of nitric oxide, muscarinic receptors, and the ATP-sensitive K^+ channel in mediating the effects of acetylcholine to mimic preconditioning in dogs. Circ Res 1993;73:1193-1201.
30. Galiè N, Guarnieri C, Ussia GP, et al. Limitation of myocardial infarct size by nicorandil after sustained ischemia in pigs. J Cardiovasc Pharmacol 1995;26:477-484.
31. Tomai F, Crea F, Gaspardone A, et al. Ischemic preconditioning during coronary angioplasty is prevented by glibenclamide, a selective ATP-sensitive K^+ channel blocker. Circulation 1994;90:700-705.
32. Ikonomidis JS, Shirai T, Weisel RD, et al. "Ischemic" or adenosine preconditioning of human ventricular cardiomyocyte is protein C dependent. Circulation 1995;92(suppl I):1-12.
33. Speechly-Dick ME, Grover GJ, Yellon DM. Does ischemic preconditioning in the human involve protein kinase C and the ATP-dependent K^+ channel? Studies of contractile function after simulated ischemia in an atrial in vitro model. Circ Res 1995;77:1030-1035.
34. McCullough JR, Normandin DE, Conder ML, et al. Specific block of the antiischemic actions of cromakalim by sodium 5-hydroxydecanoate. Circ Res 1991;69:949-958.
35. Hu K, Duan D, Li GR, et al. Protein kinase C activates ATP-sensitive K^+ current in human and rabbit ventricular myocytes. Circ Res 1996;78:492-498.
36. Grover GJ, Baird AJ, Sleph PG. Lack of a pharmacologic interaction between ATP-sensitive potassium channels and adenosine A1 receptors in ischemic rat hearts. Cardiovasc Res 1996;31:511-517.
37. Murry CE, Jennings RB, Reimer KA. Preconditioning with ischemia: a delay of lethal cell injury in ischemic myocardium. Circulation 1986;74:1124-1136.
38. Menasché P, Kevelaïtis E, Mouas C, et al. Preconditioning with potassium channel openers: a new concept for enhancing cardioplegic protection? J Thorac Cardiovasc Surg 1995;110:1606-1614.
39. Menasché P, Mouas C, Grousset C. Is potassium channel opening an effective form of preconditioning before cardioplegia? Ann Thorac Surg 1996;61:176+4-1768.
40. Pignac J, Bourgouin J, Dumont L, et al. Cardioplegia and the K^+ channel modulator aprikalim (RP 52891): improved cardioprotection in isolated ischemic rabbit hearts. Can J Physiol 1994;72:126-132.
41. Sugimoto S, Puddu PE, Monti F, et al. Pretreatment with the adenosine triphosphate-sensitive potassium channel opener nicorandil and improved myocardial protection during high-potassium cardioplegic hypoxia. J Thorac Cardiovasc 1994; 108:455-66.
42. Sugimoto S, Iwashiro K , Monti F, et al. The risk of myocardial stunning is decreased concentration-dependently by Katp channel activation with nicorandil before high K^+ cardioplegia. Int J Cardiol 1995;48:11-25.
43. Sugimoto S, Puddu PE, Monti F, et al. Activation of ATP-dependent K^+ channels enhances myocardial protection due to cold high potassium cardioplegia: a force-frequency relationship study. J Mol Cell Cardiol 1995;27:1867-1881.

44. Shigematsu S, Sato T, Abe T, et al. Pharmacological evidence for the persistent activation of ATP-sensitive K^+ channels in early phase of reperfusion and its protective role against myocardial stunning. Circulation 1995;92:2266-2275.
45. Maskal SL, Cohen NM, Hsia PW, et al. Hyperpolarized cardiac arrest with a potassium-channel opener, aprikalim. J Thorac Cardiovasc Surg 1995;110:1083-1095.
46. Hearse DJ. Activation of ATP-sensitive potassium channels: a novel pharmacological approach to myocardial protection. Cardiovascular Res 1995;30:1-17.
47. Grover GJ. Protective effects of ATP sensitive potassium channel openers in models of myocardial ischaemia. Cardiovasc Res 1994;28:778-789.
48. Sternbergh WC, Brunsting LA, Abd-Elfattah AS, et al. Basal metabolic energy requirements of polarized and depolarized arrest in rat heart. Am J Physiol 1989;256:H846-H851.
49. Inoue I, Nagase H, Kishi K, et al. ATP sensitive K^+ channels in the mitochondrial inner membrane. Nature 1991;352:244-247.
50. Wang SY, Friedman M, Johnson RG, et al. Adenosine triphosphate-sensitive K^+ channels mediate postcardioplegia coronary hyperemia. J Thorac Cardiovasc Surg 1995;110:1073-1082.
51. Lopez JR, Jahangir R, Jahangir A, et al. Potassium channel openers prevent potassium-induced calcium loading of cardiac cells: possible implications in cardioplegia. J Thorac Cardiovasc Surg 1996;112:820-831.
52. Yan GX, Yamada KA, Kléber AG, et al. Dissociation between cellular K^+ loss, reduction in repolarization time, and tissue ATP levels during myocardial hypoxia and ischemia. Circulation 1993;72:560-570.
53. Lawton JS, Sepic JD, Allen CT, et al. Myocardial protection with potassium-channel openers is as effective as St-Thomas' solution in the rabbit heart. Ann Thorac Surg 1996;62:31-39.
54. Cohen NM, Damiano RJ, Wechsler AS. Is there an alternative to potassium arrest? Ann Thorac Surg 1995;60:858-863.
55. Yao Z, Gross GJ. Effects of the Katp opener bimakalim on coronary blood low, monophasic action potential duration and infarct size in dogs. Circulation 1994;89:1769-1775.
56. Lawton JS, Harrington GC, Allen CT, et al. Myocardial protection with pinacidil cardioplegia in the blood-perfused heart. Ann Thorac Surg 1996;61:1680-1688.
57. Galiñanes M, Shattock MJ, Hearse DJ. Effects of potassium channel modulation during global ischemia in isolated rat hearts with and without cardioplegia. Cardiovasc Res 1992;26:1063-1068.
58. Grover GJ, Dwonczyk S, Parham CS. The protective effects of cromakalim and pinacidil on reperfusion function and infarct size in isolated rat hearts and anesthetized dogs. Cardiovasc Drugs Ther 1990;15:465-474.
59. Irie H. Experimental studies on ischemic injury and reperfusion injury in the sarcoplasmic reticulum. The myocardial protective effect of nicorandil. Jpn Circ J 1998;52:563-569.
60. Hosoda H, Sunamori M, Suzuki A. Effect of pinacidil on rat hearts undergoing hypothermic cardioplegia. Ann Thorac Surg 1994; 58:1631-1636.
61. Qiu Y, Galiñanes M, Hearse DJ. Protective effect of nicorandil as an additive to the solution for continuous cardioplegia. J Thorac Cardiovasc Surg 1995;110:1063-1072.
62. Menasché P, Tronc F, Nguyen A, et al. Retrograde warm blood cardioplegia preserves hypertrophied myocardium: A clinical study. Ann Thorac Surg 1994;57:1429-1435.
63. Mizumara T, Nithipatikom K, Gross GJ. Bimakalim, a ATP-sensitive potassium channel opener, mimics the effects of ischemic preconditioning to reduce infarct size, adenosine release, and neutrophil function in dogs. Circulation 1995;92:1236-1245.
64. Mizumara T, Gross GJ. The cardioprotective effect of nicorandil, a Katp channel opener nitrate is blocked by glyburide in dogs. J Mol Cell Cardiol 1995;27:A24.
65. Mizumara T, Nithipatikom K, Gross GJ. Effects of nicorandil and glyceryl trinitrate on infarct size, adenosine release, and neutrophil infiltration in the dog. Cardiovasc Res 1995;29:482-489.

66. Akimitsu T, Gute DC, Korthuis RJ. Ischemic preconditioning attenuates postischemic leukocyte adhesion and emigration: Role of adenosine and ATP-sensitive potassium channels. Circulation 1994 90;(suppl I): A2561 (abstract).
67. Sawa Y, Matsuda H, Shimazaki Y, et al. Evaluation of leukocyte-depleted terminal blood cardioplegic solution in patients undergoing elective and emergency coronary artery bypass grafting. J Thorac Cardiovasc Surg 1994;108:1125-1231.
68. Auchampach JA, Maruyama M, Cavero I, et al. Pharmacological evidence for a role of ATP-dependent potassium channels in myocardial stunning. Circulation 1992;86:311-319.
69. Videbaek LM, Aalkjaer C, Hughes AD. Effect of pinacidil on ion permeability in resting and contracted resistance vessels. Am J Physiol 1990; 259:H14-H22.

In: Mentzer, R.M., Jr., Kitakaze, M., Downey, J.M., Hori, M, eds. Adenosine, Cardioprotection and Clinical Application. Kluwer Academic Publishers, Norwell, MA, USA, 1997.

19. Anti-ischemic Effects of the ATP-sensitive Potassium Channel Opener During Coronary Angioplasty

Satoshi Saito
Tsuneo Mizumura
Tadateru Takayama
Junko Honye
Masahito Moriuchi
Yukio Ozawa
Katsuo Kanmatsuse

Introduction

Since Gross and co-workers[1] found that glibenclamide completely blocked the infarct size-reducing effect afforded by ischemic preconditioning in canine hearts, it has been widely known that the ATP-sensitive potassium (K_{ATP}) channel activation plays an important role in myocardial protection against ischemia-reperfusion injury in several species, and a number of laboratories have demonstrated that K_{ATP} channel openers such as nicorandil,[2] bimakalim,[3] and aprikalim[1] mimic the cardioprotective effect of ischemic preconditioning.

Nicorandil, which is a hybrid between K_{ATP} channel openers and nitrates, was originally developed as a potent vasodilator and is currently used for the treatment of patients with angina pectoris in Japan and some European countries. In addition to its antianginal action, nicorandil has been reported to be cardioprotective in several animal models of ischemia-reperfusion injury. Initially, Lamping et al.[2] demonstrated that intravenously administered nicorandil markedly reduced infarct size in canine hearts. Since Gross et al.[1] demonstrated that glibenclamide abolished the infarct size-reducing effect of ischemic preconditioning which is a powerful endogenous cardioprotective mechanism, the K_{ATP} channel activation has been thought to be important to protect myocardium against ischemia, and a number of laboratories have shown that the K_{ATP} channel is involved in the infarct size-reducing effect of ischemic preconditioning in several species. In humans, Deutch et al.[4] initially reported that, in the two successive balloon inflation (90 seconds each) separated by a 5-minute reperfusion period, the ST-segment elevation of electrocardiogram in the second inflation became significantly smaller as compared to that of the first inflation. This phenomenon has been considered as an ischemic preconditioning in human myocardium, and PTCA seems to be favorable clinical model of ischemia-reperfusion injury in human being. Recently, Tomai et al.[5] showed that this attenuation of ST-segment elevation in the second inflation was completely blocked in patients who were pretreated with glibenclamide. More recently, we[6] determined if nicorandil attenuates the ST-segment elevation of ECG during the similar PTCA procedure as described below.

Study Methodology

The subjects of the study were 10 patients undergoing one-vessel coronary angioplasty. All patients had clinical angina pectoris and normal left ventricular function on left ventriculography. Following coronary arteriography via the femoral artery route, coronary angioplasty was performed with a balloon catheter (2.0 - 3.5 mm diameter) that was passed over 0.014 inch diameter flexible and steerable Doppler guidewire (FloWire, Cardiometrics, Mountain View, CA). Intracoronary electrocardiogram (icECG) was used to monitor the signs of regional myocardial ischemia during angioplasty. The electrocardiographic indicator of myocardial ischemia was the magnitude of ST-segment elevation at 80 msec after the J point on the icECG during the 30-second balloon inflation. In five patients, oxygen saturation of the blood sampled from the great cardiac vein and coronary flow velocity was concurrently measured during the angioplasty procedure. The protocol consisted of two 30-second balloon inflations at a 5-minute interval. Aortic blood pressure, heart rate, icECG, great cardiac vein oxygen saturation (S_VO_2), and coronary flow velocity were monitored and recorded continuously throughout the procedure. After the first balloon inflation, patients received 0.1 mg/kg of nicorandil administered intravenously over 2 minutes. The second balloon inflation was then performed 3 minutes after the drug administration. Electrocardiographic changes were analyzed in 10 patients who had neither visible collateral circulation on coronary arteriography nor evidence of collateral flow on the coronary flow velocity measurement both during control and nicorandil balloon inflations. The time course of ST-segment elevation on icECG before (control) and after nicorandil administration is shown in Figure 19-1, and the representative case

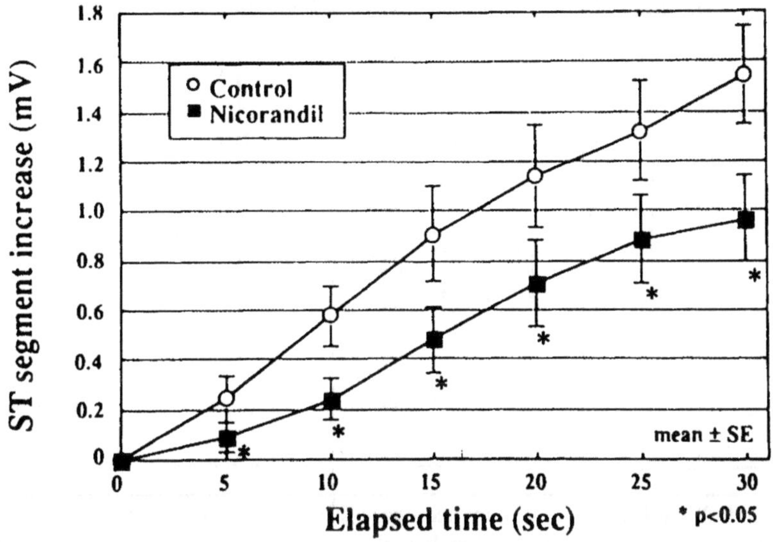

FIGURE 19-1. The time course of ST-segment elevation before (control) and after intravenous nicorandil administration (nicorandil) in 10 patients with angina pectoris who showed no evidence of collateral on both coronary angiogram and flow velocity measurement. An asterisk indicates that the response during inflation after nicorandil is significantly different from that obtained during control inflation ($p < 0.05$).

is shown in Figure 19-2. The magnitude of ST-segment elevation at 30 seconds following inflation is significantly reduced after nicorandil administration as compared with the control balloon inflation. In some patients undergoing LAD angioplasty, S_VO_2 was recorded (Fig. 19-3). S_VO_2 gradually decreased when the balloon was inflated and then rapidly increased to values greater than those baseline conditions soon after the balloon deflation There was no significant difference in S_VO_2 profile before and after the nicorandil administration. LAD blood flow, measured with Doppler guidewire, ceased after the balloon inflation, both under control conditions and after nicorandil administration. After balloon deflation, coronary blood flow attained values that were greater than those measured before balloon inflation (reactive hyperemia). This typical hyperemic response appeared to be attenuated by nicorandil (Fig. 19-4 shows a representative case). Since Murry et al.[7] reported a historical observation which they called "ischemic preconditioning" in canine hearts in 1986, the mechanism of this fascinating endogenous cardioprotective phenomenon has been studied by a number of laboratories. Gross et al.[1] initially pointed out that the importance of the K_{ATP} channel activation by showing that glibenclamide blocked the infarct size-reducing effect of preconditioning in dogs without increasing infarct size by itself.

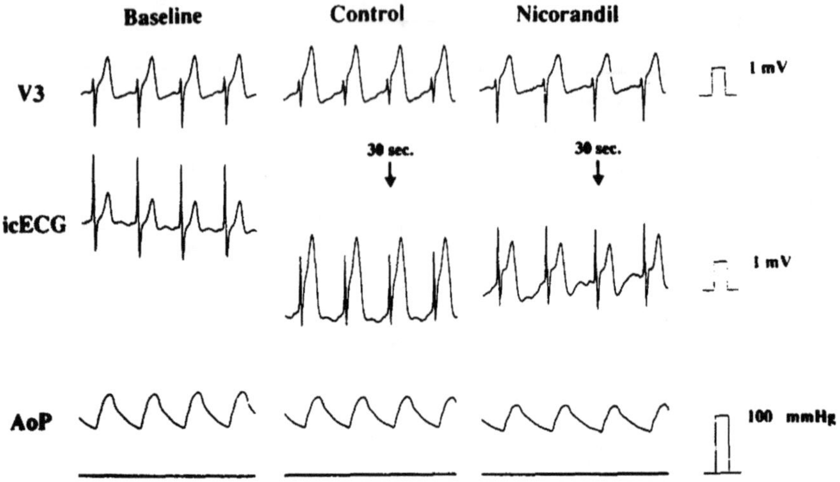

FIGURE 19-2. Surface ECG (V3), intracoronary ECG (icECG) and aortic pressure (AoP) during angioplasty on a 56-year-old male with a 85% stenotic lesion in the left anterior descending artery.

Although some controversies exist in small animals such as rabbits and rats, the K_{ATP} channel is now considered as an end effector in the mechanism of ischemic

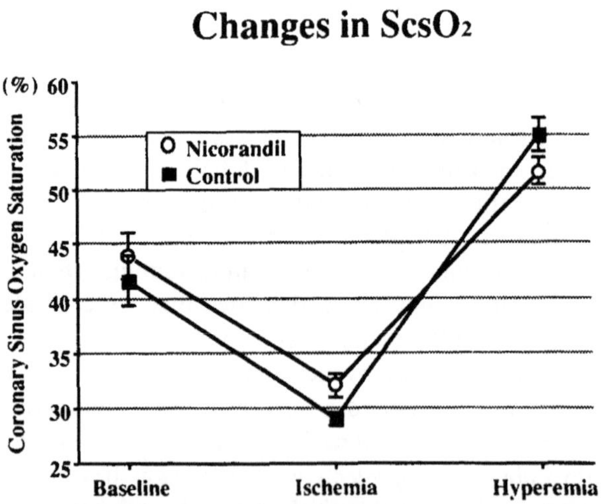

FIGURE 19-3. Changes in great cardiac vein blood oxygen saturation before and after intravenous nicorandil administration (0.1 mg/kg) in patients undergoing LAD-PTCA (n=5) measured during the inflation (ischemia) and after the deflation (hyperemia) of the balloon.

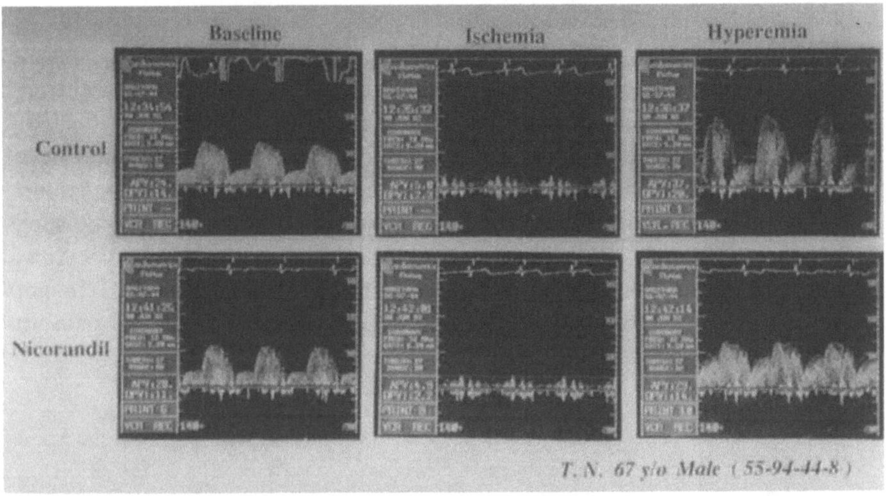

FIGURE 19-4. Left anterior descending coronary (LAD) angioplasty was performed on a 69-year-old female patient with a 90% stenotic lesion in the proximal portion. Nicorandil significantly attenuated the increase in ST-segment elevation at 30 seconds after balloon inflation.

preconditioning. Meanwhile, it has been well known that the attenuation of the magnitude of ST-segment elevation on ECG during successive balloon inflations is also recognized as an ischemic preconditioning in humans. In our study, since there were no significant changes in systemic hemodynamics and collateral blood flow before and after the nicorandil administration, the cardioprotective effect of nicorandil can be explained by its local protective action. Since nicorandil is a hybrid between K_{ATP} channel openers and nitrates, one would expect its cardioprotective effect might be a result of nitrate action. However, in animal study, Mizumura et al.[8] recently demonstrated that a nonhypotensive dose of nicorandil significantly reduced infarct size in dog hearts and this infarct size-reducing effect of nicorandil was completely reversed by glibenclamide but not by methylene blue, a selective guanulate cyclase/nitric oxide inhibitor.

Conclusion

These results indicate that this cardioprotective effect of intravenously-administered nicorandil during PTCA is directly related to the myocardial K_{ATP} channel activation and that nicorandil lowers the threshold for ischemic preconditioning in humans. In animal experiments, Mizumura et al.[9] showed that nicorandil which was started 10 min prior to the end of the 60-min occlusion and continued to the end of the 3-hr reperfusion (post treatment) also reduced infarct size in dog hearts. This indicates that the K_{ATP} channel opener may still be cardioprotective when given at the time of reperfusion in ischemia-reperfusion injury. They explained that the reduced neutrophil infiltration into the ischemic area is one of the mechanisms of this cardioprotective effect of "post-treated" nicorandil. Taken together, it is concluded that the K_{ATP} channel opener may have certain potential in several clinical settings; 1) during PTCA, to protect myocardium from ischemia caused by balloon inflation or acute coronary closure, 2) in the treatment of unstable angina pectoris or impending (evolving) myocardial infarction, 3) during the reperfusion therapy (thrombolysis or primary PTCA) of acute myocardial infarction, and 4) before or after open-heart surgery or heart transplantation.

References

1. Gross GJ, Auchampach JA. Blockade of ATP-sensitive potassium channels prevents myocardial preconditioning in dogs. Circ Res. 1992; 70: 223-233.
2. Lamping KA, Christensen CW, Pelc LR et al. Effects of nicorandil and nifedipine on protection of ischemic myocardium. J Cardiovasc Pharmacol. 1984; 6: 536-542.
3. Yao Z, Gross GJ. Effects of the K_{ATP} channel opener bimakalim on coronary blood flow, monophasic action potential duration, and infarct size in dogs. Circulation. 1994; 89:1769-1775.
4. Deutsch E, Berger M, Kussmaul WG et al. Adaptation to ischemia during percutaneous transluminal coronary angioplasty: Clinical, hemodynamic, and metabolic features. Circulation. 1990; 82: 2044-2051.
5. Tomai F, Crea F, Gaspardone A et al. Ischemic preconditioning during coronary angioplasty is prevented by glibenclamide, a selective ATP-sensitive K+ channel blocker. Circulation. 1994; 90: 700-705.
6. Saito S, Mizumura T, Takayama T et al. Antiischemic effects of nicorandil during coronary angioplasty in humans. Cardiovasc Drugs Ther. 1995; 9: 257-263.
7. Murry CE, Jennings RB, Reimer KA. Preconditioning with ischemia: A delay of lethal cell injury in ischemic myocardium. Circulation. 1986; 74: 1124-1136.
8. Mizumura T, Nithipatikom K, Gross GJ. Infarct size-reducing effect of nicorandil is mediated by the K_{ATP} channel but not by its nitrate-like properties in dogs. Cardiovasc Res. In press
9. Mizumura T, Nithipatikom K, Gross GJ. Effects of nicorandil and glyceryl trinitrate on infarct size, adenosine release, and neutrophil infiltration in the dog. Cardiovasc Res. 1995;29: 482-489.

In: Mentzer, R.M., Jr., Kitakaze, M., Downey, J.M., Hori, M, eds. Adenosine, Cardioprotection and Clinical Application. Kluwer Academic Publishers, Norwell, MA, USA, 1997.

20. Clinical Impact of Ischemic Preconditioning on Infarct Size and Coronary No-reflow Phenomenon after Successful Recanalization in the Acute Myocardial Infarction

Kazuo Komamura
Kazuhisa Kodama
Masafumi Kitakaze
Masatsugu Hori

Introduction

Now that reperfusion therapy for acute myocardial infarction is established and achieved better survival rate, attention on "no-reflow phenomenon" after complete reperfusion of epicardial coronary artery has been growing recently. In the clinical setting, no-reflow after successful thrombolysis has been visualized using coronary angiography,[1] Tl-201 SPECT[2] and myocardial contrast echocardiography.[3] Frequency of no-reflow after revascularization differs from 0.3% to 91%, according to the means of detection of no-reflow, duration of ischemia, extent of ischemia including collateral flow and extent of infarction. Although how much no-reflow counts on the prognosis of infarction remains to be determined, some impact of no-reflow on infarct size and ventricular function.[4] Clinical implication of ischemic preconditioning on myocardial infarction has been reported in terms of infarct size,[5] contractile function[6] and prognosis.[7] In the present review, we summarize the clinical impact of ischemic preconditioning on no-reflow phenomenon and infarct size using coronary vein flow measurement during the initial course of reperfused acute myocardial infarction.[8]

Materials and Methods

One hundred seven consecutive patients with evolving anteroseptal myocardial infarction were enrolled into the thrombolysis and rescue coronary angioplasty protocol of our hospital. The study group comprised the 19 patients (17 men, 2 women; mean age ± SD, 57 ± 12 years) with successful coronary revascularization who fulfilled the following criteria: 1) no history of previous myocardial infarction; 2) total occlusion of the proximal portion of the left anterior descending artery (LAD) at initial angiography and no significant (>75%) stenosis in the remaining coronary arteries; 3) no opacifiable collateral vessels on initial and follow-up angiography; 4) no use of inotropic agents, beta-adrenergic blocking agents or calcium channel blockers during the study; 5) recanalization by < 5hours of the onset of symptoms with TIMI grade 3 flow without high grade (>90%) residual stenosis; 6) neither reocclusion nor restenosis of the infarcted-related vessel on follow-up angiography. The diagnosis of acute myocardial infarction was determined on the basis of a history of chest pain that lasted > 30 min, was associated with electrocardiographic (ECG) changes suggestive of acute ischemia in at least two leads and did not respond to nitroglycerin administration. The diagnosis was subsequently confirmed by evolutional ECG changes and elevation of plasma creatine kinase activity. The ST segment-predicted risk area was determined from the initial in-hospital ECG recording. The following formula based on the number of ST segment elevations ≥0.1 mV (nST) in the standard 12 leads was used for prediction: ECG risk area = 3[1.5(nST) - 0.4] (%). This formula was validated in the Second International Study of Infarct Survival. Eligible patients underwent catheterization by the percutaneous femoral approach and received intravenous heparin, 5000U. After angiographic confirmation of total occlusion of LAD, intracoronary nitroglycerin, 0.1 mg, was subsequently administered to exclude vasospasm and intracoronary urokinase, 960,000 U, was administered during 45 to 60 min; if necessary, rescue angioplasty was performed. Successful recanalization was defined as TIMI grade 3 reperfusion. Coronary angioplasty was performed when TIMI perfusion grade was <3 or percent residual diameter stenosis was > 90%. The standard hemodynamic measurements, including systemic and right heart catheterization, were monitored throughout the procedures with catheters introduced percutaneously by way of the femoral artery and vein. The hemodynamic subset of Forrester at hospital admission was determined. The 7F coronary vein multithermistor thermodilution catheter (Wilton Webster Laboratories) was inserted percutaneously from the antecubital vein of the left arm and advanced to the great cardiac vein. Catheter position was monitored fluoroscopically during the whole procedure. Great cardiac vein flow was measured by continuous thermodilution technique. Systemic and coronary hemodynamic status was determined 60 minutes after the first angiogram when TIMI grade 3 flow was obtained, at 6, 12 and 24 hours of the onset of infarction and at follow-up. Blood from the aorta and great cardiac vein were sampled simultaneously 60 minutes after the first angiogram and at 6, 12 and 24 hours after the onset of symptoms for the determination of oxygen partial pressure and saturation. During the period of observation in CCU, creatine kinase (CK) measurement was determined to estimate myocardial damage in the acute phase. Follow-up catheterization was performed 46 ± 13 days after the onset of infarction for the determination of the coronary patency and left ventricular ejection fraction. Thallium-201 scintigraphy was performed 38 ± 11 days of the onset of infarction by a technique previously described.[8] The perfusion defect areas were weighed for the average counts in each area, and the sum of these defect areas was defined as the extent of damaged myocardium in the left ventricle, that is, "defect severity index".

Systemic hemodynamic and great cardiac vein flow measurements at baseline and collection of arterial and cardiac vein blood samples were made before thrombolysis. All patients were treated with continuous infusion of nitroglycerin (0.1 to 0.3 mg/min) for hemodynamic stabilization and with heparin infusion (3 to 7 U/min) for prevention of reocclusion during the first 24 hours after admission. Inotropic agents were not administered. In all patients with successful recanalization, systemic and coronary hemodynamic measurements and blood sampling were repeated 60 min after the first angiogram and at 6, 12 and 24 hours of the onset of symptoms. The time of reperfusion when angiography showed TIMI grade 3 flow was 30 to 60 min after the first angiogram. All patients underwent follow-up catheterization 46 ± 13 days after the onset of infarction. Neither reocclusion nor restenosis of the infarct-related vessel was proved at follow-up catheterization. Patients were classified into two groups according to the pattern of thermodilution measurements of the great cardiac vein flow: Group A included 9 patients with a decrease in great cardiac vein flow > 30 % of baseline flow during the first 24 hours of the onset of infarction; Group B included 10 patients without this observation (Table 20-1).

Results

Age, gender, hemodynamic subset on admission and time interval between the initial and repeat angiography were comparable in the two groups of patients, as were the elapsed time from the onset of infarction to reperfusion and residual coronary stenosis after reperfusion and at follow-up (Table 20-1). Four of 9 patients in Group A and 3 of 10 patients in Group B and were treated by rescue coronary angioplasty after thrombolysis (p=NS). In both groups, the thrombi were located at the proximal segment of the left anterior descending coronary artery, and there were no opacifiable collateral vessels on initial or follow-up angiography.

TABLE 20-1. Clinical Background of the 19 Study Patients

Pt.	Age/ Gender	Forrester Subset	Time to Rep.	PTCA	Res.Ste. Acute	Res.Ste. F/U	CAG Int.	ECG Risk
Group A								
1	58/M	1	3.7	-	90	50	42	12.3
2	65/M	1	2.4	+	25	25	58	16.8
3	42/M	1	4.7	-	90	90	47	12.3
4	74/M	1	2.2	+	50	0	30	21.3
5	48/M	1	1.7	+	50	50	33	25.8
6	43/M	1	2.7	-	90	90	36	12.3
7	64/M	1	4.9	-	90	90	60	21.3
8	61/M	2	5.0	+	90	90	59	16.8
9	30/M	2	3.8	-	90	25	33	17.3
mean	54		3.5		74	57	44	17.3
SD	14		1.3		25	35	12	4.7
Group B								
1	54/M	1	2.1	-	90	50	30	12.3
2	60/M	1	2.0	-	90	75	54	12.3
3	70/M	1	2.5	+	75	75	73	16.8
4	60/F	1	2.8	+	0	0	66	21.3
5	56/F	1	2.2	-	90	90	36	12.3
6	44/M	1	4.0	+	75	75	38	21.3
7	62/M	1	4.4	-	90	75	33	12.3
8	66/M	1	4.5	-	90	90	39	16.8
9	71/M	1	4.0	-	90	90	70	25.8
10	46/M	1	3.0	-	90	90	29	16.8
mean	59		3.2		78	71	47	16.8
SD	9		1.0		28	28	17	4.7

Pt. = patient; Rep = reperfusion; PTCA = percutaneous transluminal coronary angioplasty (- = no; + = yes); Res. Ste. = residual stenosis; F/U = follow-up; CAG Int. = coronary angiography interval; ECG risk = risk area derived from ECG scoring

The ECG risk area on admission did not differ between the two groups. Between the two groups, there was no differences in prevalences of coronary risk factors, i.e., hypertension, hyperlipidemia, diabetes mellitus, obesity, smoking, drinking, family history of coronary artery disease (Table 20-2). Patients taking beta or calcium blockade were not eligible for the present study. There was no differences in the number of patients taking nitrates or diuretics between the two groups (Table 20-2). Only the prevalence of antecedent angina, defined as recurrent ischemic chest pain beginning in the last week before admission, apparently diferred between the two groups (33% in Group A in contrast to 90% in Group B, Table 20-2).

TABLE 20-2. Coronary risk factors in the two groups

Pt.	HT	HLP	DM	Ob	Sm	Alco	FHx	Nit	Diu	Ang
Group A										
1	+	-	+	+	-	+	-	+	-	+
2	-	-	-	-	+	-	+	-	-	-
3	-	-	+	+	+	+	-	-	-	-
4	+	+	-	-	+	+	-	-	-	+
5	-	-	-	-	-	+	+	-	-	-
6	-	-	-	+	+	+	-	+	-	+
7	+	-	-	+	-	-	+	-	+	-
8	-	+	-	-	+	-	-	-	-	-
9	-	-	-	-	+	-	-	-	-	-
	33%	22%	22%	44%	67%	56%	33%	22%	11%	33%
Group B										
1	+	-	+	+	+	-	-	-	-	-
2	-	-	-	-	-	+	+	-	-	+
3	-	+	+	+	+	-	-	-	-	+
4	-	-	-	-	+	+	+	-	-	+
5	+	+	+	-	+	+	-	+	-	+
6	+	-	-	-	-	+	-	-	-	+
7	+	-	-	-	+	-	-	-	-	+
8	-	-	-	-	-	-	+	-	-	+
9	+	-	+	+	+	+	-	-	-	+
10	-	-	-	-	+	-	+	-	-	+
	50%	20%	40%	30%	70%	50%	40%	10%	0%	90%

Pt. = patient; HT = hypertension; HLP = hyperlipidemia; DM = diabetes mellitus; Ob=obesity; Sm = smoking; Alco = alcohol intake; FHx = family history of coronary artery disease; Nit = nitrates; Diu = diuretics; Ang = previous angina

After reperfusion, no patient had recurrent infarction or prolonged angina, congestive heart failure or cardiac arrest during the in-hospital period. Heart rate and systolic and mean arterial blood pressures in both groups were unchanged throughout the study, and there was no significant difference between the two groups in each variable at any time point. Pulmonary capillary wedge pressure decreased significantly after reperfusion in both groups (14.4 ± 6.0 to 12.1 ± 4.2 mmHg in Group A; 14.4 ± 8.3 to 10.7 ± 4.8 mmHg in Group B, $p<0.05$), and thereafter it was unchanged during the study. There was no difference in capillary wedge pressure between the two groups. At follow-up left ventriculography, systemic hemodynamic variables were also similar between the two groups. In Group B, mean great cardiac vein flow did not change during the study period. However by definition, in Group A, great cardiac vein flow gradually decreased by 26 ± 13 mL/min (mean ± SD) or 44 ± 17 % from the postreperfusion flow (58 ± 15 mL/min) during the first 24 hours of the onset of infarction. Coefficient of the regression equation for analysis of significance over time between the two groups was significant indicating that great cardiac vein flow evolved over time differently in Group A than in Group B (Fig. 20-1).

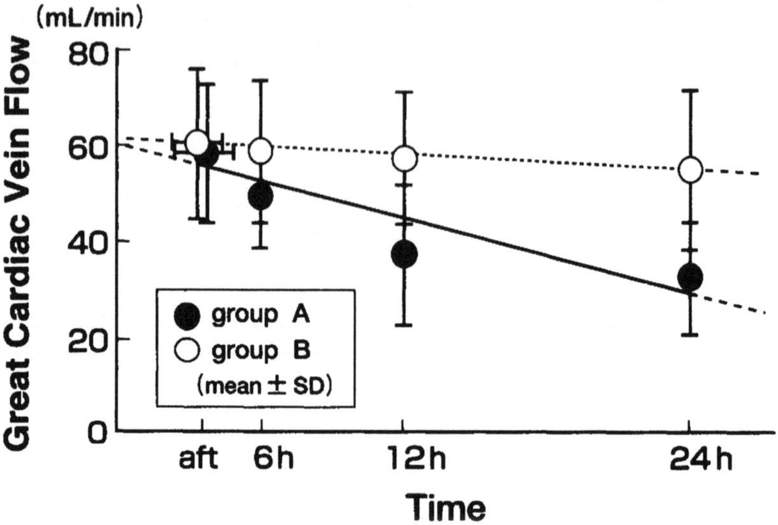

FIGURE 20-1. Serial changes in great cardiac vein flow in Groups A and B. The solid line represents the linear regression for Group A, the dashed line that for Group B. The regression equation for analysis of significance over time between the two groups was y = 60.7-1.32+1.05Dt, where t = time; D dummy variable, i.e. 0 if Group A, 1 if Group B. The time course in Group A was significantly different from that in Group B ($p<0.001$). aft = 60 min after the initial angiogram; 6h, 12h and 24h = 6, 12 and 24 hour, respectively, after the onset of infarction.

The mean myocardial oxygen extraction was gradually decreased in Group A by 0.25 ± 0.13 or 38 ± 15% from the postreperfusion value of 0.64 ± 0.11. Coefficient of the regression equation for analysis of significance over time between the two groups was significant indicating that oxygen extraction in Group A evolved over time in a manner different from that in Group A. In Group B, oxygen extraction did not change during the study.

After reperfusion in Group B, mean coronary vessel resistance remained unchanged throughout the study. Group A demonstrated gradual increases in coronary vessel resistance by 1.60±1.59 from 1.52±0.28 mmHg∗min/mL during the first 24 hours of the onset of infarction. Coefficient of regression equation for analysis of significance over time between the two groups was significant indicating that coronary vessel resistance in Group A evolved over time in a manner different from that in Group B.

Indices of myocardial damage during the course of infarct progression: total CK release and peak time of CK activity were determined in the acute phase. In

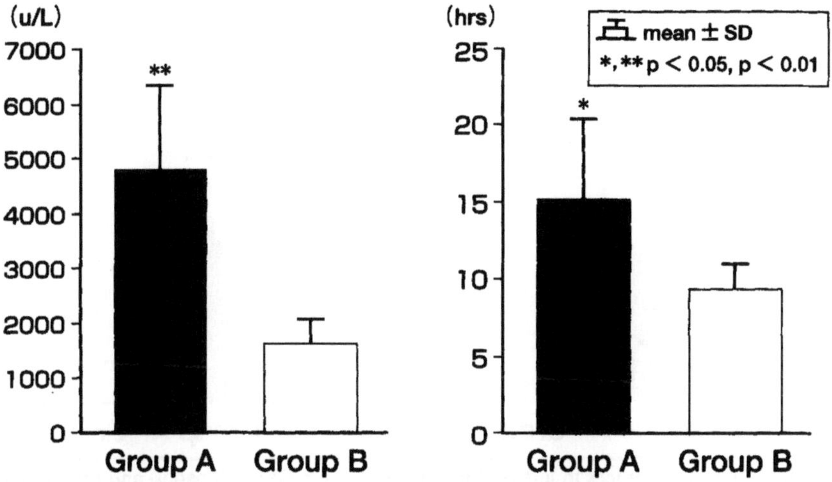

FIGURE 20-2. Differences in total CK release (left panel) and peak time of CK activity (right panel) between Groups A and B. Group A had a significantly larger (p<0.01) CK release and a later peak time of CK activity (p<0.05) compared with Group B.

Group B, total creatine kinase release was smaller (1615 ± 479 vs. 4801 ± 1544U/L, p<0.01) and peak time of creatine kinase activity was earlier (10 ± 2 vs. 15 ± 5 hours, p<0.05) than those in Group A (Figure 20-2). Group B showed a significantly higher global ejection fraction than that of Group A (63 ± 15% vs. 36 ± 7%, p<0.01). Ejection fraction was measured at follow-up catheterization, when systemic hemodynamic variables were comparable between the two groups. Group B had a significantly (p<0.01) smaller defect severity index than that of Group A (247 ± 261 vs 1091 ± 366 U, p<0.01, Fig. 20-3).

Conclusion

The term "No-reflow phenomenon" is firstly described in the article of Klug et al. on cerebral ischemia-reperfusion in 1966. Then, Kloner et al. defined "no-reflow" as the inability to perfuse previously ischemic myocardium, even when blood flow has been restored to the large arteries supplying the tissue.[9] In their study, electron microscopic analysis revealed severe capillary damage, including the presence of large endothelial blebs in the lumen of the vessels, areas of regional endothelial edema, reduced pinocytic vesicles and endothelial gaps. Microscopic hemorrhage was observed within the no-reflow area. Rouleaux formation of erythrocytes within vessels was common, but intraluminal fibrin thrombi or platelets rarely were observed. Occasionally, swollen myocytes appeared to be compressing capillaries.

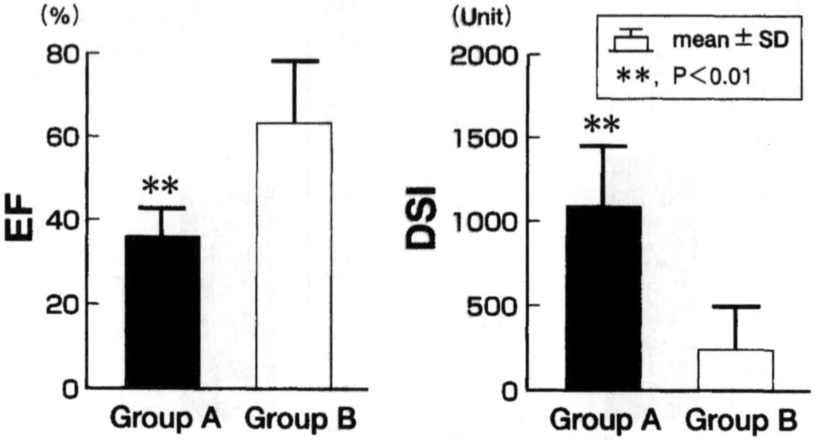

FIGURE 20-3. Differences in left ventricular ejection fraction (left panel) and thallium-201 defect severity index (right panel) between Groups A and B. Group A had a significantly lower ($p<0.01$) ejection fraction and a larger ($p<0.01$) defect size compared with Group B.

Kloner et al. concluded that no reflow was associated with anatomic damage to the endothelial cells and occurred after the onset of irreversible damage to the myocytes. Furthermore, they claimed that no-reflow was secondary event that occurs after myocyte death. However, Ambrosio et al.[10] has suggested that the no-reflow phenomenon may worsen over time. Areas with delayed impairment of flow were located within zones of contraction band necrosis and were characterized by intravascular neutrophils and erythrocyte stasis. Similar exacerbation of no-reflow has also been observed using positron emission tomography by Jeremy et. al.[11]

There is now evidence that perfusion abnormalities such as no-reflow occur in patients after thrombolytic therapy for acute myocardial infarction. Schofer et al. used a dual isotope scintigraphic technique in which thallium-201 and technetium-99m microalbumin aggregates were injected before and after thrombolysis in order to assess perfusion.[2] Before thrombolysis both isotopes revealed perfusion defects were still present. In most patients studied 2 to 4 weeks after initial thrombolysis perfusion defects persisted. This data suggests that the no-reflow phenomenon occurs in man and persists for at least several weeks after infarction.

In the present study, there are several possible mechanisms of decreased great cardiac vein flow after reperfusion. 1) Metabolic demand of reperfused myocardium might decrease because disappearance of ischemia may attenuate sympathetic nerve stimulation. However, heart rate and aortic pressure did not change in either patient group throughout the study. 2) Epicardial coronary spasm after recanalization may decrease coronary blood flow. In this case, oxygen extraction after recanalization was decreased in our patients, and there was no evidence of recurrent ischemia during the study. 3) Coronary microvascular injury in reperfused myocardium may decrease great cardiac vein flow. Leukocyte plugging and platelet aggregation[12] are often observed during reperfusion and are suggested to cause the disturbances of microcirculation. In experimental obstruction of coronary microcirculation,[13] microvascular embolization decreased oxygen extraction with massive releases of lactate and decreased coronary blood flow. These situations correspond well with our observations. Functional microvascular disturbances, such as capillary compression by myocardial tissue edema, myocardial ischemia contracture, endothelial cell swelling and increases in vasomotor tone, are also possible causes of microvascular injury after reperfusion. In previous clinical studies,[2-4] myocardial imaging by contrast echocardiography or thallium-201 scintigraphy was used to prove the presence of a no reflow zone. In the present study, we used no index of myocardial perfusion in the acute phase of infarction and measured only coronary venous flow and coronary vessel resistance. Ambrosio et al.[10] have shown that no reflow zones are characterized by abrupt vascular occlusion at both small arteriolar and venular levels and absence of capillary filling. Kloner et al.[14] revealed progressive microvascular damage after reperfusion characterized by neutrophil migration into the vessel wall and erythrocyte stasis. Furthermore, these abnormalities were associated with reduced vasodilator reserve. Another pathologic study[15] demonstrated progressive infarct extension during reperfusion. Experimental studies[11,13] of no reflow demonstrated a progressive decrease in myocardial perfusion. Our results are consistent with those findings. The progressive reduction in great cardiac vein flow strongly suggests progressive impairment of antegrade flow. Because we did not measure white blood cell count in the coronary venous blood, we could not confirm that there was leukocyte plugging in the ischemic myocardium. However, white blood cell count in the peripheral blood was higher in Group A than in Group B (15667 ± 2872 vs. 11300 ± 2177/mL, $p<0.05$), raising the possibility that the inflammatory response to ischemia might be one difference between the groups.

There is no definite evidence that reduction of the no-reflow phenomenon will limit the extent of myocardial death. Reducing of eliminating no-reflow might enhance the healing of an infarct, facilitating the removal of necrotic debris. Reducing the low-reflow phenomenon might hasten the return of postischemic dysfunction and should allow better delivery of pharmacologic agents to the peri-infarction tissue. Also, improving flow into the peri-infarct tissue or into the infarct itself might, by increasing tissue turgor, help prevent thinning and dilation of the infarcted and ischemic segment.

In conclusion, salvage of myocardial infarction by early successful thrombolysis could not be observed in the patients demonstrating progressive decreases in great cardiac vein flow. Those patients appeared to have inadequate myocardial reperfusion on a microvascular basis, which is associated with a much larger infarction. Antecedent angina may have beneficial effects on the no reflow phenomenon or infarct size limitation, or both.

References

1. Feld H, Lichtenstein E, Schachter J et al. Early and late angiographic findings of the "no-reflow" phenomenon following direct angioplasty as primary treatment for acute myocardial infarction. Am Heart J 1992;123:782-784.
2. Schoffer J, Montz R, Mathey DG. Scintigraphic evidence of the "no reflow" phenomenon with positron emission tomography. J Am Coll Cardiol 1985;5:593-598.
3. Ito H. Tomooka T, Sakai N et al. Lack of myocardial perfusion immediately after successful thrombolysis: a predictor of poor recovery of late ventricular function in anterior myocardial infarction. Circulation 1992;85:1699-1705.
4. Ito H, Iwakura K, Oh H et al. Temporal changes in myocardial perfusion patterns in patients with reperfused anterior wall myocardial infarction. Their relation to myocardial viability. Circulation 1995;91:656-662.
5. Ottani F, Galvani M, Ferrini D et al. Prodromal angina limits infarct size: A role for ischemic preconditioning. Circulation 1995;91:291-297.
6. Speechly Dick ME, Grover GJ, Yellon DM. Does ischemic preconditioning in the human involve protein kinase C and the ATP-dependent K+ channel? Studies of contractile function after simulated ischemia in an atrial in vitro model. Circ Res 1995;77:1030-1035.
7. Kloner RA, Shook T, Przyklenk K et al. Previous angina alters in-hospital outcome in TIMI 4: A clinical correlate to preconditioning. Circulation 1995;91:37-45.
8. Komamura K, Kitakaze M, Nishida K et al. Progressive decreases in coronary vein flow during reperfusion in acute myocardial infarction: Clinical documentation of the no reflow phenomenon after successful thrombolysis. J Am Coll Cardiol 1994;24:370-377.
9. Kloner RA, Ganote CE, Jennings RB. The "no-reflow" phenomenon after temporary coronary occlusion in the dog. J Clin Invest 1974;54:1496-1508.
10. Ambrosio G, Weisman HF, Mannisi JA et al. Progressive impairment of regional myocardial perfusion after restoration of postischemic blood flow. Circulation 1989;80:1846-1861.
11. Jeremy RW, Links JM, Becker LC. Progressive failure of coronary flow during reperfusion of myocardial infarction: Documentation of the no reflow phenomenon with positron emission tomography. J Am Coll Cardiol 1985;5:593-598.
12. Engler RL, Schmid-Sconbein GW, Pavelec RS. Leukocyte capillary plugging in myocardial ischemia and reperfusion in the dog. Am J Pathol 1983;65:248-255.
13. Hori M, Inoue M, Kitakaze M et al. Role of adenosine in hyperemic response of coronary blood flow in microembolization. Am J Physiol 1986;(Heart Circ Physiol 19):H509-H518.
14. Kloner RA, Giacomelli F, Alker KJ et al. Influx of neutrophils into the walls of large epicardial coronary arteries in response to ischemia/reperfusion. Circulation 1991;84:1758-1772.

15. Farb A, Kolodgie FD, Jenkins M et al. Myocardial infarct extension during reperfusion after coronary artery occlusion: Pathologic evidence. J Am Coll Cardiol 1993;21:1245-53.

In: Mentzer, R.M., Jr., Kitakaze, M., Downey, J.M., Hori, M, eds. Adenosine, Cardioprotection and Clinical Application. Kluwer Academic Publishers, Norwell, MA, USA, 1997.

INDEX

MIX
Papier aus verantwortungsvollen Quellen
Paper from responsible sources
FSC® C105338

If you have any concerns about our products,
you can contact us on
ProductSafety@springernature.com

In case Publisher is established outside the EU,
the EU authorized representative is:
Springer Nature Customer Service Center GmbH
Europaplatz 3, 69115 Heidelberg, Germany

Printed by Libri Plureos GmbH
in Hamburg, Germany